Critical Thinking, Clinical Reasoning, AND Clinical Judgment

A PRACTICAL APPROACH

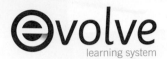
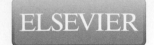
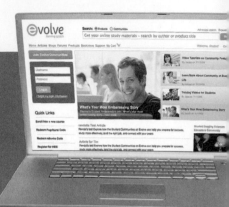

Critical Thinking, Clinical Reasoning, AND Clinical Judgment

A PRACTICAL APPROACH

Rosalinda Alfaro-LeFevre, RN, MSN, ANEF

President
Teaching Smart/Learning Easy
Stuart, Florida
www.AlfaroTeachSmart.com

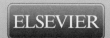

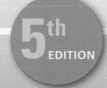

5th EDITION

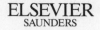

3251 Riverport Lane
St. Louis, MO 63043

CRITICAL THINKING, CLINICAL REASONING, AND   ISBN: 978-1-4377-2776-0
CLINICAL JUDGMENT: A PRACTICAL APPROACH

Notices

Knowledge and best practice in this field are constantly changing. As new research and experience broaden our understanding, changes in research methods, professional practices, or medical treatment may become necessary.

Practitioners and researchers must always rely on their own experience and knowledge in evaluating and using any information, methods, compounds, or experiments described herein. In using such information or methods they should be mindful of their own safety and the safety of others, including parties for whom they have a professional responsibility.

With respect to any drug or pharmaceutical products identified, readers are advised to check the most current information provided (i) on procedures featured or (ii) by the manufacturer of each product to be administered, to verify the recommended dose or formula, the method and duration of administration, and contraindications. It is the responsibility of practitioners, relying on their own experience and knowledge of their patients, to make diagnoses, to determine dosages and the best treatment for each individual patient, and to take all appropriate safety precautions.

To the fullest extent of the law, neither the Publisher nor the authors, contributors, or editors, assume any liability for any injury and/or damage to persons or property as a matter of products liability, negligence or otherwise, or from any use or operation of any methods, products, instructions, or ideas contained in the material herein.

Library of Congress Cataloging-in-Publication Data
Alfaro-LeFevre, Rosalinda.
  Critical thinking, clinical reasoning, and clinical judgment : a practical approach / Rosalinda
Alfaro-LeFevre.—5th ed.
    p. ; cm.
  Rev. ed. of: Critical thinking and clinical judgment / Rosalinda Alfaro-LeFevre. 4th ed. c2009.
  Includes bibliographical references and index.
  ISBN 978-1-4377-2776-0 (pbk. : alk. paper)
  I. Alfaro-LeFevre, Rosalinda. Critical thinking and clinical judgment.   II. Title.
  [DNLM: 1. Nursing Process.   2. Clinical Competence.   3. Decision Making.   4. Judgment.
WY 100.1]
  610.73—dc23
                                                                                    2011041975

Executive Content Strategist: Lee Henderson
Associate Content Development Specialist: Julia Curcio
Publishing Services Manager: Jeff Patterson
Project Manager: Clay S. Broeker
Design Direction: Paula Catalano

Printed in the United States

Last digit is the print number: 9   8   7   6   5   4   3   2   1

Dedication

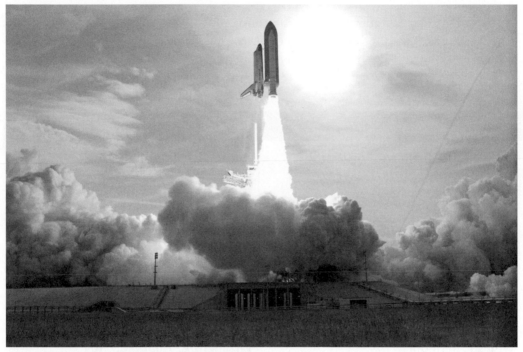

Source: NASA Images Gallery. www.nasa.gov.

Living in Florida, we saw many magnificent shuttle launches through the years. Each time, we marveled at the beautiful sight and thought about the astronauts' courage and expertise. We also were keenly aware of the all the men and women who worked together to achieve space flight.

This book is dedicated to the astronauts who flew, the astronauts who gave their lives, and the many people at NASA who showed that no matter how complex the challenges are, amazing things happen when everyone works toward common goals. I cannot think of a better group to demonstrate the importance of having a spirit of inquiry and a passion for learning—both key critical thinking characteristics. If you ask questions and are committed to finding answers and working as a team, human ingenuity can be limitless. (See page 146 for medical applications gained directly or indirectly from NASA space flights.).

Advisors and Reviewers

A note of thanks: Without the timely and insightful reviews and advice of the experts listed on these pages, this book would not have been possible. The author wishes to also acknowledge the diligent work of the translators of previous editions.

UNITED STATES

Ledjie Ballard, CRNA, ARNP, MSN
Seattle, Washington

Deanne A. Blach, MSN, RN
Nurse Educator
DB Productions
Green Forest, Arkansas

Susan A. Boyer, MEd, RN, FAHCEP
Executive Director
Vermont Nurses in Partnership, Inc.
Windsor, Vermont

Hilda H. Brito, RN, BC, MSN
Director of Education
Kendall Medical Center
Miami, Florida

Ellen B. Ceppetelli, RN, MS, CNL
Director of Nursing Education
Dartmouth Hitchcock Medical Center
Lebanon, New Hampshire

Bette Case Di Leonardi, PhD, RN-BC
Consultant in Competency Management
  and Education
Chicago, Illinois

Karen Elechko, RN, MSN
Golden Memory Clinic Coordinator
Veteran Affairs Medical
  Center—Coatesville
Coatesville, Pennsylvania

Rebecca S. Frugé, RN, PhD
Director, Graduate Nursing Program
Universidad Metropolitana
San Juan, Puerto Rico

Elizabeth E. Hand, MS, RN
Emergency Cardiac Care Instructor
Hillcrest Medical Center
Tulsa, Oklahoma

Dan Hankison
CONSULTING Dragons
Stuart, Florida

Ruth I. Hansten, RN, MBA, PhD, FACHE
Principal
Hansten Healthcare PLLC
Port Ludlow, Washington
www.rrohc.com

Cheryl Herndon, ARNP, CNM, MSN
Director of Aesthetic Services
Women's Health Specialists
Jensen Beach, Florida

Robert Hess, RN, PhD, FAAN
EVP, Global Programming, Gannett
    Education, Gannett Healthcare Group
Founder, Forum for Shared Governance
Voorhees, New Jersey

Donna D. Ignatavicius, RN, MS, ANEF
Author and Consultant
President, DI Associates
Placitas, New Mexico

Sharon E. Johnson, MSN, RNC, NE-BC
Director, Home Health and Hospice
Jefferson Health System
Bryn Mawr, Pennsylvania

Nancy Konzelmann, MS, RN-BC, CPHQ
Nursing Professional Development
    Specialist
Port St. Lucie, Florida

**Kathie J. Kulikowski, MS, MSN,
    RN, CNE**
Assistant Professor
Chamberlain College of Nursing
Columbus, Ohio

Corrine R. Kurzen, RN, MEd, MSN
Author and Consultant
Lafayette Hill, Pennsylvania

Heidi Pape Laird
Systems Designer
Partners HealthCare
Boston, Massachusetts

Nola Lanham, BSN, RN
Staff Nurse, Baptist Medical Center South
Graduate Student, Jacksonville University
    College of Nursing
Jacksonville, Florida

Barbara Maxwell, MSN, MS, CNS, RN*
Associate Professor of Nursing and
    Program Coordinator
SUNY Ulster
Stone Ridge, New York

Marycarol McGovern, PhD, RN
Assistant Professor
College of Nursing
Villanova University
Villanova, Pennsylvania

Melanie McGuire, RN, BSN
Staff Nurse
Emergency Department
Paoli Hospital
Paoli, Pennsylvania

Judith C. Miller, RN, MS
Nursing Tutorial and Consulting Services
Henniker, New Hampshire

Jan Nash, PhD, MSN, RN, NEA-BC
Vice President/CNO Patient Services
Paoli Hospital
Paoli, Pennsylvania

Charles L. Nola
Aerospace Engineer
Madison, Alabama

---

*Deceased

Marilyn H. Oermann, PhD, RN, FAAN, ANEF
Professor and Chair, Adult/Geriatric
Health Division
School of Nursing
University of North Carolina at
Chapel Hill
Chapel Hill, North Carolina

Lourdes Maldonado Ojeda, EdD, RN
Dean, School of Health Sciences
Universidad Metropolitana
San Juan, Puerto Rico

Terri Sue Patterson, RN, MSN, CRRN, FIALCP
President
Nursing Consultation Services
Plymouth Meeting, Pennsylvania
www.nursingconsultation.com

William F. Perry, MA, RN
Informatics Consultant
Creekspace Informatics
Beavercreek, Ohio

Kristen D. Priddy, MSN, RNC-OB, CNS
Clinical Instructor
College of Nursing
University of Texas at Arlington
Arlington, Texas

Susan Prion, EdD, MEd, MSN, RN
Chair, Doctor of Nursing
Practice Department
School of Nursing
University of San Francisco
San Francisco, California

James Riley
President
Capario, Inc.
Santa Ana, California

Matthew Riley, MA
Owner
Behavior for Life, LLC
Kennett Square, Pennsylvania

Michael H. Riley, MBA, MSW, LPC, EMT-Paramedic
Account Manager
Praesidium, Inc.
Fort Worth, Texas

Rose O. Sherman, EdD, RN, NEA-BC, FAAN
Director, Nursing Leadership Institute
Associate Professor
Christine E. Lynn College of Nursing
Florida Atlantic University
Boca Raton, Florida

Kathleen R. Stevens, RN, EdD, ANEF FAAN
Professor and Director
Improvement Science Research Network
and Academic Center for Evidence-
Based Practice (ACE)
University of Texas Health Science
Center—San Antonio
San Antonio, Texas

Eva Tapia, MSN, RN, NP
Nursing Program Director
Pueblo Community College
Pueblo, Colorado

Carol Taylor, PhD, RN
Professor of Nursing and Medicine
Georgetown University
Washington, DC

Brent W. Thompson, PhD, RN
Associate Professor, Department of
Nursing
West Chester University of Pennsylvania
West Chester, Pennsylvania

Elizabeth M. Tsarnas, APRN, BC
Clinical Director
Volunteers in Medicine Clinic
Stuart, Florida

Theresa M. Valiga, EdD, RN,
  ANEF, FAAN
Professor and Director, Institute for
  Educational Excellence
Duke University School of Nursing
Durham, North Carolina

INTERNATIONAL

Miriam de Abreu Almeida, RN, PhD
Professor, School of Nursing
Federal University of Rio Grande do Sul
Porto Alegre, Brazil

Judy Boychuk Duchscher, RN, BScN,
  MN, PhD
Executive Director of Nursing the Future
Assistant Professor
Nursing Department
University of Calgary
Calgary, Alberta, Canada

Aiko Emoto
Professor Emeritus
Saniku Gakuin College
Chiba, Japan

Maria Teresa Luis, RN
Professor Emeritus
School of Nursing
Barcelona University
Barcelona, Spain

Jeanne Michel, RN, PhD
Adjunct Professor
Department of Nursing
Federal University of São Paulo
São Paulo, Brazil

Joanne Profetto-McGrath, PhD, RN
Vice Dean and Professor
Faculty of Nursing
University of Alberta
Edmonton, Alberta, Canada

Preface

CRITICAL THINKING: BEHIND EVERY HEALED PATIENT

I chose the opening heading to Chapter 1 for this Preface because of its significance to developing critical thinking. Critical thinking—nurses' ability to focus their thinking to achieve timely, quality outcomes—not only decides whether they succeed or fail, it makes the difference between keeping patients safe and putting them in harm's way.

In accordance with my mission, the goal of this book is to promote excellence in nursing as measured by exceptional patient and learner outcomes and nurses' job satisfaction. This includes helping students, nurses, teachers, and leaders do the following:

- Develop the critical thinking, learning, and interpersonal skills needed to partner with patients, families, communities, and one another.
- Create a culture that keeps the focus on (1) patient and caregiver safety and welfare and (2) promoting partnerships, learning, achievement, and growth.
- Help nurses and students to learn how to get patients, families, and communities actively involved in managing and improving their own health.

To achieve the above in context of the many challenges we face today, this is the most comprehensive revision since 1995. All content has been revised to help you make decisions about how to address standards, competencies, and recommendations from the Institute of Medicine, the Quality and Safety for Nursing Education organization, The Joint Commission, the National League for Nursing, and key publications on how nursing and nursing education must be transformed to meet the needs of the 21st century.[1,2,3,4]

WHO SHOULD READ THIS BOOK?

You should read this book if:

- You're a student or beginning nurse and want to be more confident and competent in making patient care decisions.
- You're a preceptor in need of strategies and tools to work together with new nurses to promote critical thinking.
- You're an educator or a leader who wants to prepare for accreditation visits or Magnet status.
- You need to prepare for standard tests like professional certification exams and the National Council Licensure Examinations (NCLEX®).

WHAT'S NEW TO THIS EDITION

Here's what's new:

- **NEW TITLE!** We now include *Clinical Reasoning* in the title to reflect more emphasis on clinical reasoning skills. The subheading, *A Practical Approach*, stresses what readers have told us for years: this book is easy to follow and gives solid, evidence-based information in an engaging way (you'll find lots of examples and strategies to promote meaningful learning).
- **NEW CHAPTER TITLES!** All titles were changed to reflect the new content and approach.
- **NEW DESIGN!** Great pains have been taken to include elements that help learners gain a sense of salience (what's most important). The box below addresses the best way to read this book.
- **NEW MAPS AND DECISION-MAKING TOOLS!** These guide learners "to think things through" to make sound decisions (e.g., making scope of practice decisions and how to delegate safely and effectively).
- **MORE EXERCISES THROUGHOUT!** *Think, Pair, Share* exercises have been added to promote deep learning through peer and expert collaboration.

THE BEST WAY TO READ THIS BOOK

The Best Way to Read This Book Is However You Choose to Read It
1. If you like the traditional approach, read it from beginning to end. You'll enjoy the narrative, logical approach, and numerous scenarios and examples designed to help you understand and remember content.
2. If you like to use your own unique approach—for example, the back to front approach (read summaries before text), the "skip around to the stuff that looks interesting" approach, or the "read the stuff that will be on the test first approach"— here are some of the features that help you focus on what's most important.

Preceding Each Chapter
- **This Chapter at a Glance:** Allows you to scan major headings.
- **Prechapter Self-Tests:** Help you focus on learning outcomes and decide where you stand in relation to what needs to be learned.

Following Each Chapter
- **Critical Thinking Exercises:** Direct you to use content, helping you clarify understanding and move information into long-term memory.
- **Key Points/Summary:** Give a detailed summary of the most important content.

Other Features You Need to Know About
- **Critical Moments:** Give simple strategies that can make a BIG difference in results.
- **Other Perspectives:** Offer interesting (and sometimes amusing) points of view.
- **Response Key:** When appropriate, you get example responses for Critical Thinking/Clinical Reasoning Exercises to help you evaluate your responses. (All exercises

---

THE BEST WAY TO READ THIS BOOK—cont'd

that have an example response are marked with an asterisk.) This is called a response key, rather than an answer key, to avoid implying that there's only one right answer to each question. In some cases, a variety of responses are acceptable. (Great minds don't always think alike!) The point of the exercises isn't necessarily to come up with one right response; rather, the point is to get in touch with the thinking that led you to your response and to be able to evaluate and correct your thinking as needed.

Reading Efficiently

However you choose to read, keep in mind the following steps, which provide an organized and efficient way to master content.

- **Survey:** Scan the abstract, major headings, tables, and illustrations.
- **Question:** Turn major headings into questions.
- **Read:** Read, taking notes and answering your questions.
- **Review, Recite, and Reread:** Review the chapter (or your notes), reciting key content out loud, and then ask yourself, "What's still not clear here?" Read the sections you don't understand again, and raise questions to ask in class or discuss with your peers.

Here's the big picture of how content is organized:

- **Chapters 1 and 2 build the foundation for developing critical thinking, clinical reasoning, and clinical judgment.** Here, with specific examples and strategies, you learn exactly what it takes to improve your ability to think your way through nursing and personal challenges.

- **Chapters 3 and 4 help you gain the knowledge and skills required to succeed in six common nursing situations:** (1) clinical reasoning and judgment, (2) moral and ethical reasoning, (3) research and evidence-based practice, (4) teaching ourselves, (5) teaching others, and (6) test taking. Beginning students sometimes like to jump to Chapter 4, where *teaching others, teaching ourselves,* and *taking tests* are discussed, before reading other chapters. This is a good example of making learning meaningful. Read what you're most interested in first.

- **Chapter 5 helps you develop specific clinical reasoning skills by working with case scenarios that are based on real incidents.*** In this section, you gain deep understanding of nursing process skills, such assessing systematically, identifying patient-centered outcomes, and setting priorities. You learn not only *how* to accomplish these skills, but *why* they are essential to developing sound clinical reasoning and judgment.

---

*Names and some facts changed to give anonymity.

- **Chapter 6 helps you develop communication, interpersonal, teamwork and self-management skills** (e.g., managing your time, dealing with conflict). When you know how to communicate effectively, manage your emotions, organize your time, and build positive relationships with patients and team members, you spend less time getting sidetracked by interpersonal and "human nature" problems—and more time fully engaged in progress. Here, in the section on *Preventing and Dealing with Mistakes Constructively*, you also learn how to meet quality and safety standards and keep patients, caregivers, and yourself safe. The skills in this section are often considered to be leadership skills. Today, every nurse must be a leader. Advocating for your patients, yourself, your peers, and your community requires highly developed interpersonal and communication abilities.

Because of the depth and breadth of content, you can use this book to guide a specific course or as an adjunct to other courses. You get the best results if you begin to use it in beginning courses and continue to refer to as you progress through various stages of learning. You may even consider making parts of the book required reading *before* starting nursing school, when motivation to learn about nursing is high. For example, students can benefit greatly from reading Chapter 1 and the sections on teaching, learning, and test taking in Chapter 4.

Here's a summary of new content:

- How to think like a nurse to give patient- and family-centered care.
- Making patient and caregiver safety and welfare top priority in all thinking and interactions, including:
  - Taking responsibility for being "a safety net" when helping coworkers, anticipating what they may need and pitching in to prevent mistakes (e.g. "I think that glove is contaminated, so let me get you a new one," or "Here's a new needle.").
  - Maintaining nursing surveillance (points out that patient situations and systems are constantly changing and monitoring for safety and improvement).
- The idea that developing skilled communication—listening and speaking in ways that promote clarity and mutual understanding—is as important as developing clinical skills.
- Developing inquisitiveness, self-efficacy,* and a passion for lifelong learning.
- Using simulation and debriefing to promote critical thinking
- More information on:
  - Using the nursing process as a critical thinking tool and developing habits that promote safe, effective clinical reasoning
  - Paying attention to context and learning pattern recognition
  - Moving to a predictive model—*Predict, Prevent, Manage, Promote*—rather than using a more reactive *Diagnose and Treat* approach

---

*A sense of confidence about one's ability to accomplish personal and professional goals.

- The importance of thinking ahead, thinking-in-action, and thinking-back (reflective practice)
- Using preceptors to help novices develop clinical reasoning skills
- How personality, upbringing, and culture affect thinking and teamwork
- Using critical thinking indicators and the 4-circle CT model
- Developing and evaluating specific outcomes
- How multidisciplinary practice and health information technology affect thinking
- Developing informatics skills (accessing, using, and creating electronic records)
- Applying principles of research and evidence-based practice and exploring ways to seek out answers
- The roles of logic, intuition, and creativity
- Making sure your documentation reflects critical thinking
- How to promote and evaluate critical thinking in diverse nurses
- The importance of role modeling among learners, colleagues, leaders, and educators
- How to make educated guesses and pass standard tests on the first try (includes NCLEX practice questions).

WHAT'S THE SAME ABOUT THIS EDITION

The following features are retained from previous editions:
- Brain-based learning principles are applied (using strategies that get your brain plugged into learning).
- You get practical information and strategies in a concise format (gives theory, strategies, and exercises to apply content).
- To ensure up-to-date, cutting edge information, all content was reviewed by clinical and educational experts.
- A frame of reference is given to put your thinking into words and dialogue about reasoning with students, nurses, educators, and leaders.
- HMO (Help Me Out) cartoons, based on real incidences, address the funny things that happen to caregivers and receivers. If you have a story to share, please contact me at www.AlfaroTeachSmart.com.

Additional Benefits. Once again, you get access to Evolve resources, as listed on the page facing the title page.

ASSUMPTIONS AND PROMISES

Before I Began to Write This Book, I Made Some Assumptions:
- You want to learn.
- Your time is valuable, and you don't want to waste it.
- You like to learn the most important things first.
- You learn better when you're motivated, know why information is relevant, and choose your own way of learning.
- You know yourself best, so it's inappropriate for me to tell you how to think.
- You feel a sense of accomplishment when you gain the knowledge and skills that help you be more independent.

Because of These Assumptions, I Promise to:
- Let you know what's most important.
- Use lots of examples and present information in a usable way.
- Give the "reasons behind the rules."
- Encourage you to choose what works for you.
- Help you develop the skills required to be a better thinker, independent learner, and more effective nurse.

A Word About Patients, Clients, Stakeholders, and "He/She." To reflect that patients and clients are *individuals* with unique needs, values, perceptions, and motivations, whenever possible a fictitious name or "someone," "person," "consumer," or "individual" is used (instead of "patient" or "client"). The term *stakeholder* is now used when talking about *all the individuals and groups* who have a vested interest in how care is given. (Examples of *stakeholders* include patients, significant others, caregivers, and insurance companies.) *He* and *she* are used interchangeably to avoid the awkwardness of using "he/she."

PLEASE TELL US WHAT YOU THINK

We want to hear your struggles and concerns. Whether you're a student, staff nurse, leader, or educator, if you have a problem with something, it's likely that others do too. Your problems are our opportunities to learn, improve, and help others with similar issues. Please let me know what you think.

Rosalinda Alfaro-LeFevre, RN, MSN, ANEF
www.AlfaroTeachSmart.com/mailer1.cfm

REFERENCES

1. Benner, P., Sutphen, M., Leonard, V., Day, L. (2009). *Educating nurses: A call for radical transformation*. San Francisco: Jossey-Bass.
2. Committee on the Robert Wood Johnson Foundation Initiative on the Future of Nursing at the Institute of Medicine. (2010) *The future of nursing: Leading change, advancing health*. Washington, DC: National Academic Press.
3. National League for Nursing. (2008) NLN Think Tank on Transforming Clinical Nursing Education. Retrieved January 19, 2011, from www.nln.org/facultydevelopment/pdf/think_tank.pdf.
4. National Organization for Associate Degree Nursing. (2010). Response to Carnegie Foundation Report. Position statement. Retrieved January 19, 2011, from https://www.noadn.org/.

Acknowledgements

I want to thank my husband, Jim, for his love, support, and sense of humor and fun. I also want to thank the rest of my family and the following people for their ongoing support and contribution to my personal and professional growth: Heidi Laird, Ledjie Ballard, Terri Patterson, Grace and Frank Nola, Charlie Nola, Chuck and Pat Morgan, Loraine Locasale, Dan Hankison, Karen Smith, Virginia McFalls, Bill Perry, Carol Taylor, Terry Valiga, Mary Ann Rizzolo, Annette Sophocles, Melani McGuire, Maria Sophocles, Barbara Cohen, Patti Cleary, Ruth Hansten, Nancy Konzelman, Hilda Brito, Michael Ledbetter, Robin Carter, the Villanova College of Nursing Faculty, and the past and present staff nurses of Paoli Hospital, Paoli, Pennsylvania. I can't thank those of you who have been willing to advise and give so freely of your time and expertise enough.

My special thanks go to the following people at Elsevier: Lee Henderson, Executive Content Strategist; Kristin Geen, Executive Content Strategist; Julia Curcio, Associate Content Development Specialist; Jamie Horn, Senior Content Development Specialist; Clay Broeker, Senior Project Manager; and the sales and marketing staff for their vital roles in making this book successful.

Rosalinda Alfaro-LeFevre RN, MSN, ANEF
www.AlfaroTeachSmart.com

Contents

CHAPTER 3
Clinical Reasoning and Clinical Judgment, 66

CHAPTER 4
Ethical Reasoning, Evidence-Based Practice, Teaching Others, Teaching Ourselves, and Test-Taking, 128

CHAPTER 5
Practicing Clinical Reasoning Skills: Applying the Nursing Process, 164

CHAPTER 6
Developing Interpersonal, Teamwork, and Self-Management Skills, 216

RESPONSE KEY FOR EXERCISES IN CHAPTERS 1 TO 5, 266

APPENDIXES

GLOSSARY, 298

INDEX, 302

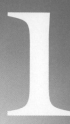

What Are Critical Thinking, Clinical Reasoning, and Clinical Judgment?

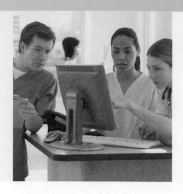

This chapter at a glance ...

Decide where you stand in relation to the following learning outcomes.

Learning Outcomes

After completing this chapter, you should be able to:

1. Describe critical thinking (CT), clinical reasoning, and clinical judgment in your own words, based on the descriptions in this chapter.
2. Give at least three reasons why CT skills are essential for students and nurses.
3. Explain (or map) how the following terms are related to one another: critical thinking, clinical reasoning, clinical judgment, decision-making, problem-solving, and nursing process.
4. Identify four principles of the scientific method that are evident in CT.
5. Compare and contrast the terms *problem-focused thinking* and *outcome-focused thinking.*
6. Clarify the term *critical thinking indicator* (CTI).
7. Use CTIs, together with the 4-circle CT model, to identify five CT characteristics you'd like to improve.
8. Explain why knowing the nursing process is needed for clinical reasoning and passing the NCLEX® and other standard tests.
9. Identify the relationships among healthy workplaces, learning cultures, safety cultures, and CT.
10. Compare and contrast the terms *thinking ahead, thinking-in-action,* and *thinking back.*

CRITICAL THINKING: BEHIND EVERY HEALED PATIENT

A powerful quote from an online BLOG sets the stage for this chapter: "Behind every healed patient is a critical thinking nurse."[1]

Critical thinking—your ability to focus your thinking to get the results you need in various situations—makes the difference between whether you succeed or fail. Whether you need to set patient priorities, figure out how to collaborate with a difficult team member, or develop a plan of care, critical thinking—deliberate, informed thought—is the key.

The journey to developing critical thinking starts with having a good understanding of what it IS. Too many nurses believe that critical thinking is like an "amorphous blob" that you can't describe—something that you're "just supposed to *do*."[2] This approach is not helpful. You must be specific about exactly what's involved when thinking critically in various contexts.

Thinking is a skill, just like music or tennis. It flows and changes depending on current conditions, and it requires gaining specific knowledge, skills, experience, and hands-on practice.

This chapter helps you begin the journey to improving thinking in two steps: (1) First, you learn why health care organizations and nursing schools stress the need for critical thinking. (2) Second, you examine exactly what critical thinking is and how it relates to clinical reasoning and clinical judgment.

CRITICAL THINKING: NOT SIMPLY BEING CRITICAL

Before going on to examine what critical thinking in nursing entails, it's important that you realize one thing: critical thinking doesn't mean simply being critical. It means not accepting information at face value without carefully evaluating it. Consider the following description:

Critical thinking clarifies goals, examines assumptions, uncovers hidden values, evaluates evidence, accomplishes actions, and assesses conclusions. "Critical" as used in "critical thinking" implies the importance or centrality of thinking to an issue, question, or problem of concern. It does not mean "disapproval" or "negative." Nurses often use critical thinking to imply thinking that's critical to be able to manage specific problems. For example: "We're working with our nurses to develop the critical thinking needed to identify people at risk for infection early."

There are many positive uses of critical thinking—for example, formulating workable solutions to complex problems, deliberating about what courses of action to take, or analyzing the assumptions and quality of the methods used in scientifically arriving at a reasonable level of confidence about a hypothesis. Using critical thinking, we might evaluate an argument—for example, whether it's worthy of acceptance because it is valid and based on true premises. Upon reflection, we may evaluate whether an author, speaker, or Web page is a credible source of knowledge on a given topic. **Source:** Adapted from http://en.wikipedia.org/wiki/Critical_thinking. Retrieved January 6, 2011.

RULE

Critical thinking—which centers not only on answering questions, but also on questioning answers—requires various types of thought (e.g., creative, reflective, and analytical thinking).[3] It also requires specific skills such as questioning, probing, and judging.

REWARDS OF LEARNING TO THINK CRITICALLY

Learning what critical thinking is—what it "looks like" and how you "do it" when circumstances change—helps you:

- **Gain confidence**, a trait that's crucial for success; lack of confidence is a "brain drain" that impedes thinking and performance.
- **Be safe and autonomous**, as it helps you decide when to take initiative and act independently, and when to get help.
- **Improve patient outcomes and your own job satisfaction** (nothing's more rewarding than seeing patients and families thrive because you made a difference).

    Yet thinking isn't "like it always was." Health care delivery is increasingly complex and dynamic, requiring very specific thinking and workplace skills (Box 1-1). Consider how the following points relate to the importance of developing sound thinking skills:

- A high-performance workplace requires workers who have a solid foundation in thinking skills, and in the personal qualities that make workers dedicated and trustworthy.[4]
- In all settings, nurses must take on new responsibilities, collaborate with diverse individuals, and make more independent decisions.
- Critical thinking is the key to preventing and resolving problems. If you can't think critically, you become a part of the problems.
- Nurses' roles within the context of the entire workforce, the nursing shortage, societal issues, and new technology continue to evolve. As a nurse, you must be a key player in designing and implementing more effective and efficient health care systems.[5,6]
- The complexity of care today requires knowledgeable individuals who are thought-oriented rather than task-oriented. For the public to value the need for nurses, we must change our image from being simply "a caring, helpful hand" to one that shows that we have specific knowledge that's vital to keeping patients safe and helping them get and stay well. We must "wear not only our hearts, but also our brains on our sleeves."[7]
- Critical thinking is crucial to passing tests that demonstrate that you're qualified to practice nursing—for example, the National Council Licensure Examination (NCLEX), the Canadian Nurse Registered Examination (CNRE), and other certification exams.

■ Patients and families must be active participants in making decisions; as the saying goes, "Nothing about me, without me." Knowing how to advocate and how to teach and empower patients and families to manage their own care requires highly developed critical thinking and interpersonal skills.

■ Critical thinking skills are key to establishing the foundation for lifelong learning, a healthy workplace, and an organizational culture that's more concerned with reporting errors and promoting safety than "pointing fingers" and "blaming" (Box 1-2).

BOX 1-1   KEY LEARNING AND WORKPLACE SKILLS

To succeed in the workplace and as learners, you must know how to:
• Be a self-starter and take initiative, ownership, and responsibility.
• Work independently and in groups to solve problems and develop plans.
• Teach yourself and others; advocate for yourself and others.
• Use resources: allocate time, money, materials, space, and human resources.
• Establish positive interpersonal relationships: work on teams, lead, negotiate, and work well with diverse individuals.
• Access, evaluate, and use information (organize and maintain files, interpret and communicate information, use computers to process data, and apply information to current situations.
• Assess social, organizational, and technologic systems.
• Apply professional and ethical standards to guide decision-making.
• Monitor and correct performance; design and improve systems.
• Use technology: select equipment and tools; apply technology to tasks; maintain and troubleshoot equipment.

Accomplishing the Above Requires You to Have the Following:
• Basic skills: reading, writing, speaking, listening, mathematics
• Thinking skills: knowing how to learn, reason, and think creatively, generate and evaluate ideas, see things in the mind's eye, make decisions, and solve problems
• Personal qualities: responsibility, self-esteem, self-confidence, self-management, sociability, and integrity

---

HOW THIS BOOK HELPS YOU IMPROVE THINKING

To keep your interest and help you understand and remember what you read, this book is designed based on principles of brain-based learning.[8,9] The following section explains brain-based learning and how this book helps both novices and experts improve thinking.

Brain-Based Learning

Brain-based learning uses strategies that help your brain get "plugged in to learning." For example:

> ## BOX 1-2 HEALTHY WORKPLACE AND SAFETY AND LEARNING CULTURES
>
> **Healthy Workplace Environment**
> Healthy workplace standards form the foundation for a climate that fosters critical thinking by providing an atmosphere that's respectful, healing, and humane. These standards stress the need for: (1) effective communication, (2) true collaboration, (3) effective decision-making, (4) appropriate staffing, (5) meaningful recognition, and 6) authentic leadership. A safe and respectful environment requires each standard to be maintained, because studies show that you don't get effective outcomes when any one standard is considered optional.
>
> **Safety Culture**
> When a group has a culture of safety, everyone feels responsible for safety and pursues it on a regular basis. Patient safety is top priority. To identify main causes of mistakes and build systems to prevent them, there's more concern about reporting errors than placing blame. Nurses, physicians, and technicians look out for one another and feel comfortable pointing out unsafe behaviors (e.g., when hand sanitation has been missed or when safety glasses should be worn). Safety takes precedence over egos or pressures to complete tasks with little help or time. The organization values and rewards such actions.
>
> **Learning Culture**
> In a learning culture, teaching and learning are key parts of daily activities. Everyone is encouraged to create learning opportunities and share information freely. Leaders, teachers, and staff are approachable and promote self-esteem and confidence by treating learners with kindness and showing genuine interest in them as people. Learners are encouraged to feel that they belong to the team. Teaching strategies are tailored to individuals, not tasks. Promoting research and improving care quality is "everyone's job."
>
> **References**
> American Association of Critical Care Nurses. Healthy work environments initiatives. Retrieved Jan 11, 2011, from: http://www.aacn.org/WD/HWE/Content/hwehome.pcms?menu=Practice&lastmenu=
> The Joint Commission. National Patient Safety Goals. Retrieved Jan 11, 2011, from: http://www.jointcommission.org/PatientSafety/NationalPatientSafetyGoals/
> Hand, H. (2006). Promoting effective teaching and learning in the clinical setting. *Nursing Standard*, 20(39), 55-63.

Source: Copyright 2011 by R. Alfaro-LeFevre. www.AlfaroTeachSmart.com.

1. **You learn best when there's logical progression of content** and you're engaged by a conversational style that gives lots of examples, strategies, and exercises to help you apply content to the "real world."
2. **Gaining deep understanding requires intensive analysis,** which means thinking about the same topics in various ways.
3. **Understanding and retaining what you read requires that you make learning meaningful** by using your own unique way of processing how content relates to you personally, rather than trying to memorize a bunch of facts.
4. **Humor reduces stress, keeps your interest, and helps you learn.**

5. **Thinking is like any skill (e.g., music, art, athletics)**—We each have our own styles and innate or learned capabilities. We can all improve by gaining insight, acquiring instruction and feedback, and deliberately working on the skills in real and simulated situations.

Organized for Novices and Experts

Whether you're a novice or an expert, the following organization helps you connect with what you already know, and move on to developing the complex skills you need to succeed today.

■   **This chapter and Chapter 2 build the foundation for developing critical thinking, clinical reasoning, and clinical judgment.** Here, with specific examples and strategies, you learn exactly what it takes to improve your ability to think your way through nursing and personal challenges.

■   **Chapters 3 and 4 help you gain the knowledge and skills required to succeed in six common nursing situations:** (1) clinical reasoning and judgment, (2) moral and ethical reasoning, (3) research and evidence-based practice, (4) teaching ourselves, (5) teaching others, and (6) test-taking. Beginning students sometimes like to jump to Chapter 4, where *teaching others, teaching ourselves,* and *taking tests* are discussed, before reading other chapters. This is a good example of making learning meaningful. Read what you're most interested in first.

■   **Chapter 5 helps you develop specific clinical reasoning skills by working with case scenarios that are based on real incidents.** In this section, you gain a deep understanding of nursing process skills, such as assessing systematically, identifying patient-centered outcomes, and setting priorities. You learn not only *how* to accomplish these skills, but *why* they are essential to developing sound clinical reasoning and judgment.

■   **Chapter 6 helps you develop communication, interpersonal, teamwork, and self-management skills** (e.g., managing your time). When you know how to communicate effectively, manage your emotions, organize your time, and build positive relationships with patients and team members, you spend less time getting sidetracked by interpersonal and "human nature" problems—and more time fully engaged in progress. Here, in the section titled *How to Prevent and Deal with Mistakes Constructively,* you also learn how to meet quality and safety standards and keep patients, caregivers, and yourself safe. The skills in this section are often considered to be leadership skills. Today, every nurse must be a leader. Advocating for your patients, yourself, your peers, and your community requires highly developed interpersonal and communication abilities.

You'll find many helpful Internet resources throughout this book. For direct links to all listed URLs, go to http://evolve.elsevier.com/Alfaro-LeFevre/CT.

WHAT'S THE DIFFERENCE BETWEEN THINKING AND CRITICAL THINKING?

The main difference between thinking and critical thinking is *purpose and control.* Thinking refers to any mental activity. It can be "mindless," like when you're daydreaming or doing routine tasks like brushing your teeth. Critical thinking is controlled and purposeful, using well-reasoned strategies to get the results you need.

CRITICAL THINKING: SOME DIFFERENT DESCRIPTIONS

Critical thinking is a complex process that changes depending on context—what you're trying to accomplish. For this reason, there is no one *right* definition for critical thinking. Many authors (including me) develop their own descriptions to complement and clarify someone else's (which is, by the way, a good example of thinking critically: critical thinking requires you to "personalize" information—to analyze it and decide what it means to you rather than simply memorizing someone else's words). Think about the following synonym and commonly seen descriptions.

A Synonym: Reasoning

A good synonym for critical thinking is *reasoning. Reasoning* is a good synonym because it implies careful, deliberate thought (as compared to *thinking,* which can be random and uncontrolled). Today, schools stress "four *R*s": reading, 'riting, 'rithmetic, and *reasoning.*

Common Critical Thinking Descriptions

Consider the following commonly seen descriptions of critical thinking:

- "Knowing how to learn, reason, think creatively, generate and evaluate ideas, see things in the mind's eye, make decisions, and solve problems"[10]
- "Reasonable, reflective thinking that focuses on what to believe or do"[11]
- "The ability to solve problems by making sense of information using creative, intuitive, logical, and analytical mental processes … and the process is continual"[12]
- "The process of purposeful, self-regulatory judgment … the cognitive engine that drives problem solving"[13]
- "Thinking about your thinking, while you're thinking, to make it better, more clear, accurate, and defensible"[14]
- "Knowing how to focus your thinking to get the results you need (includes using logic, intuition, and evidence-based practice)"[15]

CRITICAL THINKING, CLINICAL REASONING, AND CLINICAL JUDGMENT

The terms *critical thinking, clinical reasoning,* and *clinical judgment* are often used interchangeably. But there is a slight difference in how nurses use these terms:

- **Critical thinking**—a broad term—includes reasoning both outside and inside of the clinical setting. Clinical reasoning and clinical judgment are key pieces of critical thinking in nursing.
- **Clinical reasoning**—a specific term—usually refers to ways of thinking about patient care issues (determining, preventing, and managing patient problems). For reasoning about other clinical issues (e.g., teamwork, collaboration, and streamlining work flow), nurses usually use the term *critical thinking*.
- **Clinical judgment** refers to the result (outcome) of critical thinking or clinical reasoning—the conclusion, decision, or opinion you make.

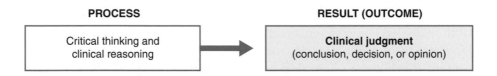

American Nurses Association (ANA) standards state that the nursing process—*assessment, diagnosis, outcome identification, planning, implementation,* and *evaluation*—serves as a critical thinking model that promotes a competent level of care[16] (discussed in depth in Chapters 3 and 5).

To clarify your understanding of the relationship of critical thinking to reasoning inside and outside of the clinical setting, study Figure 1-1. This figure also highlights requirements of ANA standards, Quality and Safety Education for Nurses (QSEN), and Institute of Medicine (IOM) competencies.

Applied Definition

To understand critical thinking in the clinical setting—a setting that's challenging, complex, and regulated by laws and standards—study the following definition.

Applied Definition

Critical thinking in nursing—which includes clinical reasoning and clinical judgment—is purposeful, informed, outcome-focused thinking that:
- **Is guided by standards, policies, ethics codes, and laws** (individual state practice acts and state boards of nursing).
- **Is based on principles of nursing process, problem-solving, and the scientific method** (requires forming opinions and making decisions based on evidence).
- **Focuses on safety and quality,** constantly re-evaluating, self-correcting, and striving to improve.
- **Carefully identifies the key problems, issues, and risks involved,** including patients, families, and key stakeholders in decision-making early in the process.*
- **Applies logic, intuition, and creativity** and is grounded in specific knowledge, skills, and experience.

- **Is driven by patient, family, and community needs,** as well as nurses' needs to give competent efficient care (e.g., streamlining charting to free nurses for patient care).
- **Calls for strategies that make the most of human potential** and compensate for problems created by human nature (e.g., finding ways to prevent errors, using technology, and overcoming the powerful influence of personal views).

*Stakeholders are the people who will be most affected (patients and families) or from whom requirements will be drawn (e.g., caregivers, insurance companies, third-party payers, health care organizations).

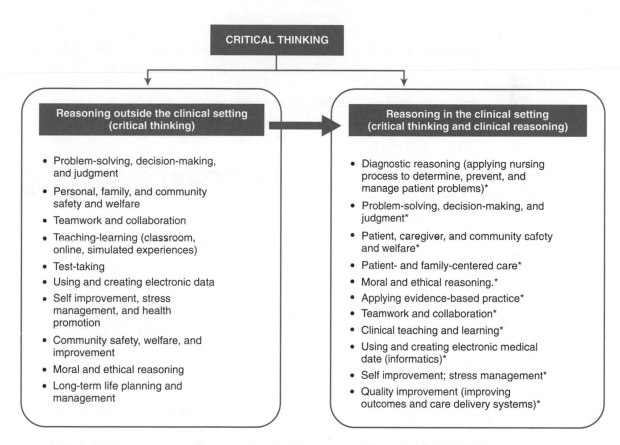

CRITICAL THINKING

Reasoning outside the clinical setting (critical thinking)

- Problem-solving, decision-making, and judgment
- Personal, family, and community safety and welfare
- Teamwork and collaboration
- Teaching-learning (classroom, online, simulated experiences)
- Test-taking
- Using and creating electronic data
- Self improvement, stress management, and health promotion
- Community safety, welfare, and improvement
- Moral and ethical reasoning
- Long-term life planning and management

Reasoning in the clinical setting (critical thinking and clinical reasoning)

- Diagnostic reasoning (applying nursing process to determine, prevent, and manage patient problems)*
- Problem-solving, decision-making, and judgment*
- Patient, caregiver, and community safety and welfare*
- Patient- and family-centered care*
- Moral and ethical reasoning.*
- Applying evidence-based practice*
- Teamwork and collaboration*
- Clinical teaching and learning*
- Using and creating electronic medical date (informatics)*
- Self improvement; stress management*
- Quality improvement (improving outcomes and care delivery systems)*

*Relates to ANA practice standards, The Joint Commission Standards, Quality and Safety Education for Nurses competencies, and Institute of Medicine competencies

FIGURE 1-1 The above shows that *critical thinking* is an "umbrella term" that includes many aspects of reasoning inside and outside of the clinical setting. The terms *clinical reasoning, critical thinking, problem-solving,* and *decision-making* are often used interchangeably. Your ability to reason *outside of the clinical setting* affects your ability to reason *in the clinical setting*. (Source: Copyright 2011 by R. Alfaro-LeFevre. www.AlfaroTeachSmart.com.)

PROBLEM-FOCUSED VERSUS OUTCOME-FOCUSED THINKING

Problem-focus thinking and outcome-focused thinking are closely related. You must have excellent problem-solving skills to get the results you need. But, keep the following points in mind.

■ **There are many ways to solve a problem.** There are quick fixes, "one-size-fits-all" solutions, temporary and long-term solutions, and solutions that are satisfactory but could be better. Outcome-focused thinking aims to fix problems in ways that get you *the best results.*

■ **Sometimes there are so many problems that the best approach may be to focus on *outcomes* rather than *problems.*** For example, if you work on a team with many interpersonal problems, your manager might say, "We have a long history of problems, and it will take forever to fix them. I want to see us all working as a team. I'm asking you to put the problems aside and get agreement on roles, responsibilities, and behavior, so that our patients get good care and we enjoy coming to work."

RULE

Critical thinking requires excellent problem-solving skills, as well as the ability to look ahead and decide exactly what outcomes (results) must be achieved.

WHAT ABOUT COMMON SENSE?

Some people believe that critical thinking is simply *common sense,* something that can't be taught. However, this belief is grounded on superficial understanding of what critical thinking is and how you get common sense. Although some people are born with common sense, a lot of it is *learned from experience.* You can put someone with great common sense in a new or stressful situation, and you're likely to see behaviors that don't seem at all sensible. Think about the following scenario.

Scenario
CRITICAL THINKING: SIMPLY COMMON SENSE?

As an evening supervisor, I stopped to check on a new graduate who was in charge for the first time. She appeared to be "in over her head," nervous and running around. Calmly, I asked how things were going. She replied, "Fine, except for the man in Room 203. His temperature was 104° an hour ago. We drew blood cultures, gave aspirin, and started him on antibiotics." I asked, "What's the temperature now?" She replied, "He's not due until 8 pm" (3 hours later). It seemed common sense to me that you would check the temperature more frequently when it was that high. Wanting to set a collaborative tone, I stressed the need to check it more frequently, and asked her to keep me informed. I also made sure I came back frequently to see how things were going. At the time, I believed this nurse had no common sense, but she went on to be an excellent clinician with a track record of success. She was simply inexperienced, nervous, and overwhelmed in a new situation. She may even have been subconsciously defending an oversight.

Common sense may be innate, but it also comes from knowledge, experience, and an ability to focus on what's important. What may be common sense to you, based on your upbringing, schooling, or experience, may not be so to someone else. If you encounter someone who seems to have no common sense, don't jump to conclusions. Dig a little deeper to determine the real problems: Is there a knowledge, confidence, communication, or organizational skills problem? Is the person simply inexperienced or stressed by a new environment? Has the person become complacent? Could a learning disability be contributing to the problem? Like critical thinking, common sense often can be taught if you determine the underlying problems and do something about them.

Scenario
CRITICAL THINKING: SIMPLY COMMON SENSE?—cont'd

WHAT DO CRITICAL THINKERS LOOK LIKE?

Research shows that most critical thinkers have high foreheads and furrowed brows, probably because of all the thinking they do. If you're not questioning this statement, then you're not thinking critically about what you're reading. When I ask, "What do critical thinkers look like?" I mean, "What characteristics do we see in someone who thinks critically?" Consider the following description:

"**The ideal critical thinker** is habitually inquisitive, self-informed, trustful of reason, open-minded, flexible, fair-minded in evaluation, honest in facing personal biases, prudent in making judgments, willing to reconsider, clear about issues, orderly in complex matters, diligent in seeking relevant information, reasonable in selecting criteria, focused in inquiry, and persistent in seeking results that are as precise as the subject and the circumstances of inquiry permit."[17]

CRITICAL THINKING INDICATORS (CTIs)

Studying *behavior*—what good thinkers *do and say*—helps you get a picture of what critical thinkers "look like." The next page shows personal critical thinking indicators (CTIs). CTIs are brief descriptions of behaviors/attitudes usually seen in individuals who are critical thinkers). These behaviors are called *critical thinking indicators* because they *indicate* characteristics of critical thinkers. To gain an understanding of these indicators, review the box and rate where you stand in relation to each indicator, using the following 0 to 10 scale:

0 = This indicator is not easy for me

10 = This indicator is pretty much a habit for me

As you evaluate yourself, keep in mind that no one is perfect—there's no ideal critical thinker who demonstrates *all* of the characteristics. Realize that even the best thinkers' characteristics vary, depending on circumstances such as confidence level and previous experience. What matters are *patterns of behavior* over time (is the behavior usually evident?). Remember that some of you, due to your nature, will be harder on yourselves than others (and vice versa). If you have some trusted friends, peers, or family members, ask them how they see your behavior. Ask them to focus on *usual patterns of behaviors* (not single incidents), and to give you specific examples. The results of this exercise may reaffirm or surprise you.

PERSONAL CRITICAL THINKING INDICATORS (CTIs)

<u>PERSONAL CTIs</u> are brief descriptions of behaviors, attitudes, and qualities often seen in individuals who are critical thinkers.

- **SELF-AWARE:** Identifies own learning, personality, and communication style preferences; clarifies biases, strengths, and limitations; acknowledges when thinking may be influenced by emotions or self-interest.
- **GENUINE/AUTHENTIC:** Shows true self; demonstrates behaviors that indicate stated values.
- **EFFECTIVE COMMUNICATOR:** Listens well (shows deep understanding of others' thoughts, feelings, and circumstances); speaks and writes with clarity (gets key points across to others).
- **CURIOUS AND INQUISITIVE:** Asks questions; looks for reasons, explanations, and meaning; seeks new information to broaden understanding.
- **ALERT TO CONTEXT:** Looks for changes in circumstances that warrant a need to modify approaches; investigates thoroughly when situations warrant precise, in-depth thinking.
- **ANALYTICAL AND INSIGHTFUL:** Identifies relationships; expresses deep understanding.
- **LOGICAL AND INTUITIVE:** Draws reasonable conclusions (if this is so, then it follows that …because…); uses intuition as a guide; acts on intuition only with knowledge of risks involved.
- **CONFIDENT AND RESILIENT:** Expresses faith in ability to reason and learn; overcomes problems and disappointments.
- **HONEST AND UPRIGHT:** Looks for the truth, even if it sheds unwanted light; demonstrates integrity (adheres to moral and ethical standards; admits flaws in thinking).
- **AUTONOMOUS/RESPONSIBLE:** Self-directed, self-disciplined, and accepts accountability.
- **CAREFUL AND PRUDENT:** Seeks help as needed; suspends or revises judgment as indicated by new or incomplete data.
- **OPEN AND FAIR-MINDED:** Shows tolerance for different viewpoints; questions how own viewpoints are influencing thinking.
- **SENSITIVE TO DIVERSITY:** Expresses appreciation of human differences related to values, culture, personality, or learning style preferences; adapts to preferences when feasible.
- **CREATIVE:** Offers alternative solutions and approaches; comes up with useful ideas.
- **REALISTIC AND PRACTICAL:** Admits when things aren't feasible; looks for useful solutions.
- **REFLECTIVE AND SELF-CORRECTIVE:** Carefully considers meaning of data and interpersonal interactions; asks for feedback; corrects own thinking; alert to potential errors by self and others; finds ways to avoid future mistakes.
- **PROACTIVE:** Anticipates consequences; plans ahead; acts on opportunities.
- **COURAGEOUS:** Stands up for beliefs; advocates for others; doesn't hide from challenges.
- **PATIENT AND PERSISTENT:** Waits for right moment; perseveres to achieve best results.
- **FLEXIBLE:** Changes approaches as needed to get the best results.
- **HEALTHY:** Promotes a healthy lifestyle; uses healthy behaviors to manage stress.
- **IMPROVEMENT-ORIENTED (SELF, PATIENTS, SYSTEMS):** SELF—Identifies learning needs; finds ways to overcome limitations, seeks out new knowledge. PATIENTS—Promotes health; maximizes function, comfort, and convenience. SYSTEMS—Identifies risks and problems with health care systems; promotes safety, quality, satisfaction, and cost containment.
  NOTE: The above is the ideal—no one is perfect.

Table 1-1 gives examples of what critical thinking is and what it's *not*. Box 1-3 (on the next page) shows how other authors describe critical thinking traits. These traits were incorporated into the CTIs using simpler terms.

TABLE 1-1	CRITICAL THINKING: WHAT IT IS AND WHAT IT IS NOT	
Critical Thinking	**Not Critical Thinking**	**Example of Critical Thinking**
Organized and explained well by using words, examples, pictures, or graphics	Disorganized and vague	Persisting until you find a way to make your ideas easy to understand; using examples and illustrations to facilitate understanding
Critical for the sake of improvement, new ideas, and doing things in the best interest of the key players involved	Critical for the sake of attacking without being able to suggest new ideas and alternatives; critical for the sake of having it your way	Determining key players affected, and then looking for flaws in the way something is done and figuring out ways to achieve the same outcomes more easily or better
Inquisitive about intent, facts, and reasons behind an idea or action; thought- and knowledge-oriented	Unconcerned about motives, facts, and reasons behind an idea or action; task-oriented, rather than thought-oriented	Raising questions to deeply understand what happened, why it happened, and what was being attempted when it happened
Sensitive to the powerful influence of emotions, but focused on making decisions based on what's morally and ethically the right thing to do	Emotion-driven	Finding out how someone feels about something, then moving on to discuss what's morally and ethically right
Communicative and collaborative with others when dealing with complex issues	Isolated, competitive, or unable to communicate with others when dealing with complex issues	Seeking multidisciplinary approaches to planning care as indicated by client needs

BOX 1-3 HOW OTHER AUTHORS DESCRIBE CRITICAL THINKING TRAITS

Scheffer and Rubenfeld's Habits of the Mind[1]
- **CONFIDENCE:** Assurance of one's reasoning abilities
- **CONTEXTUAL PERSPECTIVE:** Consideration of the whole situation, including relationships, background, and environment relevant to some happening
- **CREATIVITY:** Intellectual inventiveness used to generate, discover, or restructure ideas. Imagining alternatives.
- **FLEXIBILITY:** Capacity to adapt, accommodate, modify, or change thoughts, ideas, and behaviors
- **INQUISITIVENESS:** An eagerness to know, demonstrated by seeking knowledge and understanding through observation, and thoughtful questioning to explore possibilities and alternatives
- **INTELLECTUAL INTEGRITY:** Seeking the truth through sincere, honest processes, even if the results are contrary to one's assumptions and beliefs
- **INTUITION:** Insightful sense of knowing without conscious use of reason
- **OPEN-MINDEDNESS:** A viewpoint characterized by being receptive to divergent views and sensitive to one's biases
- **PERSEVERANCE:** Pursuit of a course with determination to overcome obstacles
- **REFLECTION:** Contemplation upon a subject, especially on one's assumptions and thinking for the purposes of deeper understanding and self-evaluation

Facione's Critical Thinking Dispositions[2]
- **TRUTHSEEKING:** A courageous desire for the best knowledge, even if such knowledge fails to support or undermines one's preconceptions, beliefs, or self-interest
- **OPEN-MINDEDNESS:** Tolerance of divergent views; self-monitoring for possible bias
- **ANALYTICITY:** Demanding the application of reason and evidence; alert to problematic situations; inclined to anticipate consequences
- **SYSTEMATICITY:** Valuing organization; focusing; being diligent about problems of all levels of complexity
- **CRITICAL THINKING SELF-CONFIDENCE:** Trusting one's own reasoning skills; seeing oneself as a good thinker
- **INQUISITIVENESS:** Curious and eager to acquire knowledge and learn explanations even when the applications of the knowledge are not immediately apparent
- **MATURITY:** Prudence in making, suspending, or revising judgment; awareness that multiple solutions can be acceptable; appreciation of the need to reach closure even in the absence of complete knowledge

Paul and Elder's Intellectual Traits[3]
- **INTELLECTUAL HUMILITY:** Consciousness of limits of your knowledge; willingness to admit what you don't know
- **INTELLECTUAL COURAGE:** Awareness of the need to face and fairly address ideas, beliefs, or viewpoints to which you haven't given serious hearing
- **INTELLECTUAL EMPATHY:** Consciousness of the need to imaginatively put yourself in the place of others to genuinely understand them
- **INTELLECTUAL AUTONOMY:** Having control over your beliefs, values, and inferences; being an independent thinker
- **INTELLECTUAL INTEGRITY:** Being true to your own thinking; applying intellectual standards to thinking; holding yourself to the same standards you hold others; willingness to admit when your thinking may be flawed
- **CONFIDENCE IN REASON:** Confidence that, in the long run, using your own thinking and encouraging others to do the same gets the best results
- **FAIR-MINDEDNESS:** Awareness of the need to treat all viewpoints alike, with awareness of vested interest

[1]Scheffer, B., Rubenfeld, M. (2000). A consensus statement on critical thinking in nursing. *Journal of Nursing Education,* 39(8), 353.
[2]Facione, P. *Critical thinking: What it is and why it counts* (2010 update). Retrieved June 1, 2010, from http://www.insightassessment.com/pdf_files/what&why2007.pdf
[3]Paul, R., Elder, L. *Valuable intellectual traits.* Retrieved December 4, 2010, from http://www.criticalthinking.org/articles/valuable-intellectual-traits.cfm.

WHAT'S FAMILIAR AND WHAT'S NEW?

We understand something best by comparing it with things we already know: How is it the same, and how is it different? Let's examine what's familiar and what's new about critical thinking.

What's Familiar

Problem-Solving. Knowing specific problem-solving strategies is a key part of critical thinking. For example, if you're caring for someone after heart surgery, you must know strategies to prevent and treat complications. Be aware, however, that using *problem solving* interchangeably with *critical thinking* can be a "sore subject." *Problem-solving* is missing the important concepts of prevention, creativity, improvement, and aiming for the best results. Even if there are no problems, you should be thinking creatively, asking, "What could we do better?" and "How can we prevent problems before they happen?"

Analyzing. Although being analytical is important, critical thinking requires more than analyzing. It requires coming up with new ideas (right-brain thinking) and judging the worth of those ideas (left-brain thinking). Some overly analytical people suffer from "analysis paralysis," over-thinking problems when they should be taking action.

Decision-Making. *Decision-making* and *critical thinking* are sometimes used interchangeably. Making decisions is an important part of critical thinking.

Scientific Method. This is an excellent tool for critical thinking, as it has been well studied and applies the following principles of scientific investigation:

- **Observing:** Continuously observing and examining to collect data, check for changes, and gain understanding
- **Classifying data:** Grouping related information so that patterns and relationships emerge
- **Drawing conclusions** that follow logically: "If this is so, then...."
- **Conducting experiments:** Performing studies to examine hypotheses (hunches or suspicions) and identify ways to improve
- **Testing hypotheses (hunches):** Determining whether we have factual evidence to support our hunches, assumptions, or suspicions

What's New

Emotional Quotient (EQ). EQ—the ability to recognize and manage your own emotions and help other do the same— is as important to critical thinking as IQ (intelligence quotient).

So-Called "Soft Skills" Aren't Soft. For years, we called communication and interpersonal skills the "soft skills" of nursing, implying that clinical skills such as managing intravenous lines are the most important skills. We now know that communication and interpersonal skills such as engaging patients, dealing with difficult people, and resolving conflicts are crucial to critical thinking. These types of skills take considerable knowledge and practice and must be as good as clinical skills.[18,19]

Right and Left Brain Thinking. Critical thinking requires right-brain thinking (generating new ideas) and left-brain thinking (analyzing and judging the worth of those ideas).

Maximizing Human Potential. We're only just beginning to identify ways to maximize the human potential to think critically. For example, new brain imaging techniques show us what parts of the brain are being used in various thinking and tasks, helping us learn how individuals use their brains. People survive brain injuries that used to be fatal, and we continue to learn from their rehabilitation. For example, some people who have had strokes cannot speak, but they can sing words. We're learning how to use brain techniques not only to learn, but also to promote healing, stress reduction, and wellness.

Mapping as a Strategy to Teach and Learn. Maps and decision trees created by experts guide seasoned and new nurses. Maps developed by learners promote deep personal understanding. They help learners make connections between concepts and information in their own unique way. You can find the "how to's" of concept mapping in Appendix A.

Changing How We View Mistakes. We now know that being allowed to make mistakes in safe situations (e.g., simulations) is a powerful way to learn. Experts also agree that "to err is human" and that most errors happen because of multiple factors and system problems (e.g. look-alike drugs or inadequate staffing or staff preparation). Humans are vulnerable to making mistakes due to "human factors" (e.g., stress, fatigue, information overload). Reducing errors related to human factors (e.g., using computers and decision support systems) is now the norm.[20]

"What-if" Scenarios—Being Prepared. Today, we have greater emphasis on developing detailed policies and procedures to address "what-if" scenarios (e.g., bioterrorism or pandemics) and be prepared.

Evidence-Based Thinking Stressed. Clinicians are expected to provide evidence that supports opinions, solutions, and courses of action. We must be confident when we're asked questions like, "What evidence do you have that this will work?" or "What data are you using to support that this is the problem or that this is a good solution?"

Measuring Outcomes (Results). Critical thinking makes it necessary to develop very specific ways to measure progress and results. For example, in the case of pain management, you don't ask a general question like, "Are you more comfortable?" You ask, "Can you rate your pain on a scale of 0 to 10, with 0 meaning pain-free, and 10 meaning the worst possible pain?"

Collaborative Thinking. The workforce is diverse. We must find ways to facilitate "meetings of the minds" to get the collaborative approaches we need today.

Relating on a "Human Level" Matters. Understanding personal interests and passions and showing your "human side" helps build the relationships needed for critical thinking.

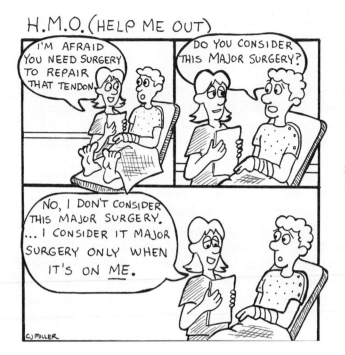

Showing your human side and using humor can help you connect with patients.

4-CIRCLE CT MODEL: GET THE PICTURE?

Whereas CTIs give verbal descriptions of behaviors that promote critical thinking, the 4-circle CT model shown on the inside front cover *creates a picture* of what critical thinking involves. Study the four circles. Note that critical thinking (CT) requires a blend of CT characteristics, theoretical and experiential knowledge, interpersonal skills, and technical skills. Realize that the top circle—CT characteristics—corresponds with the CTIs listed on page 12. In the next chapters, we'll address the other circles in more depth. For now, remember that if you develop the CT characteristics and attitudes in the *top* circle (e.g., confidence, resilience, and being proactive), developing the skills in the other *three* circles of the model will be easier.

THINKING AHEAD, THINKING-IN-ACTION, AND THINKING BACK (REFLECTING)

Critical thinking is contextual, which means it changes depending on circumstances. The saying "one size doesn't fit all" applies. Let's finish this chapter by addressing the importance of looking at critical thinking from three perspectives: *thinking ahead, thinking-in-action,* and *thinking back (reflective thinking).*

Consider the following descriptions, and think about the differences in each circumstance.

1. **Thinking Ahead:** Anticipating what might happen and being proactive by identifying what you can do to be prepared. For novices, thinking ahead is difficult and sometimes restricted to reading procedure manuals and textbooks. An important part of being proactive is asking questions like "What can I bring with me to help jog my memory and stay focused and organized?"

2. **Thinking-in-Action:** Rapid, dynamic reasoning that considers several things at once, making it difficult to describe. For example, suppose you find your stove on fire. As you spring into action, your mind races, thinking about many things at once (How can I put this out? Where's the fire extinguisher? Should I call the fire department?). Thinking-in-action is highly influenced by previous knowledge and hands-on experience. To keep safety first, in all important situations, keep experts nearby who have extensive experiential knowledge stored in their brains. If you encountered a fire, wouldn't you like to have a fireman standing at your side? Thinking-in-action is prone to "knee-jerk" responses and decisions. To use the fire example again, an untrained person may throw water on a grease fire, which can make it worse.

3. **Thinking Back (Reflective Thinking):** Analyzing the reasoning you used to look for flaws, gain more understanding, and correct and improve it. Experienced nurses double-check their thinking in dynamic ways during thinking-in-action. However, this doesn't replace reflective thinking that happens after the fact. Deliberate, methodical reflective thinking that happens *after the fact,* using specific strategies and tools (e.g., journaling, chart reviews, honest dialogue with others) brings new insights, more depth, and greater accuracy; you can more objectively identify "lessons learned" from experience.

Considering all three of the above phases of thinking helps you examine thinking in a holistic way. If you look only at *one phase,* you'll miss important parts of thinking.

PUTTING IT ALL TOGETHER

By now, you should have an idea of what critical thinking, clinical reasoning, and clinical judgment entail. To solidify your understanding of this chapter, take a few moments to decide where you stand in relation to "Questions to Evaluate Your CT Potential" on the next page.

Then study the instructions on completing the exercises throughout this book (page 20), and complete the end-of-chapter exercises.

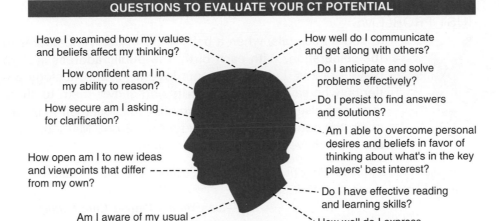

QUESTIONS TO EVALUATE YOUR CT POTENTIAL

Have I examined how my values and beliefs affect my thinking?

How confident am I in my ability to reason?

How secure am I asking for clarification?

How open am I to new ideas and viewpoints that differ from my own?

Am I aware of my usual thinking and learning habits?

How well do I communicate and get along with others?

Do I anticipate and solve problems effectively?

Do I persist to find answers and solutions?

Am I able to overcome personal desires and beliefs in favor of thinking about what's in the key players' best interest?

Do I have effective reading and learning skills?

How well do I express myself in writing?

CRITICAL MOMENTS

GOOD QUESTION!
Socrates learned more from questioning others than he did from reading books. Learn to be confident asking questions. Seek other opinions, and question deeply to gain understanding. Don't think you have to know all the answers. Simply saying "Good question!" often sparks great critical thinking.

LOOK FOR AHAS!
We say "Aha!" when we suddenly realize something or have our suspicions confirmed. We say, "Aha!" when we connect with something that was in the back of our minds but never put into words. As you read this book, look for "ahas." These moments of "light bulbs going off in your head" are energizing. They bring new ideas and stimulate you to learn more.

OTHER PERSPECTIVES

HOW TO THINK LIKE EINSTEIN
"It's not that I'm smart, it's just that I stick with problems longer."
—*Albert Einstein*

CRITICAL THINKING TRIGGERED BY POSITIVE EVENTS, NOT JUST PROBLEMS

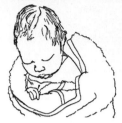

In some hospitals, when a baby is born, everyone shares in the celebration. With each birth, the public address system plays Brahms' Lullaby. Patients love it—even oncology patients, who say it lifts their spirits and allows them to share someone else's joy. Parents who have just lost their baby are given the option of playing the lullaby or not. Many of them choose to have it played for their baby.

"Playing the music is a simple thing that can be done for patients and families that costs nothing and brings a great deal of pleasure."

—*Jean Young, Patient Care Manager*

Making the Most out of the Exercises in This Book

All exercises, except for the ones labeled *Think, Pair, Share*, have example responses listed in the *Response Key* beginning on page 266. Remember that these are *example* responses, not the *only* responses. You may have a response that's different but equally as good as the example. The main point is to learn by evaluating the thinking you put into completing the exercise and the content in each chapter. If you have questions about whether your responses are appropriate, check with your instructor.

Apply strategies that use your own learning style preferences (page 34). Consider drawing pictures, diagrams, and maps to make connections between concepts. If you need help with mapping, see *Concept Mapping: Getting in the "Right" State of Mind* (page 279).

When writing responses, at first be more concerned with substance than grammar (as you would if you were writing a diary). However, as you progress, apply grammar rules, and make your responses clear to others. Making your responses clear to others helps you clarify your thoughts. Following grammar rules improves clarity and gives you practice for writing other important papers and communications.

Don't be afraid to paraphrase. Paraphrasing helps you gain understanding because you explain what you read using familiar language (your own). To avoid concerns of plagiarism, cite the page numbers you're paraphrasing.

Consider how the exercises can be improved: Give suggestions to your instructor, and send them to us by clicking on "Contact Us" at www.AlfaroTeachSmart.com. If your suggestion is unique, we will post it on the Web and cite you as the contributor.

Think, Pair, Share

This strategy promotes efficient, cooperative learning, and has three main steps: (1) Think about a question or issue independently, jotting down three thoughts or questions that seem important to you. (2) Pair off with a partner:

discuss what you each jotted down; write down things your partner listed that you did not; together with your partner, choose 1 to 3 of the most important points you want to share with the group. (3) Share these in a group discussion. You can find a template for completing *Think, Pair, Share* exercises at www.AlfaroTeachSmart.com or http://evolve.elsevier.com/Alfaro-LeFevre/CT.

Think, Pair, Share was developed by Frank Lyman at the University of Maryland. For more on this strategy, visit http://www.eazhull.org.uk/nlc/think,_pair,_share.htm

Critical Thinking Exercises

Example responses are on page 266.

1. When you form an opinion, you draw a conclusion from *facts* (evidence).
   a. What's the difference between facts and opinions?
   b. How can you determine if an opinion is valid?
2. What is the relationship between achieving outcomes and identifying problems, issues, and risks involved?
3. What is the relationship between CTIs (page 12) and behavior?
4. Compare and contrast the traits of confidence, critical thinking self-confidence, and confidence in reason listed in Box 1-3 (page 14)
5. If you are in a new or uncomfortable situation, what is likely to happen to your ability to demonstrate the CTIs (page 12)?
6. What do the following "five Cs" (context, confident, courage, curious, committed) have to do with critical thinking?
7. Why is it important to consider thinking from the following perspectives: *thinking ahead*, *thinking-in-action*, and *thinking back?*

Think, Pair, Share

With a partner, in a group, or in a journal entry:

1. Complete the following sentences, and then compare your responses with those of others:
   • If I were to explain to someone else what critical thinking is, I would say that…
   • I do my best thinking when…
   • I do my worst thinking when…
2. Study Table 1-1 (page 13). Discuss times when you've experienced some of the descriptions listed under "Not Critical Thinking." How did it affect your thinking?
3. Consider the CTIs listed on page 12. Identify five indicators that are especially challenging for beginning nurses.

4. Discuss your thoughts on the *Other Perspectives* and *Critical Moments* in this chapter.
5. Study *Key Brain Parts Involved in Thinking* in Appendix B. Decide how thinking ability would be affected by brain damage in the frontal lobe or hippocampus.
6. Discuss the implications of the *Critical Moments* and *Other Perspectives* on page 19.
7. Decide where you stand in relation to outcomes in the chapter opener.

KEY POINTS/SUMMARY

- Thinking critically doesn't mean simple criticism. It means not accepting information at face value without evaluating whether is factual and reliable.
- *Critical thinking* is like an "umbrella term" that includes the terms *clinical reasoning* and *clinical judgment*. Figure 1-1 maps the relationships among key aspects of reasoning inside and outside of the clinical setting.
- This book applies brain-based learning, using strategies that help you get your brain "plugged in" to learning.
- Because critical thinking (CT) changes with context and is a complex process, there's no one right definition—there are several that complement and clarify one another.
- Having a healthy workplace, a learning culture, and safety culture forms the foundation for developing CT skills. (Box 1-2, page 5).
- CT in nursing makes patient and caregiver safety and welfare top priorities.
- *Critical thinking* refers to purposeful, focused, informed, results-oriented thinking in any situation. The term is often used interchangeably with *clinical reasoning, clinical judgment, problem-solving,* and *decision-making*.
- Reasoning in the clinical setting is challenging, complex, and regulated by laws, standards, and policies and procedures.
- Page 8 (Applied Definition) delineates the major points of critical thinking, clinical reasoning, and clinical judgment.

- Pages 15 to 16 summarize what's familiar and what's new about CT.
- CT requires right-brain thinking (generating new ideas) and left-brain thinking (analyzing and judging the worth of those ideas).
- Communication and interpersonal skills such as engaging patients, knowing how to collaborate, and resolving conflicts are crucial to CT.
- Page 12 shows personal CTIs—behaviors that demonstrate characteristics that promote CT. Ability to demonstrate these behaviors varies, depending on circumstances such as familiarity with the people and situations at hand. These are the behaviors that you should work to develop.
- The 4-circle CT model shown on the inside front cover gives you "a picture" of what it takes to think critically. If you develop CT characteristics (top circle), you will easily develop skills related to the other circles.
- CT is like any skill (e.g., music, art, athletics). We each have our own styles and innate or learned capabilities. We can all improve by gaining awareness, acquiring instruction, and consciously practicing to improve.
- Because CT is contextual (it changes with circumstances), consider it from three different perspectives: thinking ahead, thinking-in-action, and thinking back (reflective thinking).
- Scan this chapter to review all highlighted rules.

REFERENCES

1. *Behind every healed patient is a critical thinking nurse.* Retrieved January 6, 2011, from http://www.medplusstaffing.cc/blog/?p=188.
2. Hansten, R. (January 2011). E-mail communication.
3. Darlington, R. *How to think critically.* Retrieved January 6, 2011, from http://www.rogerdarlington.co.uk/thinking.html.
4. Secretary's Commission on Achieving Necessary Skills (SCANS). *Learning a living: A blueprint for high performance.* U.S. Department of Labor. Retrieved January 4, 2011, from http://wdr.doleta.gov/SCANS/lal/.
5. Institute of Medicine. *Robert Wood Johnson Foundation Initiative on the Future of Nursing.* Retrieved January 6, 2011, from http://www.iom.edu/Activities/Workforce/Nursing.aspx.
6. Institute of Medicine. *The future of nursing: Leading change, advancing health.* Retrieved October 6, 2010, from http://www.nap.edu/catalog/12956.html.
7. Gordon, S. (2006). What do nurses really do? *Topics in Advanced Nursing eJournal,* 6(1). Retrieved January 6, 2011, from http://www.medscape.com/viewarticle/520714.
8. *Brain-based learning.* Retrieved January 8, 2011, from http://www.funderstanding.com/content/brain-based-learning.
9. Caine, R., Caine, G. (2002). *Making connections: Teaching and the human brain.* Reading, MA: Addison-Wesley.
10. Secretary's Commission on Achieving Necessary Skills (SCANS). *Learning a living: A blueprint for high performance.* U.S. Department of Labor. Retrieved January 4, 2011, from http://wdr.doleta.gov/SCANS/lal/.
11. Ennis, R., Milman, J. (1985). *Cornell tests of critical thinking: Theory and practice.* Pacific Grove, CA: Midwest Publications.
12. Snyder, M. (1993). Critical thinking: A foundation for consumer-focused care. *The Journal of Continuing Education in Nursing,* 24(5), 206-210.
13. Facione, P. *Critical thinking: What it is and why it counts.* (2010 update). Retrieved January 1, 2011, from http://www.insightassessment.com/pdf_files/what&why2007.pdf.
14. Paul, R., Elder, L. (2005). *Critical thinking: tools for taking charge of your learning and your life* (2nd ed.). Upper Saddle River, NJ: Prentice Hall.
15. Alfaro-LeFevre, R. (In press). *Applying nursing process: The foundation for clinical reasoning* (8th ed.). Philadelphia: Lippincott Williams & Wilkins.
16. American Nurses Association. (2010). *Nursing scope and standards of performance and standards of clinical practice* Washington, DC: American Nurses Publishing.
17. *The Delphi Report.* (1990). Retrieved January 14, 2011, from www.insightassessment.com/pdf_files/DEXadobe.PDF.
18. Arnold, E., Boggs, K. (2011). *Interpersonal relationships: Professional communication skills for nurses.* St. Louis: Saunders.
19. Pagana, K. D. (2010). *The nurse's communication advantage: How business-savvy communication can advance your career.* Indianapolis: Sigma Theta Tau International.
20. Institute of Medicine. (2000). *To err is human: Building a safer health system.* Washington, DC: National Academies Press. Retrieved January 5, 2011, from http://www.nap.edu/openbook.php?record_id=9728&page=1.

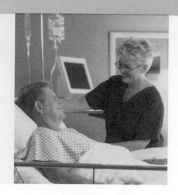

How to Develop Critical Thinking

This chapter at a glance ...

PRECHAPTER SELF TEST

Decide where you stand in relation to the following learning outcomes.

Learning Outcomes

After completing this chapter, you should be able to:

1. Explain three main steps to improving thinking.
2. Explain the relationship between effective/skilled communication and critical thinking.
3. Describe how personality, learning style, upbringing, and culture affect thinking.
4. Identify strategies to develop your emotional intelligence (EI).
5. Explain why building trust and following a code of conduct are key to promoting critical thinking.
6. Discuss how human habits influence critical thinking.
7. Address how answering the questions listed on the inside back cover promotes critical thinking.
8. Identify the roles of logic, intuition, and trial and error in critical thinking.
9. Determine your progress toward developing critical thinking indicators (CTIs) related to knowledge and intellectual skills.
10. Decide where you stand in relation to gaining the skills in the 4-circle CT model shown on the inside front cover.
11. Identify three key ways of evaluating nurses' critical thinking skills.

GAINING INSIGHT AND SELF-AWARENESS

A first-grade teacher I know tells this great story: "One of my kids came into class looking very pleased with himself. Pointing to the middle of his forehead, he announced, 'I just realized that I can read my own mind!'" Another of my friends talks to herself all the time. When asked, "Why are you talking to yourself?" she replies, "Because I'm the only one who makes any sense around here."

Many people have little understanding of their own thinking, and even *less* understanding of how *others* think. Although I can't promise that reading this chapter will stop you from talking to yourself, it *will* help you gain insight into how and why you think the way you do … and how and why *others* think the way *they* do. These insights are major steps in helping you develop critical thinking abilities.

As you read this chapter, keep the following in mind:

- Thinking is a skill like any other (e.g., music, art, athletics).
- As with any skill, we each have our own styles, and innate and learned capabilities.
- Improving thinking requires three main steps: (1) Gain insight and self-awareness. (2) Get agreement on a code of conduct (see next page) and what critical thinking entails. (3) Make the choice to develop the attitudes, knowledge, and skills required to focus your thinking to get the results you need.

Let's start with the first step, gaining insight and self awareness: Why do you think and learn the way you do?

HOW YOUR PERSONALITY AFFECTS THINKING

Personality plays a major role in how you think and learn. Your personality determines what information you notice and recall, the way you make decisions, and how much structure and control you like. Connecting with your own particular personality's needs helps you understand how and why you think the way you do. It helps you get in touch with your talents and blind spots and find ways to improve. Understanding personality types different from your own helps you realize how and why *others* think the way they do. Armed with this information, you can facilitate "meetings of the minds."

To better understand your personality and thinking style, study Do You Know What to Do When Someone Turns Blue? and Box 2-1 (What's Your Thinking Style) on the following pages. Think about where you and others who are close to you "fit into" the various styles described on those pages. Keep in mind that no one style is better than another. They are all good styles, with specific strengths and limitations. What's important is that you know that there are distinct style differences and that you (1) connect with your own style, celebrating your strengths and working to overcome limitations and (2) learn to connect with people with styles that are different from your own, respecting their need to approach things in their *own* way. Box 2-2 lists the benefits of being sensitive to personality types.

Text continued on p. 31

HEALTH TEAM CODE OF CONDUCT

As a member of this group/team, I agree to work to make the following a part of my daily routine.

1. **To keep patient and caregiver safety and welfare as the primary concern in all interactions, including:**
   - Being vigilant and monitoring for care practices that increase risks of errors
   - Remembering that no one is perfect and that all humans are vulnerable to making mistakes
   - Taking responsibility for being "a safety net" when helping co-workers, anticipating what they may need, and pitching in to prevent mistakes (e.g., "I think that glove is contaminated; let me get you a new one." or "Here's a new needle.")
   - Making it a team principle that "If we witness unethical or unsafe practices, it's our responsibility to address it" (first directly with the person, then through policies and procedures if needed).

2. **To promote empowered partnerships by:**
   - Valuing your time and the contribution you make to the team/group.
   - Accepting the diversity in our styles—recognizing that you know yourself best and should be allowed to choose your own approaches.
   - Promising to be honest, and treating you with respect and courtesy.
   - Promoting independence and mutual growth by applying the Platinum Rule (Treat others as *they* want to be treated, not assuming they have the same desires *you* do).*
   - Listening openly to new ideas and other perspectives.
   - Attempting to walk a mile in your shoes.
   - Committing to resolving conflict without resorting to using power.
   - Taking responsibility for my own emotional well-being (if I feel bad about something, it's my responsibility to do something about it).
   - Ensuring that we both:
     - Stay focused on our joint purpose and responsibilities for achieving it.
     - Make decisions together as much as possible.
     - Realize that we're accountable for the outcomes (consequences) of our actions.
     - Have the right to say no, so long as it doesn't mean neglecting responsibilities.

3. **To foster open communication and a positive work environment by:**
   - Addressing specific issues and behaviors.
   - Acknowledging/apologizing if I've caused inconvenience or made a mistake.
   - Doing my "homework" before drawing conclusions.
   - Maintaining confidentiality when I'm used as a sounding board.
   - Using only ONE person as my sounding board before I decide to either give feedback
   - or drop the issue.
   - Validating any rumors I hear.
   - Redirecting co-workers who are talking about someone to speak directly
   - to the person.
   - Addressing unsafe or unethical behavior directly and according to policies.
   - Offering feedback as indicated:
     - Within 72 hours, using "I' statements ("I feel ..." rather than "You make me feel ...")
     - Describing behaviors and giving specific examples
     - Limiting discussion to the event at hand and not discussing past history and telling you honestly and openly the impact of the behavior

4. **To be approachable and open to feedback by:**
   - Taking responsibility for my actions and words.
   - Taking time to reflect on what was said, rather than blaming, defending, or rejecting.
   - Asking for clarification of the perceived behaviors.
   - Remembering that there's always a little bit of truth in every criticism.
   - Staying focused on what I can learn from the situation.

*Retrieved January 11, 2011, from www.alessandra.com/abouttony/aboutpr.asp.
Source: Copyright 2011 by R. Alfaro-LeFevre. www.AlfaroTeachSmart.com

DO YOU KNOW WHAT TO DO WHEN SOMEONE TURNS BLUE?

Here's a theory that gives new meaning to turning blue, red, white, or yellow (no, it doesn't mean becoming cyanotic, inflamed, shocky, or jaundiced). Psychologist Taylor Hartman uses colors to represent personality types.* (By the way, he says you can't really *turn* one color or another—you are what you are *born*.) Hartman believes that each of us, from birth, is blessed with a core motive—a drive to approach life from a certain perspective. Using colors as labels, here's how he describes four distinct personality types:

REDS have a drive for power. They know how to take charge and make things happen. Red strengths are that they are confident, determined, logical, productive, and visionary. However, they can be bossy, impatient, arrogant, argumentative, and self-focused.

BLUES are driven to achieve intimacy. They love getting to know people well, have strong feelings, and like talking about the daily details of life. Blues are creative, caring, reliable, loyal, sincere, and committed to serving others. On the flip side, they can be judgmental, worry-prone, doubtful, and moody, and often have unrealistic expectations.

WHITES strive for peace. They're independent, contented people who ask little of those around them. Whites are insightful, flexible, tolerant, easygoing, patient, and kind. But Whites tend to avoid conflict at all costs, are indecisive, are silently stubborn, and may "explode" because they hold things in until there are so many things bothering them that just one more problem pushes them over the edge.

YELLOWS are driven to have fun and enjoy the moment. They wake up happy, know how to enjoy life in the present moment, and are simply fun to be around. Yellows are outgoing, enthusiastic, optimistic, popular, and trusting. However, they tend to avoid facing facts and can be impulsive, undisciplined, disorganized, and uncommitted.

Applying the *Color Code* principles helps you connect with inner drives that often lie dormant, waiting to be harnessed in positive ways. Armed with this knowledge, you can make better "people decisions," like how to nurture a team or get along with difficult people. Imagine how you could apply this theory to help a group come together to give a presentation. You might get a productive, visionary Red to coordinate and lead the project; a caring, detail-oriented Blue to do the handouts; a peace-loving, insightful White to be a "human suggestion box" (no one's afraid to approach a White); and a fun-loving Yellow to make sure that the class is more than serious stuff (a little fun, humor, and refreshment make it an enjoyable, memorable, learning experience).

Think about what could happen in the above situation if you switched some of those personalities and tasks around! *The Color Code* facilitates a crucial first step to improving thinking—understanding how and why we think the way we do (and how and why others think they way they do). These are challenging times that require us to think and work in teams. Applying these principles helps us spend less time spinning wheels and more time "in gear," fully engaged in progress. **To take the Color Code test, or order the book**, go to www.ColorCode.com. For a CEU article on this topic, go to www.nurse.com/ce/CE236.

*Summarized from Hartman, T. (1998). *The color code*. New York: Scribner.
Source: Adapted from Alfaro-LeFevre, R. (1998). *Do you know what to do when someone turns blue?* Nursing Spectrum Nurse Wire (www.nurse.com).

BOX 2-1   WHAT'S YOUR THINKING STYLE? (MYERS-BRIGGS TYPE)*

EXTROVERT
Thinks out loud
Draws energy from being with people

INTROVERT
Thinks inside
Draws energy from being quiet

Sensate
Perceives the world discretely through the five senses
Looks for facts

Intuitive
Perceives the world overall
Looks for meaning

Thinking
Uses objective data
Seeks just decisions

Feeling
Uses subjective data
Seeks fair decisions

Judging
Orders the environment
Likes to plan

Perceiving
Keeps things flexible and open
Likes to be spontaneous

*Data from www.humanmetrics.com/#Jtype. You can find various style inventories at www.humanmetrics.com.

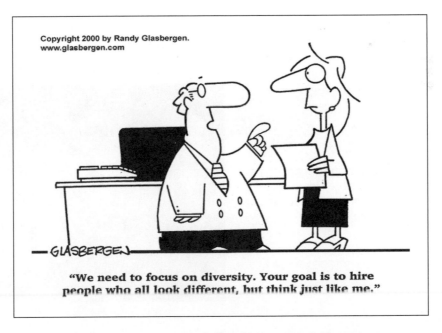

Reprinted with special permission from www.glasbergen.com.

BOX 2-2 BENEFITS OF BEING SENSITIVE TO PERSONALITY TYPES

Partnering and Team Building
- Helps diverse personalities come together with understanding and respect, promoting solid relationships
- Keeps the focus on common goals, improving quality and efficiency
- Helps identify strategies to reduce and resolve conflicts
- Facilitates collaboration and makes the most of individual and team talents

Performance and Retention
- Promotes critical thinking (people think better when they understand and trust one another)
- Reduces stress, allowing more brainpower for finding solutions
- Increases self-confidence by providing style-specific strategies
- Promotes an environment that nurtures professional and personal growth

Consumer and Patient Satisfaction
- Facilitates communication with "difficult" patients and families
- Improves outcomes by helping you tailor approaches to consider different personalities' wants and needs

Patients and families feel understood, empowered, and motivated by receiving care that's "in sync" with their own specific styles

You are born with unique and inherited personality traits. Your birth order, gender, upbringing, and culture also affect your personality and learning preferences.

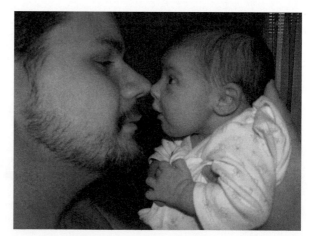

CONNECTING WITH YOUR LEARNING STYLE

Your ability to connect with your preferred learning style makes the difference between learning efficiently (feeling energized and capable and wanting more) and wasting time (feeling tired, useless, and frustrated). Many people believe they are poor learners. However, the reality is that they're simply unaware of their own learning preferences. For example, a friend once said: "What I like best about computers is that I never was a good learner … but with computers, it doesn't matter because I just have to figure things out for myself … and I'm good at that." Learning is *figuring things out for yourself.* When you figure things out for yourself, it's *learning at its best* because you "own the material and make it yours." You understand deeply, and your brain retains more.

RULE

There are no right or wrong ways to learn. There are only *differences.* Connecting with your preferred style helps you identify strategies to learn efficiently in your own way. When you figure things out *in your own way,* you're thinking critically. Page 34 gives strategies for various learning preferences.

SELF-EFFICACY: BELIEVE IN YOURSELF

Self efficacy—having a strong sense that you're capable of accomplishing all that you must do to achieve your goals—greatly affects your ability to gain the knowledge and skills needed for critical thinking. Today, independent learning in a complex world is the norm. We must all be self-sufficient. People with a strong sense of efficacy tend to challenge themselves, recover more easily from setbacks, and put forth a high degree of effort to meet commitments. On the other hand, people with a poor sense of efficacy believe they can't be successful. They're less likely to make a concerted, extended effort and may see challenging tasks as threats to avoid. These people often have low aspirations, which may result in disappointing academic and clinical performances and become a self-fulfilling prophecy.[1]

Developing self-efficacy takes considerable self-coaching, as noted in the following quote:

> *"You must be your own coach. If you don't talk to yourself and give yourself pep talks, start now. Time was, only crazies talked to themselves; now, you miss the boat if you don't. Our minds are tricky things. We can't give in to self doubt or negativity. We must focus on the positives, as learning and performance depend on it."*[2]
> —Jean T. Penny, PhD, ARNP

If you have a low sense of self-efficacy, don't feel bad about it. Many of the challenges you face are common to others in your situation. It's not just YOU! Problems with self-efficacy can often be overcome through formal or informal coaching. Having a sensible coach to help you put things in perspective—to help you identify why you feel this way, how to use your strengths, and what strategies can help you handle learning challenges—can significantly affect your ability to succeed.

EFFECTS OF BIRTH ORDER, UPBRINGING, AND CULTURE

Your birth order—whether you were the first born who was expected to lead or the "baby" who had few responsibilities—impacts on how you think, as does your parents' "parenting style." If you were raised by strict, authoritarian parents who insisted that you "do as you are told, without asking questions," it's likely that you'll find it difficult to approach teachers or leaders to discuss problems, ask for feedback, or offer suggestions. Some of you need to muster courage to overcome deep-seated insecurities that come from lessons learned as a child.

Where you grew up and the culture you embrace also affects thinking. For example, in some countries, questioning teachers is considered rude. However, when students ask questions, everyone learns.

MALE VERSUS FEMALE THINKING

Male versus female thinking is a common topic in journals, in the media, and on the Internet.[3] Women are often considered to be intuitive, creative, and able to multitask. Men are often viewed as being focused, logical, and methodical.

Studies show that structurally, male and female brains are different.[4,5] There are also male-female biological differences. Males and females tend to be raised differently from one another. Yet, we can't make assumptions, as there are many creative males and logical females. Just remember that we each have a unique brain and upbringing, that there often are male and female tendencies, and that we should be careful about pushing our own expectations onto others. This is especially important as more males enter into nursing—a historically female profession.[6] Think about the wisdom in the following e-mail from a colleague.

"My doctoral research opened my eyes to the struggles of male nursing students. Men learn differently from women, have different backgrounds on entering nursing school, and have different experiences once in school. Men are less likely to be assigned to female patients in med-surg units. Their peers, and sometimes their instructors, seek them out to help with moving and positioning patients. Some men feel they must be "extra" professional to avoid misconceptions by patients. Men approach teamwork differently from what they experience in nursing. They tend to address issues directly, whereas women often talk around issues and avoid the person with whom they have a conflict. Learning to care is a big deal for guys. Men are socialized to not express emotion. Yet when we teach therapeutic communication, what do we expect? We want them to maintain eye contact and use touch to show connection. We want interactive responses that show engagement—'really?' 'uh huh,' head nods, and, of course, reflective restatements. We talk about maintaining an open posture without crossing our arms, and leaning in to show attention. But, what are normal male responses to conversation? They may rest against the wall with arms crossed and respond to patients' concerns with humor. Too often, instructors regard this type of communication as inattentive, unconnected, and not therapeutic (because that's not how we females interact). Men may be just as connected and therapeutic in their approaches. We have to be careful not to judge their performance based on our female expectations."[7]

EMOTIONAL INTELLIGENCE (EI)

Being aware of your emotional intelligence—your ability to recognize emotions and make them work in positive ways—may be even more important than IQ (cognitive intelligence quotient). Studies estimate that IQ accounts for only 4% to 25% of successful job performance.[8,9] You may be intellectually smart, but you must also be able to recognize and manage your emotions. To develop good working relationships, you must be sensitive to others' emotions and learn how to work through difficult communications. If not, your great ideas and intentions will be lost in emotional issues.

Developing EI enhances critical thinking because how you feel about something significantly affects how you think. Many people aren't aware of deep, strong feelings. Clarifying your own emotions and giving them the attention they deserve helps you adjust your behavior, be more logical, and improve results. Clarifying what other people think and feel is just as important. You have to "name emotions to tame them" (Box 2-3). Pay attention to facial expressions, as they are the best reflection of emotions (Figure 2-1).

BOX 2-3 DEVELOPING EMOTIONAL INTELLIGENCE (EI)

Definition: Knowing how to recognize and manage emotions to get positive results.
1. **Connect with emotions.** Put your feelings into words and, through dialogue, help others to do the same ("I feel ... because ..." If you're trying to connect with others' emotions, ask "What are your thoughts and feelings on this?"). Never assume you know what someone else is feeling. Never expect others to know what you're feeling.
2. **Accept true feelings** for what they are. No one's to blame for what he or she feels.
3. **Learn mood management.** Recognize the importance of connecting with how emotions are affecting thinking. Learn to manage feelings like anger, anxiety, fear, and discouragement.
4. **Don't be too concerned with isolated events.** Patterns of behavior are what matter. Don't sweat the small stuff.
5. **Keep in mind that emotions are "catching."** If you're depressed, you may trigger depression in someone else. If you're enthusiastic, you may trigger enthusiasm.
6. **Pay attention to stress levels.** When the going gets rough, take time out, focus on the positives, find a sense of humor, play a game, or take a walk.

Recommended: Consortium for Research on Emotional Intelligence in Organizations: http://www.eiconsortium.org/; Daniel Goleman Web site: www.danielgoleman.info/blog.

STRATEGIES FOR LEARNING PREFERENCES

LEARNING PREFERENCE
Observers (Visual Learners)

Learn best by watching. For example, you'd rather watch someone give an injection before reading the procedure.

STRATEGIES TO PROMOTE LEARNING

Sit in the front of the room, so you stay focused on the teacher, not on what's going on around you.

Visualize procedures in your mind's eye, rather than trying to follow individual steps.

In skills labs, don't go first. Rather, watch your classmates and take a later turn.

Ask for observational experiences.

Take lots of notes, draw maps, and use a highlighter. Recopy your notes when you're studying.

When learning new terms or concepts or trying to remember something, write them on "sticky notes" and put them where you'll see them frequently (e.g., the bathroom mirror, the computer).

Preview chapters by scanning headings and illustrations.

Doers (Kinesthetic Learners)

Learn best by moving, doing, experiencing, or experimenting. For example, you'd rather play with a syringe and inject a dummy before reading the procedure.

Start by doing (e.g., play with equipment before reading about how to use it) because it will make observing, reading, and listening more meaningful.

Be sure you know the risks of *doing without much knowledge*, and find ways to minimize them (e.g., if you're playing on the computer, make sure you can't inadvertently erase a file).

When taking notes, use arrows to show relationships.

Draw boxes and circles around key concepts; use arrows when you make diagrams and maps.

Pace up and down while reciting information to yourself; ride a bicycle while listening to an instructional tape.

Make tapes with the information you're trying to learn, and play them while exercising (e.g., riding a bike), or read while riding a stationary bike.

Write key words in the air; use your fingers to help you remember (bend the forefinger as you memorize a concept, and then bend the next for the next concept, and so on).

Change positions frequently while studying; take frequent short breaks involving activity.

Study in a rocking chair; play background music.

Ask if you can do assignments in an active way (e.g., create a poster, be part of a discussion group).

Listeners (Auditory Learners)

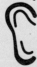

Learn best by hearing. For example, you learn best when you can listen without worrying about taking notes.

Whisper as you read, listening to your words (especially important when reading test questions).

Listen in class without taking notes, focusing on understanding what the teacher says, and then copy someone else's notes.

Tape classes and listen to the tapes two or three times before exams.

Ask if you can give an oral report or hand in an audiotape for extra credit.

Memorize by making up songs or rhymes.

Study with a friend, so you talk about the information.

Tape yourself as you read key information out loud, and then listen to the tapes.

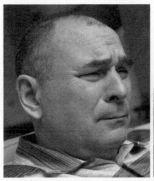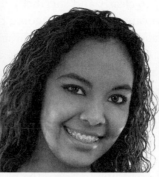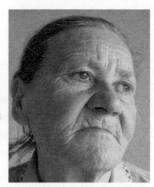

FIGURE 2-1 Facial expressions are the best indicators of emotions. What emotions do you read in these photos?

COMMUNICATING EFFECTIVELY

If you said, "Name one skill we should all work on to improve thinking," I would reply, "Communicating effectively."

> **RULE**
>
> **All critical thinking depends on the quality of communication—*mutual exchange* of information.** Communication problems are a major cause of mistakes and adverse outcomes (e.g., falls, injuries, and care omissions).[10] You must be able to understand others and be understood by others to gain the information and insight you need to think critically and keep patients safe.

Keep in mind that communication means more than talking and listening. It means paying attention to both verbal and nonverbal messages, and developing skills that promote the *mutual exchange* of the most important facts, thoughts, and feelings. Also remember that communication is usually based on more than one interaction, and is highly influenced by messages sent by behavior over time. For example, you may be committed to giving good patient care, but if you constantly arrive late for work, you send a different message.

> **RULE**
>
> **Developing your communications skills is as important as developing your clinical skills.** Because communication is a challenging two-way process that involves *mutual exchange* of verbal and nonverbal messages, it requires developing specific skills that enable you to: (1) give information in ways that others readily understand what you have to say, (2) use specific strategies to encourage others to express what they think and feel, and (3) listen in ways that help you gain deep understanding of the facts, thoughts, and feelings that are being conveyed to *you*.

Developing the ability to clearly and succinctly communicate with patients, families, and all levels of the health care team is an ongoing challenge. Today, you must not only be a good listener and speaker, you have to determine the best channel of communication to use to meet your goals (e.g., face-to-face, phone, or electronic messages). There are a wide variety of communication channels. Adapting your style to meet others' communication preferences promotes timely exchange of information (many of us have learned to text message only because it's the way our families, patients, and clients best respond).

A key nursing competency today is being able to promote open expression of ideas and to encourage communication among patients and caregivers.

Communication, especially in stressful situations, requires specific strategies aimed at promoting mutual understanding between the person giving the information and the person receiving it. Throughout this book, you have many opportunities to practice specific communication skills in context of various challenges (e.g., giving change-of-shift hand-off reports, dealing with conflict, addressing complaints, and giving and taking feedback). You'll examine powerful scenarios and strategies that show the difference between skilled versus unskilled communication. For now, think about the lessons learned from the following scenario, based on a real incident.

Scenario
COMMUNI-CATION: WHAT'S WRONG AND WHAT'S RIGHT?

Parents bring a young boy to the emergency department with a painful broken arm. They're greeted by Jane, the nurse who decides which patients will be seen first. As Jane puts a splint on the child, she announces, "It will be at least 4 hours before he'll be seen." The parents ask, "Should we go somewhere else?" Jane replies, "Well, there will be a fee for this." Upset by her son's injury, the mother angrily shouts. "Four hours is unacceptable!" Jane calls security, who stands by on call. The mother announces, "This is humiliating! We're leaving!" As the parents go out the door, Bob, another nurse, pulls them aside and says, "Write a letter to Risk Management about this … this was BADLY handled."

The parents write a letter describing their bad experience. They also point out how much it meant to have Bob's kindness and concern. They wonder if Jane was just having a bad day. A few weeks later, they receive a call from the hospital explaining that due to privacy issues, not much could be said. But, the caller did say one thing: "Jane will not be having any more bad days at our hospital."

What went wrong with the communications in this scenario? How might it have been handled differently? What went *right*?

COMMUNICATION STRATEGIES THAT PROMOTE CRITICAL THINKING

The following gives powerful communication strategies that promote critical thinking.
Aim for mindful communication.[11] This means clearing your mind of "clutter" and staying focused on the present moment. With mindful communication, your goal is

to gain a keen awareness of the situation, the information you gain, and the interaction of those engaged in the communication. To be mindful, pause before engaging in a communication and from time to time during the communication to allow yourself to get centered.

Examine your "personal story" about the communication you're about to have.[12] What are your thoughts and feelings? Do you have preconceptions? What assumptions and judgments have you made? What's your confidence level? What can you do to be more objective and positive about the communication? Staying objective, overcoming bad feelings, focusing on the present, and expressing the desire for positive outcomes improve the quality of communication.

Consider how the other person may perceive both you and the situation. Think about cultural differences and communication preferences. What can you do to make the other person more comfortable? Use clear, concise, simple language.

Evaluate your stress level, and that of the other person. Choose the right time and place.

Explain that your intent is not to judge, but to understand (e.g., "I'm not here to judge. I just want to understand what's going on.").

Listen first. Work to understand the thoughts and feelings that others are expressing before trying to get them to understand *you*.

Use strategies that help you see other points of view.
- Ask for clarification (e.g., "Can you clarify further?" or "Help me understand what the most important issues are.").
- Use phrases like, "From your way of looking at it" or "From your perspective."
- Repeat back what you hear, using your own words (e.g., "You're saying … Is that correct?").

Listen empathetically (with the intent of understanding the other person's way of looking at the situation). This is called imagining what it's like to "walk a mile in someone else's shoes," and can be done by taking the following steps:[13]
1. Clear your mind of thoughts about how you view the situation or concerns about how you're going to respond.
2. Focus on listening to the person's feelings and perceptions.
3. Rephrase the feelings and perceptions as you understand them to be (e.g., "I realize that you're frustrated and angry.").
4. Detach and come back to your own frame of reference.

Apply strategies that help you get accurate and comprehensive information.
- Use open-ended questions (those requiring more than a one-word answer). For example, "How do you feel about leaving tomorrow?"
- Avoid closed-ended questions (those requiring only a one-word answer). For example, "Are you ready to leave tomorrow?"
- Use exploratory statements that lead the person to expand on specific issues. For example, "Tell me more about …"
- Don't use leading questions (those that lead someone to a desired answer). For example, "You don't smoke, do you?"
- Put body language into words. For example, "You looked a little sad …"

- Use silence. Allow the person time to gather his thoughts.
- Record the information you gathered, and then look to see what's missing and check for inconsistencies.
- Ask the person to keep a log or diary, or keep one yourself. When you write things down, feelings often become clear and patterns emerge.

Use strategies that help you get your point across:
- Wait until the person is ready to listen.
- When voicing an opinion, use phrases that convey that you're voicing an opinion, rather than dictating what is so (e.g., "From my way of looking at it … From my perspective …").
- Ask the person to paraphrase what you've said (e.g., "I need to know you understand. Explain to me what I just said.").

Demonstrate behaviors that send messages like *I'm responsible*, *I can be trusted*, and *I want to do a good job*. For example, keep promises, be punctual, accept responsibility, and respect others' time.

When you may have caused inconvenience, made a mistake, or offended someone, offer a sincere apology, taking accountability (e.g., "I should have been more aware, and I'm sorry this happened".).

Respect others' territory. Ask permission (e.g., "May I listen to your chest?" rather than, "Sit up and let me listen to your chest").

Keep an open mind, and practice your listening skills (see the following shaded section).

Listening: A Lost Art?

"Not listening to each other separates us from family, friends, co-workers. We have not learned to listen and truly hear with empathy. We listen to prepare our responses, whether to tell our own story or to offer advice…. Most of us are preoccupied with the rush of our own lives and give little thought to the needs of others to be heard. We listen as though we are expected to respond. When we want to be there for someone, we listen for where we can help. When we are spoken to heatedly, we become defensive and either talk back heatedly or withdraw."[14]

Receptive Listening: Promoting Self-Awareness and Professional Growth

As part of a year-long nurse residency program at Dartmouth Hitchcock Medical Center in New Hampshire, facilitators trained in Receptive Listening (listening without valuing, judging, helping, or changing) meet monthly in 90-minutes sessions with small groups of new nurses. Nurses report that this type of listening creates a safe environment that contributes to their self-awareness, renewal, learning, problem-solving, and sense of belonging and connectedness to the organization. Receptive Listening has also shown direct benefits to patients in an unpublished doctoral study. For more information, e-mail rceppete@comcast.com.[15]

BUILDING RELATIONSHIPS

From dealing with patients to dealing with peers and professionals, building trust in relationships is crucial to getting the results you need. Without trust, you're likely to have superficial—rather than meaningful—discussions, as people are afraid to speak their minds. Improving thinking requires honest, open dialogue—something that only happens when there's trust between the two people.

RULE

People think best when they like and trust one another. The first step to building trust is agreeing to a code of conduct and making roles and responsibilities clear. Be sensitive to style differences, and follow the *Platinum Rule* ("Treat others as they want to be treated"), rather than the *Golden Rule* ("Do unto others as you would have them do unto you").[16] This changes your thinking from "This is what I want, so I'll give everyone the same thing" to "Let me first understand what others want so I can give it to them."

PRECEPTORS, MENTORS, AND EMPOWERED PARTNERSHIPS

Think about the following quotes:

"Early in my career, I was powerfully influenced by a nursing instructor who saw potential in me that I did not recognize. Under the watchful, yet caring, tutelage of this person, I began to find my professional self."[17]

—*Patricia Thompson, RN, EdD*

"Expert nurses are made, not born. Remember your first code, your first day in charge, the sadness with the death of your primary patient, or feeling alone? These experiences are all common to the novice nurse. The perception of the experience, as well as what is brought forward to future career events, can be shaped by an experience with a mentor."[18]

—*Margaret M. Ecklund, RN, MS, CCRN*

Most nurses can identify people in their lives who have impacted on their thinking. Often, these individuals are parents, teachers, co-workers, or friends. Today, because we know the value of improving thinking and performance through on-the-job partnerships, many organizations assign preceptors or mentors to help students and novice nurses. Preceptors and mentors are nurses with exemplary skills whose role it is to teach, nurture, and empower new nurses on a one-to-one basis. Learning how to be a mentor (acquiring the skills needed to nurture novices) and how to be a "mentee" (knowing how to learn from a more experienced person) is an important step in clinical learning. When choosing mentor-novice partnerships, it's important to give thought to the pair's "fit." When matched well, mentors experience the reward of making a difference in someone else's life. Under competent, caring guidance from a well-matched mentor, novices "spread their wings." If matched poorly, for example, if the two nurses are very different thinkers or personalities, the end result can be frustration, disappointment, and damaged spirits on both sides. Remember that mentoring isn't a "one size fits all" situation. Build empowered partnerships, pay attention to personal style differences, and address these early (see *Developing Empowered Partnerships* in Chapter 6).

FACTORS INFLUENCING CRITICAL THINKING ABILITY

Have you ever found yourself saying, "I just wasn't thinking" or "This really got me thinking—I came up with some great ideas"? We all feel this way at one time or another. Our ability to think well varies, depending on personal factors and the circumstances that are present at the time. This section addresses personal and situational factors that influence thinking.

Personal Factors Influencing Thinking

In addition to learning styles, personality, birth order, culture, upbringing, and male versus female differences as described earlier, think about how the following personal factors influence your thinking.

Fair-Mindedness and Moral Development. People who are fair-minded and have a mature level of moral development are more likely to think critically. It makes sense that those who are keenly aware of their own values, have a good sense of right and wrong, and approach situations with an attitude of "I must consider all viewpoints and make decisions in the key players' best interests" already are critical thinkers.

Age/Maturity. Age often correlates with critical thinking ability: The older you get, the better a thinker you become. There are two logical reasons for this: (1) Moral development usually comes with maturity. (2) Most older people have had more opportunities to practice reasoning in various situations. Realize, however, that sometimes older nurses are rigid and set in their ways—in this case, age impedes critical thinking.

Dislikes, Prejudices, and Biases. These are subtle but powerful factors that hinder critical thinking. If you don't recognize these factors—put them out on the table, so to speak—and overcome them, you're unlikely to think critically in situations where you have to function in spite of your dislikes, prejudices, and biases.

Self-Confidence. For the most part, as addressed earlier, self-confidence aids thinking. If you aren't confident, you use much of your brain power worrying about failure, reducing the energy available for productive thinking. *Occasionally* self-confidence hinders critical thinking; some people become overly confident and believe they can't be wrong or have little to learn from others.

Knowledge of Problem-Solving, Decision-Making, Nursing Process, and Research Principles. Because critical thinking is based on many of these same principles, familiarity with the methods enhances critical thinking.

Early Evaluation and Reflection. When you make it a habit to evaluate early—reflecting on your thinking and checking whether your information is accurate, complete, and up-to-date—you can make corrections early. You avoid making decisions based on outdated, inaccurate, or incomplete information. This is a combination of *thinking-in-action* and *reflective thinking*, as described in Chapter 1.

Past Experience. Most authors view *experience as an enhancing factor*, since you remember best what you learn from experience. If, however, your past experience is a bad one, it may be an inhibiting factor. For example, if a mother had a bad experience breast-feeding her firstborn child, it may be difficult for her to think clearly about breast-feeding subsequent children.

Effective Writing Skills. When you learn how to make yourself clear in writing, you learn to apply critical thinking principles like identifying an organized approach, deciding what's relevant, and focusing on others' perspectives.

Effective Reading and Learning Skills. Because critical thinking often requires that you use resources independently, you must know how to read and learn well. Having effective reading skills doesn't mean knowing how to read rapidly. It means knowing how to read efficiently, identifying what's important, and drawing conclusions about what the material implies.

Situational Factors Influencing Thinking

Anxiety, Stress, and Fatigue. Anxiety and stress, often the first to drain your brain power, make concentration difficult. When you're fatigued, you're already operating on a "low battery." A low anxiety level, however, like being a little nervous about a test, can promote critical thinking by motivating you to prepare.

Awareness of Risks. Usually this is an enhancing factor. When you know the risks, you think more carefully (you "think before acting"). Sometimes awareness of the risks can increase anxiety to a level that impedes critical thinking. For example, most of us remember how hard it was to think critically when we gave our first injection.

Knowledge of Related Factors. The more you know about a situation, the better you'll be able to reason. For example, you might know about diabetes, but if you don't *know the person* you're going to teach about diabetes—the person's lifestyle, desires, and motivations—you'll be unlikely to design a plan that the person will follow.

Awareness of Resources. Awareness of resources is the key to thinking critically. No one knows everything. You must know where to get reliable help (from human and other information resources).

Positive Reinforcement. Positive reinforcement promotes critical thinking by building confidence and focusing on what's being done *right*.

Negative "Talk." Focusing too much on what could go wrong impedes thinking, as it drains your confidence and takes your attention away from what you need to do *right*.

Evaluative or Judgmental Styles. An evaluative or judgmental style impedes critical thinking. When you think someone is judging or evaluating you, you spend more brain power worrying about what the *other person* is thinking than what *you* are thinking.

Presence of Motivating Factors. Having motivating factors (things that make you *want* to think critically) entices you to get your brain "in gear." For example, think how motivated you are to learn something when a teacher says, "You must know this because it will be on the test, and you'll run into it a lot in the clinical setting."

Time Limitations. This can be an enhancing or impeding factor. Time limitations can be motivating factors—deadlines stimulate us to get things done. If there's too little time, however, you may make decisions more quickly than you'd like and come up with less than satisfactory answers. It's interesting to note that the courts give more leeway to decisions that were made in emergency situations than to those made with plenty of time for thinking.

Distractions. These impede critical thinking for obvious reasons—the more distractions, the more difficult it is to stay focused. For example, it's best to do your charting in a quiet place, where there are few interruptions and distractions.

Habits Causing Barriers to Critical Thinking

As humans, most of us have deeply ingrained habits that create barriers to critical thinking. Consider the following list, and then read on to learn more about how they impede thinking.

BARRIERS TO CRITICAL THINKING		
• Self-Focusing	• Mine-Is-Better*	• Tunnel Vision
• Choosing-Only-One	• Face-Saving*	• Resistance to Change*
• Conformity*	• Stereotyping*	• Self-Deception*

*From, Ruggerio, V. (2006). *The art of thinking: A guide to critical and creative thought* (8th ed.). New York: Longman.

Keep in mind that these habits are simply a result of human nature. Whether we realize it or not, we're all victims of these behaviors to some extent at one time or another.

Self-Focusing. Focusing on ourselves is a carry-over from primitive survival instincts. In the early days of man, humans had to be keenly centered on their own needs to survive. We still have this instinct. Critical thinking requires you to overcome this natural tendency and work to understand needs, perspectives, and challenges that are *different* from our own.

Mine-Is-Better. We tend to regard our ideas, values, religions, cultures, and points of view as being superior to others. To think critically, recognize when you are biased and have strong personal "pro" or "con" views that may influence your opinions.

Tunnel Vision. Tunnel vision is a universal problem. We see what we *expect* to see, often misinterpreting what's before us. A classic example of tunnel vision is when a psychiatric nurse fails to consider whether someone's confusion is related to a *medical problem*, and vice versa (a medical-surgical nurse fails to consider whether someone's confusion is related to a *psychiatric problem*).

Choosing-Only-One. When faced with more than one choice, we tend to choose only one. We forget to think about things like, Are there other, better choices? Can we do *both*?

Do we have to do *either*? Beginners are most vulnerable to the *choosing-only-one habit*. They tend to blindly accept that if they've chosen at least one option, they've made a good decision. They also tend to make the assumption that there must be *one best way* to do something, rather than thinking that there probably are several good ways of getting things done and that each has advantages and disadvantages, depending on circumstances. You can overcome this tendency by remembering to ask, "Must I choose only one?" or "Is this the only way?" "What approaches can we combine?"

Face-Saving. We have a strong instinct to protect our image—we try to save face. Critical thinking requires us to learn and grow. As we learn and grow, we'll make mistakes or realize that our old ways of thinking or doing things can be improved. To be a critical thinker, we must be comfortable saying things like "I'm not sure," "I was wrong," or "I have to think about that."

Resistance to Change. We all tend to resist change. Too often change is considered "guilty until proven innocent." Overcoming this barrier doesn't mean embracing every new change uncritically. It means being willing to suspend judgment long enough to make an informed decision on whether the change is worthwhile (see *Navigating and Facilitating Change* in Chapter 6).

Conformity. Although some conformity—like following policies and procedures—is *good*, there's also harmful conformity. Harmful conformity is when we conform to group thinking just to avoid being viewed as "different." Conforming without thought stifles the ability to be creative and improve. An example of harmful conformity is following policies blindly, even if there are circumstances that clearly indicate that the policy doesn't apply in *this* particular situation.

Stereotyping. We stereotype when we make fixed and unbending overgeneralizations about others (e.g., *homeless people aren't very bright*). When our minds are fixed and unbending, we're unlikely to see what's really before us. By recognizing our tendency to stereotype, we can make a conscious effort to overcome this habit.

Self-Deception. This is the subconscious forgetting of things about ourselves we don't particularly feel good about. An example of this is experienced nurses who believe that they never made learning errors or were shy, nervous, or insecure when they were beginning nurses.

Habits That Promote Critical Thinking

Developing habits that promote critical thinking is a constant "work in progress." Critical thinking requires ongoing self-reflection, self-correction, and practice. We gain experience and insight *over time*.

Consider how making the following behaviors your personal habits can bring balance to your life and promote your ability to think critically.*

*Adapted from Covey, S. (1989). *The 7 habits of highly effective people.* New York: Simon & Schuster; and Cardillo, D. *Zen and the art of nursing: Seven ways to make the most of each workday.* Retrieved January 11, 2011, from http://news.nurse.com/article/20100503/DD01/105030020

- **Be proactive and responsible for your own life.** Anticipate responses, and act before things happen.
- **Affirm your path.** Your work is important, and it's a privilege to have it. Stay focused—fully present in everything you do—and give complete attention to each action, interaction, and task.
- **Communicate effectively.** Be a good listener, working to understand other points of view, before presenting your own.
- **Begin with an end in mind.** Identify clear expected outcomes. What exactly do you want to accomplish? Make your goals and expectations explicit.
- **Know your priorities—put first things first.** Decide what's important, and stick to priorities moment by moment, day by day.
- **Think win-win.** Aim for *mutual benefit* in all human interactions.
- **Create good karma (spiritual energy that brings good things for all).** Your thoughts and actions directly impact your environment. Don't judge others or take part in gossip or negativity.
- **Stay grounded in who you are—"sharpen the saw."** Look after yourself physically, emotionally, and spiritually. Author Stephen Covey explains "sharpening the saw" this way: *A man is sawing a tree trunk for hours. The saw is dull, and the man is exhausted. Someone suggests that he might do better if he sharpens the saw. The man responds, "I don't have time" and continues to work ineffectively.*
- **Develop good learning habits, and be committed to life-long learning.** Try to learn something new every day and help others to do the same.

Critical Thinking Exercises

Example responses are on page 266.

1. According to this chapter, if you had to choose only *one* skill to develop to promote your ability to think critically, what should you choose?
2. Emotive thinking is thinking that's driven by feelings: How does this relate to critical thinking?
3. Compare and contrast the *Golden Rule* and the *Platinum Rule*.

 ### Think, Pair, Share

With a partner, in a group, or in a journal entry:

1. Discuss the following in relation to *Do You Know What to Do When Someone Turns Blue?* (page 28) and *What's Your Thinking Style?* (page 29):
   a. Your thinking style and main motive according to Myers-Briggs and Hartman's *Color Code*
   b. How your style and innate motives affect your ability to think clearly

    c. What personalities and thinking styles are difficult for you to work with … and how you can improve your ability to work with these styles

    d. How other factors such as birth order, culture, and upbringing affect how you think

    e. How you would feel about taking a personality test for your own personal knowledge versus taking one for use by your teachers at school or supervisors at work

2. Go to http://userpage.fu-berlin.de/health/selfscal.htm and consider where you stand in relation to The General Self-Efficacy Scale (a 10-item psychometric scale designed to assess optimistic self-beliefs and ability to cope with difficult life challenges).

3. Discuss the influence of feelings on your thinking. Are you ruled more by your heart than your head, or vice versa? Do you tend to focus on positives or worry about the negatives? What difference does that make? Identify at least one thing you can do to improve your ability to have balanced thinking (thinking that considers both "heart" and "head," recognizes negatives, and focuses on positives to motivate and build confidence).

4. Consider Communication Strategies That Promote Critical Thinking (pages 36 to 38), and answer the following questions.
   - What strategies are new to you?
   - What are the challenges involved in using the strategies?
   - Recall a time when you were frustrated by a communication. What strategies would have helped reduce the frustration?

5. Choose two of the following articles to discuss.

    Thornby, D. (2006). Beginning the journey to skilled communication. *AACN Advanced Critical Care,* 17(3), 266-271. Retrieved January 6, 2011, from http://www.aacn.org/WD/HWE/Docs/AACN17_3_266-271_HWE.pdf.

    "Male logic" and "women's intuition." Retrieved January 6, 2011, from http://neptune.spaceports.com/~words/malelogic.html.

    Vital Smarts™. (2005). *Silence kills: The Seven Crucial Conversations® for healthcare.* Retrieved January 11, 2010, from http://www.silencekills.com/Download.aspx.

    Habel, M. *Emotional intelligence helps RNs work smart.* Retrieved January 6, 2011, from http://ce.nurse.com/ce373-60/CoursePage.

    Federwisch, A. (2010). *Personal "learning style" key to educational success.* Retrieved January 6, 2011, from http://news.nurse.com/article/20100712/NATIONAL01/107120118/-1/frontpage.

6. Determine where you stand in relation to the following learning outcomes from the pre-chapter self test.

    a. Explain three main steps to improving thinking.

    b. Explain the relationship between effective/skilled communication and critical thinking.

c. Describe how personality, learning style, upbringing, and culture affect thinking.

d. Identify strategies to develop your emotional intelligence (EI).

e. Explain why building trust and following a code of conduct are key to promoting critical thinking.

f. Discuss how human habits influence critical thinking.

OUTCOME-FOCUSED (RESULTS-ORIENTED) THINKING

As addressed in Chapter 1, critical thinking and clinical reasoning is outcome-focused (results-oriented) thinking: A key first step is to determine exactly what you are trying to accomplish—exactly what *benefits* and *desired end results* you aim to achieve.

This section clarifies the relationship between goals and outcomes and explains why *focusing on outcomes* promotes critical thinking.

Goal (Intent) Versus Outcome (Result)

The terms *goal, objective,* and *outcome* are often used interchangeably because they have similar meanings. There is, however, a significant difference among these terms.

- **Goal (objective):** Indicates **general intent**, what you *aim* to do. Example: My goal (or objective) is to teach Steve about diabetes.

- **Outcome:** Indicates specific, **measurable results.** Example: After I complete my teaching, Steve will be able to demonstrate insulin injection and explain how he will keep his blood sugar within normal range through diet, exercise, and medication.

Goals are often vague, and can be idealistic. Outcomes center on *clearly observable benefits and desired ultimate results,* forcing you to be realistic and think things through from the beginning.

Clarifying outcomes takes in-depth thinking. Think about the following scenario that shows the importance and challenges of clarifying outcomes.

Scenario
CLARIFYING OUTCOMES (END RESULTS): NOT THAT SIMPLE

A group gathers to discuss building a bridge in a small town. Someone says, "Let's first be sure that we all agree on the end result." Several members consider this a dumb statement: Isn't the end result simply that the town will have a bridge? A bridge is a clear and observable outcome, right? How about if I tell you this is very limited thinking? The real end result you need to focus on is that *whoever wants to get across that bridge is able to do so.* You must pay attention to the end users—the people who will use the bridge. This means starting by asking questions like "Who will use this bridge?" "How much room will they need to get their vehicles across?" "When will there be the most traffic, and how much will that traffic weigh?" "Where is the best place for this bridge?" If these questions aren't raised in the beginning, it's likely that you'll end up with a costly, useless, inconvenient, or even dangerous bridge.

> **RULE**
>
> 1. **Determining outcomes requires you to stay centered** on the *key people who will demonstrate that the desired end result has been achieved*. In the previous scenario, the key people are those who travel the bridge. In health care, it's patients, families, clients, and consumers.
> 2. **Critical thinking and clinical reasoning requires you to ask two main questions:** (1) What exactly are the major results you need? and (2) What are the problems, issues, or risks that must be addressed to get the results? (Sometimes the results you *need* may conflict with the results you *want*. For example, you may want things done your way. But if you allow people to do things their way, you may get better results.)

Chapter 5 gives opportunities to practice determining patient-centered (client-centered) outcomes, For now, just remember that if you haven't given enough thought to exactly what *end results* you need, you aren't thinking critically. Use the following memory jog to help you remember these two terms.

> **RULE**
>
> To remember the relationship between goals and outcomes, use the following:
>
> G = G   Goals = General intent (what you hope to accomplish)
> O = O   Outcomes = Observable results (what you will examine to determine how well you accomplished your goal or objective)

CRITICAL THINKING STRATEGIES

This section first summarizes 10 questions key to critical thinking, and then it addresses using logic, intuition, and trial and error. It also points out the importance of using specific strategies such as mapping and simulation.

10 Key Questions

There are 10 key questions to ask to determine your approach to critical thinking in different situations. These are summarized on the inside back cover and addressed in detail here.

1. **What major outcomes (*observable* beneficial results) do you and key stakeholders (e.g., patient, family, care providers) expect to observe in the patient after care is complete?** Be as specific as possible. For example, compare the vague outcome in the first situation below with the more specific outcome in the second situation.

   Situation 1: Jody will be discharged home in 2 days.

   Situation 2: Jody will be discharged home in 2 days in the care of her mother, who will be able to demonstrate sterile dressing change by then.

2. **What problems, issues, or risks must be managed to achieve the major outcomes?** Identifying the problems, issues, and risks that may *impede progress* is 60% of the critical thinking challenge. Asking this question helps you prioritize. You have only so much time—assign top priority to addressing problems, issues, or risks that may impede progress toward getting results. Using the previous example, Jody's mother tells you that she knows nothing about changing sterile dressings and also wants to know how she can improve her parenting skills. If time is short, give top priority to teaching her about dressing changes, and handle the issue of how to be a better parent by giving her information on reference materials and support groups.

3. **What are the circumstances (context) in this particular patient situation?** The approach to critical thinking changes, depending on the circumstances. For example, imagine that you're in class and you're asked how to manage a patient in shock. You aren't sure, but you think you know, so it's appropriate for you to answer. If you're in the clinical setting, however, trying to manage shock based on uncertain knowledge is dangerous.

4. **What knowledge and skills are required to care for this patient?** Having discipline-specific knowledge and skills is crucial to critical thinking. For example, how can you think critically about managing cardiac pain if you don't know the causes and common treatments of cardiac pain? If you don't know what knowledge and skills are required, you probably don't know enough to get involved—get help.

5. **How much room is there for error?** When there's less room for error, we must carefully assess the situation, examine all possible solutions, and make every effort to make prudent decisions. For example, which situation below has less room for error, and how might your approach to decision-making change in each situation?

    Situation 1: You need to decide whether to give an over-the-counter antihistamine to someone who is usually in good health.

    Situation 2: You need to decide whether to give an over-the-counter antihistamine to someone with multiple chronic health problems.

    The first situation has more room for error because the person is less likely to have preexisting conditions or be taking medications that might interact with the antihistamine. The second situation requires consultation with a physician.

6. **How much time do you have?** If you have plenty of time, you can take time to think independently, using resources such as textbooks. If you don't have much time, you may need to activate the chain of command (immediately report the problem to your supervisor) to ensure timely attention. **Patient safety and welfare is number one.**

7. **What human and information resources can help?** Identifying resources (e.g., textbooks, computers, or experts) is essential to getting the information you need to think critically. For example, you don't have to know every side effect of every drug in a drug manual. Rather, know when you need detailed information. Look the drug up in a manual, or check with a pharmacist to carefully review *all* side effects.

8. **Whose perspectives must be considered?** Critical thinking requires you to consider the perspectives of all of the key players involved; otherwise you risk having conflicting purposes. For example, to develop an effective plan for home care, you must

consider the perspectives of the patient, other household members, and other key members of the health care team. Imagine what could happen if you sent a grandmother home with many brightly colored medications and everyone forgot to consider the perspective of a toddler in the home!

9. **What's influencing thinking?** Recognizing influencing factors such as personal biases helps us identify vested interests, an important step in making fair-minded choices. For example, a nurse who is strongly against abortion may avoid working in gynecology, where women's decisions might make it difficult to give objective nursing care.

10. **What must be done to monitor, prevent, manage, or eliminate the problems, issues, and risks identified in question 2 (and who's accountable for doing it)?** Getting results depends on your ability to identify specific strategies to prevent or manage problems that may be barriers to outcome achievement. For example, if you have a bedridden patient who has surgery, preventing skin breakdown is a problem that must be managed to ensure timely discharge. Deciding *who* is accountable for *what* is essential to ensure that nothing "falls through the cracks."

Using Logic, Intuition, and Trial and Error

Let's consider how logic, intuition, and trial and error relate to critical thinking.

Logic—sound reasoning that's based on facts (evidence)—is the foundation for critical thinking. It's the safest, most reliable approach. For all important decisions and opinions, make sure you can explain the logic of your thinking.

Intuition—a valuable part of thinking—is best described as "knowing something without evidence." For experts, intuitive hunches speed up problem-solving, since they have a lot of experiential knowledge in their heads. For them, thinking-in-action is rapid, dynamic, and intuitive. Novices must rely more on step by step logic. Keep in mind that sometimes things are counterintuitive—the *opposite* of what your intuition tells you. In important situations, bring logic to your thinking and look for evidence to support gut feelings. If you have no evidence to support your intuition, consider the risks of acting on intuition alone. For example, can you remember a time when you did something on your computer based on intuition and ended up with a disaster? This can also happen with patients.

Trial and error—trying several solutions until you find one that works—is risky but sometimes necessary. Use trial and error only when there's plenty of room for mistakes, when the problem can be monitored closely, and when the solutions have been logically thought through. A common example of useful trial and error is trying to determine the best way for a dressing to be applied to an awkward wound—it may take several tries before the best way is determined.

Focusing on Details and Big Picture

Whether you see yourself a "details" person or a "big picture" person, it's important to realize that critical thinking requires focusing on *both* the big picture *and* the details—the whole and the parts. Think about the following examples.

- **Mr. Martinez has cardiac problems.** He tells you he has chest pain and is afraid he might die. Treating both "the whole" (Mr. Martinez's pain and anxiety) and "the parts" (Mr. Martinez's oxygen-deprived heart) is essential to resolving the chest pain (and, perhaps, to saving his life).
- **You're trying to teach Tonya how to care for her newborn.** You're well prepared with lots of nice pamphlets. She seems interested, but she keeps yawning and doesn't seem to retain information very long. Finally you say, "Is there a better time we could do this?" She admits that she hasn't slept all night and is too tired. You come back later after Tonya's had a good rest. She learns readily. In this case, paying attention to an important detail (fatigue) helped you be a more effective teacher.

Remember to ask questions like "What's the big picture here?" "Am I considering both the parts and the whole?" and "Am I paying attention to key details?"

Drawing Maps, Diagrams, and Decision Trees

Drawing maps, diagrams, and decision trees promotes critical thinking by helping your brain grasp complex relationships. When you draw your own map, diagram, or decision tree, it helps you "personalize" information and "make it your own." When you study well-designed maps, diagrams, or decision trees, you learn more quickly, because your brain does better with "pictures" than words. Your brain handles information differently, depending on how it's presented. For example, study how the following same percentages are displayed in different ways. Which is easiest for you to grasp?

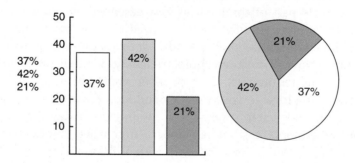

When trying to learn or teach someone something, consider questions like "How can we look at this differently?" "What is the best way to represent this information?" "Is there a table, map, diagram, or decision tree that can add to understanding?"

Clinical Simulation and Debriefing

Simulated learning experiences give safe, powerful, ways to learn problem-solving, clinical reasoning, and other critical thinking skills (e.g., juggling technical skills together with other thinking). With highly sophisticated training patient simulators, you can practice on your own or in groups, correcting mistakes in real time. Simulated learning is especially valuable for learning how to "think on your feet." When simulations are done in groups, these experiences also help you develop collaboration skills that are so important in the clinical setting.

Simulated learning is even more powerful when followed by debriefing. During debriefing, learners and teachers reflect on what happened during the simulation to critique the experience and discuss the following sorts of questions:

- What was the overall performance?
- What specifically went well?
- What needs correcting or improving?
- What thinking came into play?
- What thinking should have come into play?
- What would you have done if _____?
- What was the most important thing you learned?
- How confident are you about handling this in real situations?
- How will you handle this in real situations (e.g., handle independently, get help, what resources will help).

By using debriefing, you gain deep insight and engage in reflection that translates into actionable knowledge—key knowledge that you can use to guide decisions and actions in real situations. Debriefing is a great opportunity to discuss thinking ahead, thinking-in-action, and thinking back (reflective thinking), as addressed in Chapter 1. For both learners and teachers, knowing how promote learning with debriefing sessions is essential competency. It's as important as knowing how to learn *during* simulation.[19,20,21]

RULE

Experiential, hands-on learning is a powerful way to learn and remember. Seek out simulated and on-the-job opportunities to broaden your knowledge and skills.

Other Useful Strategies

The following summarizes other useful strategies that promote critical thinking.

Anticipate questions others might ask. These may include: "What will my instructor want to know?" "What do patients need to know?" "What will the doctor want to know?" "This helps identify a wider scope of questions that have to be answered to gain relevant information."

- **Ask, "What else?"** Change "Have we done everything?" to "What else do we need to do?" Asking "What else?" pushes you to look further and be more complete.
- **Ask, "What if?"** For example, "What if the worst happens?" or "What if we try another way?" This helps you be proactive instead of reactive. It enhances your creativity and helps you put things in perspective.
- **Ask, "Why?"** To fully understand something, you must know what it is and *why it's so*. There's a saying: "She who knows what and how is likely to get a good job. She who knows why is likely to be her boss."

Think out loud or write your thoughts down. When you put your thinking into words, you make your ideas, reasons, and logic explicit, making it easier to assess and correct yourself.

Ask an expert to think out loud. When you ask experts to think out loud, you often learn systematic approaches to solving problems and making decisions.

Look for flaws in your thinking. Ask questions like "What's missing?" and "How could this be made better?" If you don't go looking for flaws, you'll be unlikely to find them. Once you've found them, you can make corrections early.

Ask someone else to look for flaws in your thinking. This offers a "fresh eye" for evaluation and may bring new ideas and perspectives.

Paraphrase in your own words. Paraphrasing helps you understand information using a familiar language (your own).

Compare and contrast. This forces you to look closely at the *parts* of something as well as the *whole*, helping you become more familiar with both things you're comparing. For example, if I ask you to compare two different kinds of apples, you have to look closely at both of them. As a result of comparing them, you are more likely to know and remember each type of apple better.

Organize and reorganize information. Organizing information helps you see certain patterns, but it may make you *miss* others. Reorganizing it helps you see some of those other patterns. For example, compare the following groups of numbers (each group contains the same numbers, organized differently). What patterns do you see and which is easiest to remember?

   36345643   34343 656   333 44 566

Develop good habits of inquiry. Develop habits that aid in the search for the truth, such as keeping an open mind, verifying information, and taking enough time.

Revisit information. When you give something "a second pass"—coming back and studying it afresh—you'll view it differently.

Replace the phrases "I don't know" or "I'm not sure" with "I need to find out" or "Let's find out." This shows you have the confidence and ability to find answers and mobilizes you to locate resources.

Turn mistakes into learning opportunities. Share your mistakes with peers, so that everyone can learn. We all make mistakes, and we need to work together to find ways to prevent them. Mistakes are often stepping stones to maturity and new ideas. If you aren't making any mistakes, maybe you aren't trying enough new things.

CRITICAL THINKING INDICATORS FOR KNOWLEDGE AND INTELLECTUAL SKILLS

Identifying critical thinking indicators (CTIs) related to the knowledge and intellectual skills required in the clinical setting is an important starting point to developing clinical reasoning and critical thinking skills. CTIs help you answer the questions, "What do I have to know?" and "What do I have to be able to do?"

Whereas page 12 lists CTIs for personal attitudes of critical thinkers, the boxes below and on the next pages give specific CTIs for knowledge and intellectual skills that nurses must gain. Keep in mind that developing *intellectual skills* requires you to be able to *apply knowledge*. For example, *distinguishing normal from abnormal* (listed under *intellectual skills* CTIs) requires you to apply knowledge of *normal and abnormal function* (listed under *knowledge* CTIs).

To assess where you stand in relation to having the required *knowledge* and *intellectual skills CTIs*, think about each indicator listed in the boxes and rate your ability to demonstrate the behavior using the following 0 to 10 scale:

0 = I am unable to demonstrate this indicator at this time.

10 = This indicator is pretty much a habit for me.

If you're a beginner, don't be concerned about low scores when comparing yourself to the CTIs. These skills are developed on the job through practice and experience. You also get some practice developing these skills as you complete the exercises throughout the book. What's key is that groups working together have a common reference to help identify the skills you needed to practice safely and effectively (everyone should be "on the same page").

CRITICAL THINKING INDICATORS (CTIS) DEMONSTRATING KNOWLEDGE

NOTE: Requirements vary, depending on context of specialty practice (e.g., pediatrics vs. adult health care).

Clarifies Nursing Knowledge

- Nursing and medical terminology
- Nursing vs. medical and other models, roles, and responsibilities
- Scope of nursing practice (qualifications; applicable standards, laws, and rules and regulations)
- Related anatomy, physiology, and pathophysiology
- Spiritual, social, and cultural concepts
- Normal and abnormal growth and development (pediatric, adult, and gerontologic implications)
- Normal and abnormal function (bio-psycho-social-cultural-spiritual)
- Factors affecting normal function (bio-psycho-social-cultural-spiritual)
- Nutrition and pharmacology principles
- Behavioral health and disease management
- Signs and symptoms of common problems and complications.
- Nursing process, nursing theories, research, and evidence-based practice
- Reasons behind policies, procedures and interventions; diagnostic studies implications
- Ethical and legal principles
- Risk management and infection control
- Safety standards, healthy workplace standards, and principles of learning and safety cultures
- Interrelationship of health care disciplines and systems
- Reliable information resources

Continued

CRITICAL THINKING INDICATORS (CTIs) DEMONSTRATING KNOWLEDGE—cont'd

Clarifies Knowledge of Self
- ❑ Personal biases, values, beliefs, needs
- ❑ How own culture, thinking, personality, and learning style preferences differ from others'
- ❑ Level of commitment to organizational mission and values

Demonstrates
- ❑ Focused nursing assessment skills (e.g., breath sounds or IV site assessment)
- ❑ Mathematical problem-solving for drug calculations
- ❑ Related technical skills (e.g., n/g tube or other equipment management)

Source: Alfaro-LeFevre, R. (2011). *Evidence-based critical thinking indicators.* Available at www.AlfaroTeachSmart.com. All rights reserved. No use without permission.

CRITICAL THINKING INDICATORS (CTIs) DEMONSTRATING INTELLECTUAL SKILLS/COMPETENCIES

Nursing Process and Decision-Making Skills
- ❑ Communicates effectively orally and in writing
- ❑ Applies standards, principles, laws, and ethics codes
- ❑ Makes safety and infection control a priority; prevents and deals with mistakes constructively
- ❑ Includes patient, family, and key stakeholders in decision-making; teaches patient, self, and others
- ❑ Identifies purpose and focus of assessment
- ❑ Assesses systematically and comprehensively as indicated.
- ❑ Distinguishes normal from abnormal; identifies risks for abnormal
- ❑ Distinguishes relevant from irrelevant; clusters relevant data together
- ❑ Identifies assumptions and inconsistencies; checks accuracy and reliability (validates data)
- ❑ Recognizes missing information; gains more data as needed
- ❑ Concludes what's known and unknown; draws reasonable conclusions—gives evidence to support them
- ❑ Identifies both problems and their underlying cause(s) and related factors; includes patient and family perspectives
- ❑ Recognizes changes in patient status; takes appropriate action
- ❑ Considers multiple ideas, explanations, and solutions
- ❑ Determines individualized outcomes and uses them to plan and give care
- ❑ Manages risks, predicts complications
- ❑ Weighs risks and benefits; anticipates consequences and implications—individualizes interventions accordingly
- ❑ Sets priorities and makes decisions in a timely way
- ❑ Reassesses to monitor outcomes (responses)
- ❑ Promotes health, function, comfort, and well-being
- ❑ Identifies ethical issues and takes appropriate action
- ❑ Uses human and information resources; detects bias

CRITICAL THINKING INDICATORS (CTIs) DEMONSTRATING INTELLECTUAL SKILLS/COMPETENCIES—cont'd

Additional Related Skills
- ❑ Advocates for patients, self, and others
- ❑ Establishes empowered partnerships with patients, families, peers, and co-workers
- ❑ Fosters positive interpersonal relationships; addresses conflicts fairly; promotes health workplace and learning cultures
- ❑ Promotes teamwork (focuses on common goals, respects diversity; encourages others to contribute in their own way)
- ❑ Facilitates and navigates change
- ❑ Organizes and manages time and environment
- ❑ Gives and takes constructive criticism
- ❑ Delegates appropriately (matches patient needs with worker competencies; determines worker learning needs, supervises and teaches as indicated; monitors results personally)
- ❑ Leads, inspires, and helps others move toward mutually defined common goals.
- ❑ Demonstrates systems thinking (shows awareness of relationships existing within and across health care systems).

Source: Alfaro-LeFevre, R. (2011). *Evidence-based critical thinking indicators.* Available at www.AlfaroTeachSmart.com. All rights reserved. No use without permission.

Box 2-4 (on the next page) shows the results of two studies that aimed to describe critical thinking skills. This information was incorporated into the CTIs.

DEVELOPING CHARACTER—ACQUIRING KNOWLEDGE AND SKILLS

Becoming a critical thinker requires a commitment to develop character and acquire the necessary knowledge and skills. Study the four circles of the 4-circle CT model on the inside front cover. Identify some things you can do to develop your abilities in each of the four circles.

ASSESSING AND EVALUATING THINKING

Let's end this chapter by briefly addressing issues related to assessing and evaluating thinking. In context of trying to determine how someone thinks, the terms *assess* and *evaluate* are often used interchangeably, as I will use them.

Evaluating critical thinking is important for three reasons:
1. You need to know what you're doing well, and what you need to work on.
2. Your teachers and employers need to know whether you're competent to practice in the clinical setting.
3. Your ability to think critically is closely linked to safe, quality patient care.

Unlike *Star Trek's* Dr. Spock, we humans can't read minds—it's a challenge to determine what goes on in someone else's head. We are all unique, with various personalities

---

BOX 2-4 RESULTS OF TWO STUDIES DESCRIBING CRITICAL THINKING SKILLS

Scheffer and Rubenfeld*
- **Analyzing:** Separating or breaking down a whole into parts to discover their nature, function, and relationships
- **Applying standards:** Judging according to established personal, professional, or social rules or criteria
- **Discriminating:** Recognizing differences and similarities among things or situations and distinguishing carefully as to category or rank
- **Information seeking:** Searching for evidence, facts, or knowledge by identifying relevant sources and gathering objective, subjective, historical, and current data from those sources
- **Logical reasoning:** Drawing inferences or conclusions that are supported in or justified by evidence
- **Predicting:** Envisioning a plan and its consequences
- **Transforming knowledge:** Changing or converting the condition, nature, form, or function of concepts and contexts

The American Philosophical Association Delphi Report†
- **Interpretation:** Categorizing, decoding sentences, clarifying meaning
- **Analysis:** Examining ideas, identifying arguments, analyzing arguments
- **Evaluation:** Assessing claims, assessing arguments
- **Inference:** Querying evidence, conjecturing alternatives, drawing conclusions
- **Explanation:** Stating results, justifying procedures, presenting arguments
- **Self-regulation:** Self-examination, self-correction

---

*Scheffer, B., Rubenfeld, M. (2000). A consensus statement on critical thinking in nursing. *Journal of Nursing Education,* 39(8), 353.
†Facione, P. *Critical thinking: What it is and why it counts* (2010 update). Retrieved June 1, 2010, from http://www.insightassessment.com/pdf_files/what&why2007.pdf.

and thinking styles. What may seem like good thinking to *you* may seem disorganized and inefficient to someone *else*. We're still in the early stages of learning how to evaluate thinking. To help you prepare for when you're involved in either giving an evaluation or getting one, this section briefly addresses issues related to evaluating thinking.

Basic Principles of Evaluating Thinking

It takes a knowledgeable, experienced, critical thinker who is familiar with key elements of assessing reasoning to evaluate thinking.

Drawing valid conclusions about someone's thinking abilities requires focusing on *patterns over time*, not *single incidences*. For example, anyone can make a mistake, but if the person makes the same mistake several times, it's a problem.

The following are key things to consider when evaluating critical thinking abilities.

1. **Outcomes (results): Does the person usually get respectable outcomes?**
   - In the clinical setting, this means assessing the nurse's patients directly to determine level of care (e.g., Are the patients safe, comfortable, and satisfied with care?).

- In class, evaluating outcomes means analyzing completed projects (e.g., papers and presentations).

2. **Process: How does the person usually go about achieving desired outcomes?** On the whole, does the nurse usually seem organized and prepared? Be sure to consider style differences that may affect your opinion. For example, if the nurse usually gets respectable results, but seems disorganized, it may be simply a style difference between you and the nurse.

3. **Behavior: What patterns of behavior and communication do you and others observe in the person over time?** Does the nurse's usual behavior send messages of CTIs such as *being inquisitive, persistent, confident, and proactive?* If you're not sure about behavior, ask for an explanation of the *reasoning behind behavior.* For example: *Help me understand what you're trying to do … Tell me what's going on in your head … I realize I'm putting you on the spot, but take your time and try to explain your thinking … Let's talk later so that I can understand what was going on here.* To understand whether opinions and decisions are based on evidence, ask questions like "How do you know?" and "What information do you have to support this?" To determine whether someone is proactive, ask questions like "What do you expect to happen when you do this?" "What if _____ happens … how will you handle it?" and "What alternatives have you thought about?"

4. **Charting and other communication: When you review the nurse's charting and other communications, are they relevant, clear, and concise?** Does the charting help you learn more about the patient, or does there seem to be nothing but repetitive comments in all her charts? While electronic charting does have specific rules that guide what the nurse records, lapses in critical thinking can still be noted. For example, there may be a "drag and drop" field, which the nurse uses even though it's not really applicable to this particular patient. How well does the person communicate verbally and in writing?

Valid assessment of someone else's thinking depends on three things:

1. **The level of trust in the relationship** (mistrust damages communication and stunts critical thinking abilities).

2. **Mutual understanding of exactly what critical thinking behaviors will be assessed.** The person doing the assessment and the person being assessed must "be on the same page."

3. **Having many ways of looking at the person's thinking**: observing behavior, engaging in dialogue ("tell me what you're thinking right now"), assessing patient outcomes, and analyzing charting and other written communication.

Self-Assessment

Assessing your own progress is one of the most important things you can do to improve. What are you doing well? What areas do you target for improvement? What knowledge, skills, and experiences do you need to gain? Be honest. Remember that "self-deception" is a human habit that impedes thinking. Share your target areas for improvement with your instructors, peers, and supervisors. We all learn together—ask for help when you need it. This shows that you are confident and committed to improvement and keeping patients safe.

Peer Review

Because of the importance of getting others' perspectives to increase the likelihood of valid evaluations, many schools and hospitals have a *peer review* process to get input from peers and colleagues.[22] With peer review, nurses (or students) assess and judge the performance of their peers against predetermined standards (e.g., against the behaviors listed in the CTIs). By comparing what they observe in their colleagues with the predetermined standards, they form opinions about performance. Keep in mind that personal style differences sometimes makes peer review difficult. For example, someone who's a logical, step-by-step thinker may have trouble understanding a creative person who's great at multitasking.

Peer review is an efficient way of getting feedback that helps identify clinical learning needs and increases safety and care quality for patients. Yet, peer review is complex process. It involves the thoughts of several people, and sometimes there are interpersonal and other issues involved. If you are struggling with your peer review process (either giving or accepting peer review), discuss your concerns with your teachers or supervisors. Resolving these concerns often improves the peer review process.

Using Tests and Instruments

Many experts continue to work to develop valid instruments and tests to assess critical thinking skills. But evaluating what goes on in someone else's head is a complex process, and these tests and instruments are difficult to develop. While using well-developed tests and instruments may help assess some critical thinking skills, it's important to realize that tests don't always predict your ability to think critically in real situations. They indicate your ability to think critically in context of that particular instrument or test. If you do poorly on tests or instruments, think about how you do in real situations. For example, I sometimes do poorly on timed tests because I am indecisive and like to mull over the questions. However, this doesn't translate to my being indecisive *when it matters:* I was charge nurse in the intensive care unit (ICU) and a supervisor of a 300-bed hospital. I can make timely decisions in the clinical setting as well as anyone. If you have a track record of success in handling real situations, it's quite likely that you're one of those creative, complex thinkers who struggles with test-taking and needs lots of practice to develop test-taking skills (see Chapter 4).

There are many standard tests that aim to measure critical thinking. Because the results of these tests may have significant impact on the people taking the test—for example, whether students progress to graduation— these tests come under the category of high-stakes testing.[23] Before using these tests and instruments, the best-qualified people (e.g., educators) should carefully examine test plans personally and answer at least some of the questions themselves. This gives first-hand knowledge of the test and prevents the use of tests that aren't really suited to the purpose they want. From a priority perspective with students, the best standard tests to use to assess critical thinking are those that have questions that are formatted in the same way as the national state board exams (e.g., NCLEX). This increases the likelihood of predicting students' ability to pass tests like NCLEX and gives opportunities to practice "thinking in the way the test requires you to." When students have lots of practice, they gain both the knowledge and test-taking skills needed to do well when "it really counts."

To summarize, evaluating thinking is a complex issue that requires a lot of critical thinking and knowledge of testing and evaluation issues. Using several approaches to evaluating thinking increases the likelihood of drawing valid conclusions. Evaluation helps you validate your knowledge and identify areas that have to be developed. Ultimately, the aim of evaluation is to improve your ability to think critically and make a positive impact on your patients' lives.

CRITICAL MOMENTS

BOUNDARIES AND PRIORITIES—NOT GUILT
Many nurses feel guilty when they say no to requests for help. Yet, there are only so many hours in the day. Don't feel guilty about setting boundaries for what you will and will not do. You can't do it all. When going through busy or stressful periods, avoid being distracted from the major priorities in your life: Set boundaries.

CONSIDERING ALTERNATIVES GETS RESULTS
People aren't successful because they come up with one right answer or explanation. Rather, it's because they come up with many answers or explanations. To get the best results, make it a habit to look for alternative explanations, problems, or solutions.

MOTIVATION: WHAT'S IN IT FOR THEM?
Connecting with others' motivations sparks critical thinking. When trying to teach or motivate others, use the human instinct to self-focus to your advantage. Ask yourself questions like "What's in it for them?" and "How can I make this relevant and worth their time?"

FOCUSING ON OUTCOMES: IMAGINE THE FUTURE
Focusing on outcomes—the end products or results—helps you think things through and avoid "best-laid plans" problems. To think critically, put your mind in the future and imagine what things will be like on the day you reach the outcomes. For example, once I was on a program planning committee. One of our goals was to keep costs down, so we decided to skip refreshments for the afternoon break. This made sense until someone put her mind in the future and said, "I don't want to be the one to stand up in front of 100 tired, thirsty people and announce, 'There will be no refreshments during this break.'" When determining

outcomes, "think future." Imagine consequences: Exactly how will things be on the day you reach your outcome?

 ## OTHER PERSPECTIVES

HOW LITERATE ARE YOU?
"The illiterate of the twenty-first century will not be those who cannot read and write, but those who cannot learn, unlearn, and relearn."[24]

—*Alvin Toffler, author of* Future Shock

LOVE YOUR BRAIN
"I have a very weird brain. But I like it—it's the only one I have."[25]

—*Ruth Hansten, FACHE, PhD, MBA, BSN*

LEARNING PROVERB
"I hear, I forget. I see, I remember. I do, I understand."

—*Astronaut John Glenn*

IN SOME CULTURES, QUESTIONING SHOWS WEAKNESS
"I have trouble asking questions. In my culture, asking questions is discouraged and is a sign of weakness and embarrassment. What I'm working on and want to know is how to become more confident and capable asking questions. I realize it's essential to critical thinking."

—*One of my foreign workshop participants*

WORRIED ABOUT ANALYSIS PARALYSIS?
"For every person paralyzed with excessive doubt, there are 100 who have too little doubt and charge off to take action without enough reflection."[26]

—*Philip Hansten, Author of* Premature Fraculation:
The Ignorance of Certainty and the Ghost of Mantaigne.

TRIAL AND ERROR: A CONTINUOUS PROCESS
"Trial and error, the process of trying one thing and observing the outcome, and then analyzing the result and making changes, is an important learning experience. It takes a great deal of critical thinking. Call it what you want, but individuals and health care organizations must continue to interact with the world, learn from experience, and then use that experience to improve the next attempt. However, remember that trial and error is a continuous cycle. You must constantly try to improve care quality based on what you learn from experience—it isn't just a one-time thing."

—*Workshop participant, a quality improvement expert*

A 4-YEAR-OLD CRITICAL THINKER
Susie was helping her mother pour medications. As she struggled with the lid of one of the bottles, her mother said, "You can't get that off because little children like you shouldn't get medications on their own." Susie responded, "How does it know it's me?"

BE YOURSELF
Be yourself. Everyone else is taken.

—*Oscar Wilde*

SWEATING SILENCE
"As part of my teaching strategies class, I had to practice student questioning. One strategy required that I ask a question, and then remain silent until someone responded. My instructor videotaped the class and told me that under no circumstances was I to answer my own question. Soon into the class, I asked why a certain clinical activity was done. No one answered. I waited. Then waited some more. I began to sweat, but I refused to say anything. Finally, after what seemed like 2 full minutes of staring, someone spoke up. The next day I watched the video and timed the pause after my question. It was only 9 seconds! Like anyone in front of a group, teachers are uncomfortable with silence. We need to let learners think through the answer and take a chance by speaking up. Students often let the teacher answer so they then find out the 'right' answer. This lesson can be applied to all important communication. Whether we're dealing with patients, colleagues, or peers, silence is often golden."[27]

—*Brent Thompson, DNSc, RN*

"CONFIDENT VULNERABILITY" PROMOTES CRITICAL THINKING
"Developing *confident vulnerability*—showing that you're vulnerable and open to suggestions, yet confident in who you are—promotes critical thinking. If you're too confident, you don't have an open mind to different opinions or new ideas. *Confident vulnerability* is the opposite of 'the God complex' often seen in 'prima donnas' who believe they can do no wrong."[28]

—*Cheryl Herndon, ARNP, MSN, CNM*

GO OUTSIDE YOUR LEARNING BOX.
"Knowing where you fall on an inventory of learning styles shouldn't be a stumbling block to learning. For example, don't avoid sim lab experiences because you aren't a kinesthetic learner (who learns best by doing). You can strengthen your learning abilities by encouraging yourself to operate in dimensions that aren't your preference."[29]

—*Lyn DeSilets, RN-BC, EdD*

Critical Thinking Exercises

Example responses are on page 267.

1. Using your own words and giving an example, explain the relationship between *goals* and *outcomes.*
2. Critical thinking is contextual. How would your approach to critical thinking change in the following two situations?
   a. You want your committee to brainstorm about ways to improve satisfaction with surgical experiences.
   b. You want your committee to develop a policy for managing postoperative complications.
3. Identifying assumptions—recognizing things you've taken for granted without realizing it—is essential for critical thinking. Answer the following two riddles, and then check the response on page 267 to see what assumptions you made.

Riddles

   a. You're running in a race. You overtake the second person. What position are you in?
   b. Jack and Jill were found dead on the floor, surrounded by water and pieces of broken glass. There was no blood. What happened?

 ### Think, Pair, Share

With a partner, in a group, or in a journal entry:

1. Discuss what happens when you do "a," "b," and "c" below. Identify other strategies that help you see relationships, understand, and remember.
   a. Rearrange the following numbers into a pattern that helps you remember them:

   992887656780898

   b. Draw a square around the numbers "765" above, then shade the numbers 089.
   c. Underline the numbers 928 above
2. Think of someone who is a good thinker. Describe what this person does when communicating and thinking through issues.
3. Discuss how you did when you assessed your ability to demonstrate the CTIs related to knowledge and intellectual skills.

4. Share the challenges of accomplishing the strategies given in *"Zen and the Art of Nursing: Seven ways to make the most of each workday,"* available at: http://news.nurse.com/article/20100503/DD01/105030020
5. Discuss the implications of the *Critical Moments* and *Other Perspectives* on pages 59 to 61.
6. Decide where you stand in relation to achieving the outcomes in the chapter opener.

KEY POINTS/SUMMARY

- Improving thinking requires three main steps: (1) Gain insight and self-awareness. (2) Get agreement on a code of conduct and what critical thinking entails. (3) Make the choice to practice and develop the attitudes, knowledge, and skills required to focus your thinking to get the results you need.
- Gaining insight into your personal style—how and why you think and learn the way you do—is a key starting point for improving thinking.
- Connecting with your preferred styles helps you identify strategies to learn effectively in your own way. Connecting with your personality type helps you gain insight into how and why you think the way you do. Understanding personality types different from your own helps you realize how and why *others* think the way *they* do.
- Birth order, upbringing, and the culture you embrace greatly affects your thinking.
- Self efficacy—having a strong sense that you're capable of accomplishing all that you need to do to achieve your goals—greatly affects your ability to gain the knowledge and skills needed for critical thinking.
- Developing your emotional intelligence—your ability to recognize emotions and make them work in positive ways—is as important as developing your IQ.
- Without trust in relationships, you're unlikely to have meaningful dialogue, as people are afraid to speak their minds. Page 27 shows a code of conduct that promotes critical thinking.
- Human habits can either promote or impede critical thinking (pages 42 to 44).
- Using simulated learning experiences, and drawing maps, diagrams, and decision trees are all useful strategies to develop critical thinking skills.
- Goals, because they focus on *intent*, may be vague and unrealistic. Identifying observable, measurable outcomes (results) helps you be realistic and focused from the start.
- Logic—sound reasoning based on evidence—provides the foundation for critical thinking. Using intuition as a guide to look for evidence is an effective strategy that should be nurtured. Before acting on intuition alone, be sure you consider the possible risks of harm.
- Trial and error (trying several solutions until you find one that works) is sometimes risky, but sometimes a necessary approach to problem-solving.
- Developing effective communication skills significantly improves critical thinking.
- The 4-circle CT model on the inside front cover shows how critical thinking requires a blend of critical thinking characteristics, knowledge, intellectual skills, interpersonal skills, and technical skills.

- The inside back cover summarizes 10 questions to promote critical thinking in context of evidence-based practice.
- Evaluating someone else's thinking is a difficult task that requires: (1) knowledge of the many issues related to assessing thinking, (2) a common frame of reference about what CT skills are being examined, and (3) a great deal of critical thinking.
- The following are key strategies for evaluating thinking: (1) Directly assessing a nurse's patients to determine results. (2) Reflecting on how the nurse achieved those results. (3) Analyzing the nurse's patterns of behavior and communication. (4) Performing self-assessment and peer review.
- Scan this chapter to review all highlighted rules.

REFERENCES

1. Kirk, K. *Self-efficacy: Helping students believe in themselves.* Retrieved January 6, 2011, from http://serc.carleton.edu/NAGTWorkshops/affective/efficacy.html.
2. Penny, J. (June 2010). E-mail communication.
3. Burnet, M. (2007). Gender gap. *Advance for Nurses,* 9(3), 12. Retrieved December 1, 2010, from http://nursing.advanceweb.com.
4. Sabbatini, R. *Are there differences between the brains of males and females?* Retrieved January 6, 2011, from http://www.cerebromente.org.br/n11/mente/eisntein/cerebro-homens.html.
5. Schlaepfer, T., Harris, G., Tien, A., et al. (1995). Structural differences in the cerebral cortex of healthy female and male subjects: A magnetic resonance imaging study. *Psychiatry Research,* 61(3), 129-135.
6. Williams, D. *Recruiting men into nursing school.* Retrieved January 10, 2011, from http://www.minoritynurse.com/men-nursing/recruiting-men-nursing-school.
7. Anthony, A. (March 2008). E-mail communication.
8. Codier E., Kooker B. M., Shoultz J. (2008). Measuring the emotional intelligence of clinical staff nurses: an approach for improving the clinical care environment. *Nursing Administration Quarterly,* 32(1), 8-14.
9. Habel, M. *Emotional intelligence helps RNs work smart.* Retrieved January 10, 2011, from http://ce.nurse.com/ce373-60/CoursePage.
10. Vital Smarts™ (2005). *Silence kills: The Seven Crucial Conversations® for healthcare.* Retrieved January 8, 2011, from http://www.silencekills.com/Download.aspx.
11. Anthony, M., Vidal, K. (2010). Mindful communication: A novel approach to improving delegation and increasing patient safety. *The Online Journal of Issues in Nursing,* 15(2), manuscript 2.
12. Thornby, D. (2006). Beginning the journey to skilled communication. *AACN Advanced Critical Care,* 17(3), 266-271. Retrieved January 6, 2011, from http://www.aacn.org/WD/HWE/Docs/AACN17_3_266-271_HWE.pdf.
13. Covey, S. (1989). *The 7 habits of highly effective people®.* New York: Simon & Schuster.
14. Mclean, S. (2009). Digest of Nichols, M. *The lost art of listening: How learning to listen can improve relationships* (2nd ed.) New York: Guilford Press. Retrieved January 11, 2011, from http://www.creativespirit.net/learners/counseling/docu19.htm.
15. Ceppetelli, E. (2010). *Receptive listening©: A strategy to facilitate transition into practice and improve retention.* Presentation at the 2nd Annual Research & Evidence-Based Practice Symposium, Promoting Nursing's Future. November 5, Burlington, VT.
16. Alessandra, T. *The platinum rule.* Retrieved January 5, 2011, from www.alessandra.com/abouttony/aboutpr.asp.

17. Thompson, P. (2000). Mentoring power. *Reflections on Nursing Leadership*, 26(1), 7.

18. Ecklund, M. (January 2001). *Reach out and touch: Making the mentoring connection.* Retrieved January 10, 2011, from www.aacn.org.

19. Dreifuerst, K. (2009). The essentials of debriefing in simulation learning: A concept analysis. *Nursing Education Perspectives*, 30(2), 109-114.

20. Harder, N. (2010). Use of simulation in teaching and learning in health sciences: A systematic review. *Journal of Nursing Education*, 49(1), 38-44.

21. Smith, S., & Roehrs, J. (2009). High-fidelity simulation: Factors correlated with nursing student satisfaction and self-confidence. *Nursing Education Perspectives*, 30(2), 74-78.

22. Boehm, H., & Bonnel, W. (2010). The use of peer review in nursing education and clinical practice. *Journal for Nurses in Staff Development*, 26(3), 108-115.

23. National League for Nursing. (2010). *Reflection and dialogue: High-stakes testing.* Retrieved January 6, 2011, from http://www.nln.org/aboutnln/reflection_dialogue/refl_dial_7.htm.

24. Toffler, A. (2000). In S. Thorpe (ed.), *How to think like Einstein* (p. 26). Naperville, IL: Sourcebooks.

25. Hansten, R. (March 2010). E-mail communication.

26. Hansten, P. (January 2011). E-mail communication.

27. Thompson, B. (January 2010). E-mail communication.

28. Herndon, C. (February 2010). E-mail communication.

29. Federwisch, A. (2010). *Personal "learning style" key to educational success.* Retrieved January 1, 2011, from http://news.nurse.com/article/20100712/NATIONAL01/107120118/-1/frontpage.

Clinical Reasoning and Clinical Judgment

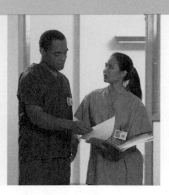

This chapter at a glance ...

Decide where you stand in relation to the following learning outcomes.

Learning Outcomes

After completing this chapter, you should be able to:

1. Map and describe key elements of critical thinking, clinical reasoning, and clinical judgment.
2. Clarify nurses' unique role in health care, including their main responsibilities related to diagnosis and management of medical and nursing problems.
3. Address how to use critical thinking indicators and the 4-Circle CT model as tools to promote critical thinking.
4. Address the relationship among patient safety goals, nursing surveillance, and critical thinking.
5. Describe *outcome-focused, evidence-based care* in your own words.
6. Explain the difference between clinical, functional, and quality of life outcomes.
7. Discuss the roles of ethics codes, standards, guidelines, and laws in making decisions.
8. Compare and contrast the *diagnose and treat* and the *predict, prevent, manage, promote* approaches.
9. Clarify the purpose of each phase of the nursing process
10. Make decisions about your scope of nursing practice.
11. Apply the "four steps" and "five rights" to delegate effectively in the clinical area.
12. Decide where you stand on the Novice to Expert continuum.

NURSES: THE GLUE AND CONSCIENCE OF HEALTH CARE

The following stresses the importance of what you learn in this chapter.

Nurses are the glue that holds care systems together. In many cases, and in many areas, nurses are the only regular, qualified health care providers available. Through their organizations, nurses are the conscience of health care systems.* Health care consumers rank nurses as being the number-one most-trusted professionals (outranking the next most trusted, pharmacists and military officers).[1] Working in complex settings—hospitals, specialized centers, home care, long-term care, schools, and communities—nurses spend more time with patients than any other professional. They monitor and manage many acute and chronic problems, and they teach patients and families to do the same. Finding that no two days are alike, nurses have challenging, rewarding jobs. They are on the frontline, making a difference in life-changing events such as trauma, surgery, childbirth, and end of life.

Your ability to think critically and develop sound clinical reasoning and judgment affects the lives of many. You must be prepared for a job that is much more than a caring presence. You must gain the knowledge and skills needed to manage resources, prevent complications, and promote physical and mental well-being in diverse patients with complex issues.

This chapter and the Chapter 4 are designed to help you acquire the knowledge and skills needed to succeed in six common nursing situations: (1) clinical reasoning and judgment, (2) moral and ethical reasoning, (3) evidence-based practice, (4) teaching others, (5) teaching ourselves, and (6) test-taking. To keep the length of the chapters manageable—to avoid asking you to do too much at one time—content is divided into two chapters. This chapter focuses on clinical reasoning and clinical judgment. Chapter 4 focuses on moral and ethical reasoning, evidence-based practice, teaching others, teaching ourselves, and test-taking.

As you read this chapter, remember that you'll have opportunities to apply this content in Chapter 5, which helps you develop clinical reasoning skills through practice with case scenarios that are based on real experiences.

GOALS AND OUTCOMES OF NURSING

To better understand nursing thinking, let's consider the question "What are the major goals and outcomes of nursing?"

---

*Summarized from Florence Nightingale International Foundation (Web Page) Retrieved January 7, 2011, from http://www.fnif.org/support.htm.

Goals of Nursing

Nurses aim to achieve the following goals in a safe and humanistic way:

1. To help people avoid illness and its complications
2. To help people—whether they are ill, injured, disabled, or well—have optimum quality of life (the best possible function, independence, and sense of well-being)
3. To continually improve patient outcomes, care delivery practices, and nurses' ability to be effective and satisfied in their jobs.

Outcomes of Nursing

Broadly speaking, the following shows the major outcomes that demonstrate the benefits of nursing care.

After receiving individualized, evidence-based care, people will demonstrate improved physical, mental, and spiritual health, as evidenced by the following:

■ Absence of (or reduction in) signs, symptoms, and risk factors of illness, disability, or injury
■ Use of behaviors and strategies that evidence shows will promote health, function, and quality of life
■ Documentation of individualized, evidence-based, state-of-the-art care

What Are the Implications?

There are three main implications of the goals and outcomes of nursing:

1. Because the conclusions and decisions we as nurses make affect people's lives, our thinking must be guided by sound reasoning—precise, disciplined thinking that promotes accurate data collection that's as complete and in-depth as the situation warrants.
2. Since our ultimate goal is for people to be able to manage their own health care to the best of their ability, we must stay focused on *patient perceptions, needs, desires, and capabilities.*
3. Because we're committed to achieving quality outcomes in a cost-effective, timely way, we must constantly seek to improve both our personal ability to give nursing care and the overall quality of health care delivery. We must continue to work to find answers to questions like "How can we achieve better outcomes?" "How can we improve satisfaction with our services?" "How can we contain costs, yet maintain high standards?" and "How can we ensure competent nursing practice and retain good nurses?"

CRITICAL THINKING, CLINICAL REASONING, AND CLINICAL JUDGMENT

As explained in Chapter 1, the terms *critical thinking, clinical judgment,* and *clinical reasoning* are often used interchangeably. Also remember that *critical thinking* and *clinical reasoning* are a process. *Clinical judgment* is the *result* of the process (the conclusion you come to, the decision you make, or the opinion you form).

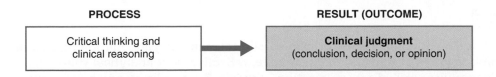

Christine Tanner, a clinical judgment expert, defines clinical judgment like this: "an interpretation or conclusion about a patient's needs, concerns or health problems, and/or the decision to take action (or not), to use or modify standard approaches, or to improvise new ones as deemed appropriate by the patient's response"[2]

Applied Definition

Let's review the applied definition from Chapter 1.

Applied Definition

Critical thinking in nursing—which includes clinical reasoning and clinical judgment—is purposeful, informed, outcome-focused thinking that:

- **Is guided by standards, policies, ethics codes, and laws** (individual state practice acts and state boards of nursing).
- **Is based on principles of nursing process, problem-solving, and the scientific method** (requires forming opinions and making decisions based on evidence).
- **Focuses on safety and quality,** constantly re-evaluating, self-correcting, and striving to improve
- **Carefully identifies the key problems, issues, and risks involved,** including patients, families, and key stakeholders in decision-making early in the process.*
- **Applies logic, intuition, and creativity** and is grounded in specific knowledge, skills, and experience.
- **Is driven by patient, family, and community needs,** as well as nurses' needs to give competent efficient care (e.g., streamlining charting to free nurses for patient care).
- **Calls for strategies that make the most of human potential** and compensate for problems created by human nature (e.g., finding ways to prevent errors, using technology, and overcoming the powerful influence of personal views).

Stakeholders are the people who will be most affected (patients and families) or from whom requirements will be drawn (e.g., caregivers, insurance companies, third-party payers, health care organizations.)

> **RULE**
>
> **Guided by nursing process principles, clinical reasoning and judgment require various ways of thinking (e.g., creative, reflective, and analytical thinking).** It also requires skilled communication—knowing how to listen and how to question, probe, and analyze—and well-developed intellectual and technical skills.

What Other Nurses Say

To get a deeper understanding of critical thinking, consider the following quotes from some of my colleagues.

> *"Improving thinking allows you to develop the most important tool you have in your toolbox: yourself. This means being clear about who you are as a person, and how your attitudes, assumptions, frames of reference, and tendencies to stereotype affect problem solving—how your personal choices and behaviors affect communication and interpersonal relationships. You also need very specific ways of looking at what CT is in context of each particular clinical setting. Too many leaders have the "amorphous blob" concept of CT and just wish people would think better, Then they decree that it's up to the managers and educators to fix the nurses!!"[3]*
>
> —*Ruth Hansten, RN, PhD, FACHE, MBA, BSN*

> *"Fostering, supporting, and rewarding critical thinking is key to recruitment and retention. If we don't encourage nurses to grow in these skills, they become frustrated, telling themselves, 'I'll just do as I'm told, try not to think too much, and not say a word'"[4]*
>
> —*Donna D. Ignatavicius, MS, RN, ANEF*

> *"Critical thinking involves using our brainpower to view and interact with the world and to act in a reflective, discerning way. It includes having intellectual curiosity, being creative, being open to new ideas, examining underlying assumptions, and considering alternative ways of thinking to make reasoned judgments that are sensitive to context."[5]*
>
> —*Theresa M. Valiga, EdD, RN, ANEF, FAAN*

> *"To think critically, look at each situation objectively, uncovering layers to get a deep understanding of what's happening. This often requires playing devil's advocate and looking at the circumstances from all angles, even those you'd rather not consider."[6]*
>
> —*Karen Elechko, RN, MSN*

> *"You begin to learn critical thinking skills in school. But you really develop your critical thinking abilities on the job with a strong mentor and experience. You get good at knowing what to look for, how to interpret signs and symptoms, and what needs to be done first."[7]*
>
> —*Melani Mcguire, RN, BSN*

Mapping Critical Thinking

Mapping critical thinking gives you another way of examining what critical thinking in nursing entails. Study Figure 3-1 (next page), which maps the relationships among key aspects of critical thinking as addressed in this chapter and the next ones. Also study Box 3-1, which summarizes conclusions drawn by Tanner after analyzing almost 200 articles.

Improving Practice and Performance

To many nurses, critical thinking simply means good problem solving. Although problem-solving skills are required, you need a broader view of critical thinking to succeed in today's competitive health care setting. If you don't have a sincere desire to improve—to find ways to broaden your knowledge and skills and to make current practices more efficient and effective—you aren't thinking critically.

Another way to describe critical thinking is a commitment to look for the best way, based on the most current research and practice findings (e.g., the best way to manage pain in a specific person or for a specific health problem). The following diagram shows how critical thinking in nursing constantly strives to improve.

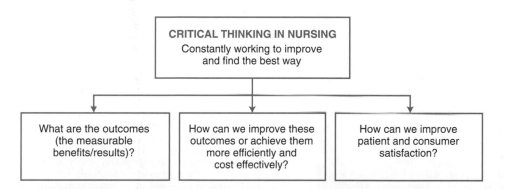

Source: Summarized from Tanner, C. (2006). Thinking like a nurse: A research-based model of clinical judgment in nursing. *Journal of Nursing Education*, 45(6), 204.

CRITICAL THINKING

Reasoning outside the clinical setting (critical thinking)	Reasoning in the clinical setting (critical thinking and critical reasoning)
• Problem-solving, decision-making, and judgment • Personal, family, and community safety and welfare • Teaching-learning (classroom, online, simulated experiences) • Teamwork and collaboration • Test-taking • Using and creating electronic data • Self improvement, stress management, and health promotion • Community safety, welfare, and improvement • Moral and ethical reasoning • Long-term life planning and management	• Diagnostic reasoning (applying nursing process to determine, prevent, and manage patient problems)* • Patient-centered care[†] • Problem-solving, decision-making, and judgment • Patient, caregiver, and community safety and welfare[†] • Moral and ethical reasoning. • Applying evidence-based practice[†] • Teamwork and collaboration[†] • Clinical teaching and learning • Using and creating electronic medical data (informatics)[†] • Self improvement; stress management, • Quality Improvement (improving outcomes and care delivery systems)[†]

Effective/skilled communication
Knowledge-based thinking
Evidence-based thinking
Standards-based thinking
Analytical thinking
Creative/imaginative thinking
Intuitive and logical thinking
Collaborative thinking
Thinking ahead
Thinking in action
Thinking back (reflective thinking)

Partnering with patients and caregivers[†]
Teaching patients and families[†]
Assessign systematically*
Clarifying outcomes*
Identifying problems, issues, and risks*
Preventing and solving problems*
Developing and implementing action plans*
Delegating appropriately[†]
Monitoring progress – evaluating outcomes*
Preventing errors – learning from them[†]
Improving performance and process*[†]

*Required by American Nurses Association Standards (2010) *Nursing scope and standards of performance and standards of clinical practice*. Washington, DC: American Nurses Publishing.
[†]Relates to Quality and Safety Education for Nurses (QSEN) and Institute of Medicine (IOM) competencies. (www.qsen.org and www.iom.edu).

FIGURE 3-1 Key elements of critical thinking. Your reasoning *outside* of the clinical setting affects your ability to reason *inside* the clinical setting. Source: Copyright 2011 by R. Alfaro-LeFevre. www.AlfaroTeachSmart.com.

CRITICAL THINKING INDICATORS AND THE 4-CIRCLE MODEL

Being familiar with critical thinking indicators (CTIs)—short descriptions of behaviors that demonstrate the knowledge, characteristics, and skills that promote critical thinking in the clinical setting—is central to developing critical thinking. If you're not familiar with CTIs, review pages 12 and 53 to 54, which address personal CTIs, knowledge CTIs, and intellectual CTIs. Keep in mind that no one is perfect or able to demonstrate all of the behaviors perfectly all the time. If you use the CTIs as a checklist, you can compare yourself with the listed indicators and decide what you do well and what needs improving. You can also use the CTIs to jog your mind about what you have to do to think critically when you're in a new or complex situation. For example, when you know that a key intellectual CTI is *assessing systematically and comprehensively*, it's likely that one of your first thoughts will be, "I need to figure out a way to assess this patient in a systematic, comprehensive way."

The 4-circle CT model on the inside front cover also helps you assess and improve your ability to think critically. Asking questions like "What parts of the circles do I need to work on most?" helps you prioritize what knowledge and experience you need to gain.

NOVICE VERSUS EXPERT THINKING

Consider the following scenario.

A car hits a young man riding his bicycle in the park. Thrown 60 feet, he lies motionless. Within minutes, two park rangers arrive. They put on latex gloves and begin to assess his injuries. An ambulance pulls up and one ranger yells, "We'll need intubation equipment!" A woman, out for a walk, looks on from a distance. A second woman, riding a bicycle, comes upon the scene. Here's how the conversation goes:

Scenario **NOVICE VERSUS EXPERT THINKING**

First woman: This is terrible. I wish the ambulance had gotten here sooner.

Second woman: Oh?

First woman: Yes. He was thrown at least 50 feet. If the ambulance had arrived sooner, they could have done more. I can't believe these two rangers didn't start resuscitation right away. They waited for this ambulance ... they should have been breathing for him.

Second woman: These rangers look like they know what they're doing. They would have started resuscitation if he needed it. This young man has been thrown so far, I'm sure they're concerned about spinal cord injuries. If they tilt his head back to start respirations, they risk severing his spinal cord—they don't want to do that unless it's absolutely necessary.

BOX 3-2　HOW NOVICES BECOME EXPERTS

According to researcher Patricia Benner, nurses go through the following stages of knowledge and expertise acquisition.*

1. **Novices:** Beginners who lack experience in specific situations (e.g., a new graduate with no experience in nursing or an experienced psychiatric nurse who is beginning to work in obstetric nursing)
2. **Advanced beginners:** Those with marginally acceptable performance based on a foundation of experience with real situations (e.g., a nurse who is in the first year of employment or the first year of a new clinical specialty)
3. **Competent:** Those with 2 or 3 years of experience in similar situations (e.g., a nurse who has practiced emergency and intensive care nursing for 2 or 3 years)
4. **Proficient:** Those with broad experience that allows meaning to be understood in terms of the big picture rather than isolated observations (e.g., a nurse who is in charge of making patient assignments)
5. **Expert:** Those with extensive experiences that enable an intuitive grasp of situations and problems (e.g., an experienced nurse who serves as charge nurse, preceptor, or member of a committee)

---

*Summarized from Benner, P. (2001). *From novice to expert*. Upper Saddle River, NJ: Prentice Hall.

The scenario on the previous page is a true story. I was the second woman on the bicycle. As I talked more with the first woman, I learned she was a student nurse. She thanked me for pointing out something she hadn't thought about. After it was all over, I realized our conversation demonstrated a common difference between expert and novice thinking: The student nurse felt a need to act immediately. As an experienced nurse, I knew the importance of *assessing before acting.*

We're all novices at one time or another. We all know what it's like to be new at something and watch an experienced professional and wonder, "Will I ever know this much?" And almost always, with time and commitment, we soon find ourselves helping someone else who looks at us and thinks, "Will I ever know this much?"

Decide where you stand in relation to being a novice or expert by studying the descriptions in Box 3-2 (above). Then study Table 3-1 (next page), which shows the differences between novice and expert thinking. If you're a novice, determine some things you can do to improve your thinking. If you're an expert, decide how you can help a novice.

PAYING ATTENTION TO CONTEXT

Paying attention to context (circumstances) is a major part of critical thinking. What works in one situation may not work in another. For example, think about the difference between working in pediatrics versus working with adults. Growth and development issues and differences in anatomy and physiology affect many aspects of care. Realize that you may be an expert nurse, but if the circumstances change and you're unfamiliar with giving care under those circumstances, you are more like a novice. Don't be afraid to say, "I'm unfamiliar with dealing with these circumstances and need help."

TABLE 3-1	NOVICE THINKING VERSUS EXPERT THINKING

Novice Nurses	Expert Nurses
• Knowledge is organized as separate facts. Rely heavily on resources (e.g., texts, notes, preceptors). Lack knowledge gained from experience (e.g., listening to breath sounds).	• Knowledge is organized and structured, making recall of information easier. Have a lot of experiential knowledge (e.g., what abnormal breath sounds are like, what subtle changes look like).
• Focus so much on actions that they tend to forget to assess before acting	• Assess and think things through before acting
• Need clear-cut rules	• Know when to bend the rules
• Hampered by unawareness of resources	• Are aware of resources and how to use them
• Hindered by the brain-drains of anxiety and lack of self-confidence	• More self-confident, less anxious, and more focused
• Have limited knowledge of suspected problems; therefore, they question and collect data more superficially	• Have a better idea of suspected problems, allowing them to question more deeply and collect more relevant and in-depth data
• Rely on step-by-step procedures. Tend to focus more on procedures than on the patient response to the procedure	• Know when it's safe to skip steps or do two steps together. Are able to focus on both the parts (the procedures) and the whole (the patient response)
• Become uncomfortable if patient needs preclude performing procedures exactly as they were learned	• Comfortable with rethinking procedure if patient needs necessitate modification of the procedure
• Follow standards and policies by rote	• Analyze standards and policies, looking for ways to improve them
• Learn more readily when matched with a supportive, knowledgeable preceptor or mentor.	• Are challenged by novices' questions, clarifying their own thinking when teaching novices

Source: Copyright 2011. www.AlfaroTeachSmart.com

Sometimes, you may be very familiar with the care, but unfamiliar with the patients. This also may require you to seek help.

> **RULE**
>
> **Patients are *individuals* who may have similar problems, but different attitudes, beliefs, and responses.** Each person and each situation has its own "unique story." Look for differences in patient responses or changes in circumstances—for example cultural, developmental, physical, or emotional differences—and adjust care as needed. When you have a deep understanding of patients' *individual circumstances*, you can avoid making assumptions and tailor care to achieve the best outcomes.

TRENDS THAT AFFECT THINKING

Health care is changing more quickly than you can say the word *computer*. Pardon the word play, but computers are one of the main reasons for rapid change. From diagnostic technology to information management and decision support, computers are at the core of many changes in health care. This section describes major changes that affect how you think and work today.

Institute of Medicine Competencies

The 2000s brought a "wake-up call" for health care consumers and providers. We experienced terrorism, hurricanes, disasters, and new diseases that threatened large populations on unprecedented scales. Institute of Medicine (IOM) studies revealed that because of reliance on outmoded systems, there were many safety and quality problems in health care.[8,9,10]

The IOM concluded that poorly designed systems set staff up to fail—regardless of how hard they tried. Four underlying reasons for inadequate care were cited:[10]

1. Growing complexity of medical science and technology
2. Increase in the number of people with chronic conditions
3. Poorly organized health care delivery systems
4. Lack of use of informatics (the use of computers to facilitate the acquisition, storage, retrieval, and use of information)

The IOM developed core competencies stating that all health care providers must be able to provide patient-centered care, work in interdisciplinary teams, employ evidence-based practice, apply quality improvement methods, and use informatics.[9] Nurse educators responded to the IOM competencies by developing the Quality and Safety Education for Nurses (QSEN) project, as described in the next section.

Quality and Safety Education for Nurses' Competencies

The QSEN goal is to prepare future nurses to gain the knowledge, skills, and attitudes needed to continuously improve the quality and safety of the health care system.[11] QSEN clarifies what the IOM competencies mean to nursing in the following way (competencies quoted from www.qsen.org):

■ **Patient-centered care:** Recognize the patient or designee as the source of control and full partner in providing compassionate and coordinated care based on respect for patient's preferences, values, and needs.

■ **Teamwork and Collaboration:** Function effectively within nursing and inter-professional teams, fostering open communication, mutual respect, and shared decision-making to achieve quality patient care.

■ **Evidence-based Practice (EBP):** Integrate best current evidence with clinical expertise and patient/family preferences and values for delivery of optimal health care.

■ **Quality Improvement (QI):** Use data to monitor the outcomes of care processes, and use improvement methods to design and test changes to continuously improve the quality and safety of health care systems.

■ **Safety:** Minimize risk of harm to patients and providers through both system effectiveness and individual performance.

If the above sounds familiar to you, it may be because we've already addressed many of these issues. Content related to IOM and QSEN competencies is integrated throughout this book. For example, patient-centered care is stressed throughout. Evidence-based practice and quality improvement are addressed in the next chapter. Chapter 6 addresses *transforming a group into a team, accessing and using information, preventing and dealing with mistakes constructively,* and other skills you need to achieve the competencies.

Safety Is Top Priority

Recognizing that safety must be top priority, new standards based on National Practice Safety Goals (NPSG) are implemented in virtually all health care organizations.[12]

Acknowledging that improvements happen when mistakes are reported—rather than hidden—regulations implementing the Patient Safety and Quality Improvement Act (PSQIA) began in 2009. PSQIA establishes a voluntary reporting system to increase the data available to assess and resolve patient safety and quality issues. To encourage the reporting and analysis of medical errors, PSQIA provides federal privilege and confidentiality protections for error reporting and patient safety information (called *patient safety work product*).[13]

RULE

Critical thinking in nursing is focused—centered on major patient issues and problems. Patient and caregiver safety and welfare must be central to all thinking in health care.

Upholding Patients' Rights and Privacy Is Law

Upholding patient's rights is guaranteed by federal and state laws. For example, patients have the right to have copies of their medical records, and to keep them private, as stated in Health Insurance Portability and Accountability Act (HIPAA) privacy laws. Other rights are upheld by health care standards. For example, patients have the right to have communication and cultural needs met. Most health care organizations have a patients' bill of rights that addresses specific rights (see example in Appendix C).

Patient- and Family-Centered Care

Acknowledging that emotional, social, and developmental support are central to allocating resources and achieving outcomes efficiently, organizations work to develop a culture of patient and family-centered care. Patients and families are viewed as key members of the health care team. This type of approach aims to shape policies, programs, facility, and staff day-to-day interactions to focus on greater patient and family satisfaction.[14]

Population-Based Care: Meeting Diverse Needs

We recognize that nurses must meet the needs of diverse patient populations (e.g., patients of certain cultures, age groups, languages, or sexual orientation.) The Joint Commission—the main accrediting body for health care organizations—has set standards for "population-based care." You can download a road map to meeting these standards entitled *Advancing Effective Communication, Cultural Competence and Patient- and Family-Centered Care: A Road Map for Hospitals* from http://www.jointcommission.org/Advancing_Effective_Communication/.

Empowering Patients: Nurses as Stewards for Safe Passage

Two important shifts in thinking are key to empowering patients and families to manage their own care:

1. Shift from "I know what's best for you" to "I want to empower you to make your own decisions."
2. Shift from "I'm here to take care of you" to "I'm here to make sure you know how to take care of yourself when I'm not here."

    Much like a ship's steward—who has the job of protecting passengers on a journey—your job as a nurse is to protect patients and help them navigate safely through the health care system. As a steward, you hold *patients' lives* in your hands, but *they* should be "at the helm," directing where they want to go. Help patients understand the concept of empowerment by saying things like "I'm here to take care of you, but even more importantly, I'm here to make sure you know how to take care of yourself when I'm not here," "Let me know when you have questions or concerns," and "Stay involved in your care—you know yourself best and will do better if you let us know what you need and want." Box 3-3 (*Speak Up* initiatives) gives an example of how patients today are encouraged to stay involved in their care and speak up when they have concerns.

    If you're unfamiliar with the process of establishing empowered partnerships, review *Developing Empowered Partnerships* (in Chapter 6).

Health Information Technology and Electronic Health Records

Health Information Technology (HIT) and Electronic Health Records (EHR) significantly affect thinking: critical thinking and clinical reasoning depend on having ready access to

---

BOX 3-3 IMPROVE SAFETY: URGE YOUR PATIENTS TO SPEAK UP

Encourage patients to become involved, informed participants on the health care team. The following simple steps are based on research that shows that patients who take part in health care decisions have improved outcomes.

- **S**peak up if you have questions or concerns, and if you don't understand, ask again. It's your body, and you have a right to know.
- **P**ay attention to the care you are receiving. Make sure you're getting the right treatments and medications by the right health care professionals. Don't assume anything.
- **E**ducate yourself about your diagnosis, the medical tests you are undergoing, and your treatment plan.
- **A**sk a trusted family member or friend to be your advocate.
- **K**now your medications and why you take them. Medication errors are the most common health care errors.
- **U**se a hospital, clinic, surgery center, or other type of health care organization that has undergone a rigorous on-site evaluation against established state-of-the-art quality and safety standards, such as that provided by The Joint Commission.
- **P**articipate in all decisions about your treatment. You are the center of the health care team.

Source: Courtesy of The Joint Commission.

accurate, organized, complete patient information. Federal initiatives push for "meaningful use" of informatics—the use of HIT to facilitate the acquisition, storage, retrieval, and use of information by all health care professionals—refers to both a goal and a process toward universal EHR for all Americans, as noted below.

Meaningful Use of Informatics: Goal and Process.[15] Goal: The purposeful flow of shared health information among patients and their care providers in order to streamline care delivery and improve overall patient care outcomes.

Process: Federal standards and incentives push all health care organizations to work toward meaningful use of HIT. The Health Information Technology for Economic and Clinical Health (HITECH) Act authorizes U.S. Health and Human Services to establish programs to improve care quality, safety, and efficiency through the use of private, secure HIT. Eligible health care professionals and hospitals can qualify for Medicare and Medicaid incentive payments when they implement certified EHR technology and use it to achieve clearly specified objectives. The Centers for Medicare and Medicaid Services (CMS) have issued regulations defining the minimum EHR requirements that providers must meet to qualify for funding, and specify standards and certification criteria for eligible EHR technology systems.

Electronic and Printed Tools

In most cases today, you use electronic or printed standard tools that affect your thinking. Standard evidence-based tools are essential to collecting complete information, communicating care, improving decision-making, promoting efficiency, preventing mistakes, and keeping everyone "on the same page." However, we're still in the early stages of streamlining EHR, and HIT is only as good as the designers make it. We also have to help "the humans" use them with active, critical minds. As with all complex computer systems, we'll continue to experience "growing pains." In some cases, using EHR has caused more complications and problems than they solved.[16]

Because computers—now extensions of humans—are only as good as they are designed, leaders and frontline nurses must be involved in planning, development, and testing of all systems. Be a critical thinker and an active voice in improving systems. If something about your EHR seems error-prone or time-consuming (e.g., having to chart the same data in more than one place), report this to your manager or educator.

> **RULE**
>
> **While EHR and decision-support tools aim to promote critical thinking, they do not *think for you*.** Keep an open active mind, look for flaws, and decide how the computer's information applies to your patients' individual circumstances, *right now*. You—not the computer—work in "real time."

Standard, interdisciplinary tools such as critical pathways (tools that outline care management for particular problems, such as postoperative care of knee surgery) and algorithms (tools that describe an ordered sequence of steps to take under specific circumstances, such as how to proceed when a patient arrives in the emergency department complaining of chest pain) are the norm. You can download an example critical pathway from http://evolve.elsevier.com/Alfaro-LeFevre/CT.

When you use well-designed, evidence-based tools and HIT, two things happen that promote critical thinking: (1) As you use the same tools over and over again in various situations, your brain creates a mental file of what's most important (e.g., what information must be collected and what to assess *first*). (2) The documentation associated with the tool gives you and the rest of the team a record you can reflect on to identify patterns and pick up omissions. But remember, tools, HIT, and EHR must be designed for specific purposes—one size doesn't fit all.

Standard Tools Prevent Miscommunication

To prevent miscommunication among caregivers, safety standards stress the need for standard communication tools. For example, the Situation, Background, Assessment, Recommendation (SBAR) tool (Box 3-4) is often used for change-of-shift reports (handoffs) and for reporting problems to physicians. Safety standards also delineate that nurses must use "Read Back" and "Repeat Back" rules as in the following rule.[12]

> **RULE**
>
> **To prevent communication errors, use "Read Back" and "Repeat Back" rules.** When you receive verbal orders or lab values, write them down and read them back to check for accuracy. When you give lab results or important communications to others, ask, "Can you repeat that back to me to be sure we're on the same page"?

BOX 3-4 SBAR (SITUATION, BACKGROUND, ASSESSMENT, RECOMMENDATION)*

NOTE: Pronounced *S-BAR* and first used by the military to promote effective communication between caregivers, the SBAR approach is recommended by patient safety experts. SBAR forms vary depending on purpose and setting. Some places use SBAR for giving handoff situations (when one nurse transfers patient care to another). Some places require SBAR forms like the one below to be completed before calling physicians about a problem.

→ **Have the chart in hand before you make the phone call, and be sure you can readily communicate all of the following information.**

S   **SITUATION:** Briefly state the issue or problem: what it is, when it happened (or how it started), and how severe it is. Give the signs and symptoms that make you concerned.

B   **BACKGROUND:** Give the date of admission and current medical diagnoses. Determine the pertinent medical history, and give a brief synopsis of the treatment to date (e.g., medications, oxygen use, nasogastric tube, IVs, code status).

A   **ASSESSMENT:** Give most recent vital signs and any changes in the following:

  ■ Mental status, neuro signs   ■ GI status (nausea, vomiting, diarrhea,
  ■ Respirations   distention)
  ■ Pulse, skin color   ■ Urine output
  ■ Comfort, pain   ■ Bleeding, drainage
                                       ■ Other: _____

R   **RECOMMENDATION:** State what you think should be done. For example:

  ■ Come see the patient now.
  ■ Get a consultation.
  ■ Get additional studies. (e.g., CXR, ABG, EKG, CBC, other)
  ■ Transfer the patient to ICU.
  ■ How frequently do you want vital signs?
  ■ If there's no improvement, by when do you want us to call you?

*Data from: Haig, K, Sutton, S., Whittington, J. (2006) SBAR: A shared mental model for improving communication between clinicians. *Journal of Quality and Patient Safety*, 32(3), 167-175. Retrieved from http://unmc.edu/rural/patient-safety/tool-time/TT1-052506-SBAR/SBAR%20shared%20mental%20model.pdf.
Source: Copyright 2011. www.AlfaroTeachSmart.com.

Time-outs Promote Group Thinking and Prevent Errors

In today's fast-paced clinical setting, many professionals are involved in giving care to one patient—there are many "cooks stirring the pot." We must ensure that "the right ingredients" go into the "pot" (the patient) at the right time." We need everyone's eyes, ears, and brains to prevent mistakes.

Time-outs, in which the entire team stops to become focused and "on the same plan of care," are now commonplace. There are two kinds of time-outs. One is routine, such as at the beginning of surgeries, when patients' identities and surgical procedures are double- and triple-checked. The other type of time-out is spontaneous. If at any time *any* team member—nurse, nursing aid, respiratory therapist, or physician—recognizes an actual or potential risk of harm to the patient, he or she is responsible for calling a time-out and pointing out his or her concern (and the rest of the team is accountable for listening and deciding how to address the concern).[17]

> **Health Care Reform Also Affects Nursing's Thinking.** Because this process is ongoing, for up-to-date information from the ANA, go to http://www.rnaction. org/site/PageServer?pagename=nstat_take_action_healthcare_reform%26auto login=true%26ct=1.

DIAGNOSE AND TREAT VERSUS PREDICT, PREVENT, MANAGE, AND PROMOTE

Care has shifted from a *diagnose and treat* (DT) approach, which implies that we wait for evidence of problems to start treatment, to a predictive model: *predict, prevent, manage, and promote* (PPMP).

PPMP is a proactive approach that aims to predict and manage risk factors *before* problems arise. PPMP is based on evidence. Thanks to research, we can often predict which people are at risk for certain problems and, if needed, begin an aggressive prevention plan. Sometimes prevention requires "treatment" (called *prophylaxis*). Think about the following examples:

- **To prevent venous thromboembolism (VTE),** the use of pulsating antiemboli stockings is standard during and after many surgeries. Because VTE has potentially fatal complications, including pulmonary embolism, VTE prevention is a major health care initiative. Hospitals use technology and evidence-based practice to reduce VTE risks. For example, Johns Hopkins Hospital developed a mandatory computer-based decision support system to facilitate specialty-specific risk factor assessment, allowing risk-appropriate VTE prophylaxis (prevention). Washington DC Veterans Affairs Medical Center designed a 7-step process that walks providers through an evidence-based risk factor assessment to determine appropriate prophylactic therapy.[18]

- **We may give an influenza vaccine** to someone with chronic lung disease and *also* vaccinate the whole family (to reduce the person's risk of contracting the virus from a family member).

- **For those with significant exposure to the human immunodeficiency virus (HIV),** treatment begins immediately, before there's evidence of the virus in the blood.

- **Sometimes taking an antihistamine for a week** *before* allergy season can reduce allergic response.

The PPMP approach requires you to do the following:

1. **Predict common problems and complications, and then develop a plan to monitor and prevent them.**[19] For example, if you're caring for someone who has just arrived in the emergency department with a heart problem, you:

   ■ Initiate nursing surveillance (the close observation of patients at risk for complications).[20] Monitor closely for early signs and symptoms that indicate increasing problems (e.g., monitor for irregular pulse, fluid in the lungs, ankle swelling, and chest discomfort).

   ■ Involve the patient in detecting and preventing complications (e.g., tell him to let you know if he has any new symptoms; tell him you will monitor his intake to be sure be sure he doesn't overload his heart with fluids).

   ■ Be prepared to manage complications in case they can't be prevented (e.g., have a fully prepared emergency cart nearby, and know how to use it).

2. **Focus on risk management:** Screen for the presence of risk factors, and identify ways to eliminate or manage them. For example, you make a home visit to assess an infant. As part of the assessment, you look for risks to the infant's safety (check where the baby sleeps, and find out if the parents are aware of possible infant hazards). If you identify risks to the baby's safety, you're responsible for making a plan to correct the situation. Failing to make a plan may be considered negligence.

3. **Encourage behaviors that promote health, optimum function, independence, and sense of well-being.** For example, explain to asthmatics that a walking or exercise program is key to promoting optimum lung function, encourage all smokers to stop, and stress the need for colonoscopy after age 50.

For more on risk management and health promotion: Go online to *Healthy People 2020 Initiatives* (www.healthypeople.gov). the Harvard Center For Risk Analysis (www.hcra.harvard.edu/), and The Centers for Disease Control and Prevention Web page (www.cdc.gov/).

4. **Use technology to reduce errors and improve accuracy and efficiency.** Ask, "What technologic advances are there to monitor this patient and prevent complications?" For example, for many years, to ensure proper placement of central venous lines, we did chest x-rays to be sure the lines were in the vein, not in the chest cavity. Now we know the importance of preventing this complication by using live ultrasound *as the line is inserted.*

The PPMP approach—predict, prevent, manage, promote—prevents complications, saves lives, prioritizes care, improves satisfaction, and contains costs.

The following scenario shows the importance of risk management and being proactive when promoting health and managing health problems.

Scenario
IMPROVE EXERCISE TOLER-ANCE: PREDICT, PREVENT, AND MANAGE DEHYDRA-TION

Living in Florida, where we have heat, humidity, and a lot of elderly people, I learned the need to manage—rather than treat—dehydration firsthand. Many health care providers tell people to walk to gain strength. Sometimes these instructions backfire, and people faint in the heat. If you or someone else is going to exercise, improve performance by pacing yourself and ensuring adequate hydration. On hot days, predict the risk of salt depletion and dehydration from sweating. Prevent dehydration and heat stroke by teaching about risk factors (obesity, alcohol or caffeine use, use of some medications like diuretics, and being very young or old will put you at risk). Teach signs of heatstroke (i.e., weakness, nausea, vomiting, chills, confusion, disorientation, hallucinations). Stress the importance of improving ability to exercise by drinking water *before* exercising (so you start out well-hydrated), wearing loose-fitting clothes, avoiding the hotter parts of the day, avoiding tea or caffeine (they act as diuretics), and replacing fluids during exercise (water is usually best). If you suspect heatstroke, manage it by cooling down the person immediately (place the person near an air conditioner, or place damp towels all over the body, especially to the temples and wrists, where blood vessels are near the skin). If the person can tolerate liquids, offer cool drinks. If the person becomes dazed, confused, or has stopped sweating, head for the emergency room because dehydration is severe, requiring immediate medical management.

Point of Care Testing Fine-Tunes Care

Today, point of care testing—testing that happens at the patients' bedside to fine-tune care—is a key part of managing certain health problems. For example, with acute brain injuries, nurses perform highly skilled neurologic assessments at least every hour. These assessments help identify subtle changes that are then used to guide how the patient is managed on an hour-by-hour basis. The management of diabetes is another example of the importance of using point of care testing to fine-tune care management.

Rapid Response Teams and Code H (Help)

Rapid response teams (RRTs) and Code H (help) are great examples of using the whole team's brain power to ensure early intervention. The complexity of care today makes it difficult for nurses to balance their patient load. If a nurse is worried that someone's condition is deteriorating, he or she calls the RRT to do an assessment. The RRT usually is staffed by nurse managers, house physicians, respiratory therapists, critical care nurses, and pharmacists.

Code H was developed after18-month-old Josie King died when her family was unable to get her the attention they felt she needed.[21] With Code H, patients, families, and visitors can trigger levels of rapid response. For example, patients and visitors can call a code number, which goes directly to hospital operators. The operators are trained to ask questions according to an algorithm. Callers who report something important, such as bleeding or chest pain, are routed immediately to the RRT. If the call is about problems like delays in getting pain medications, lack of communication, or some issue that doesn't require the RRT, the operator triggers a Code H. In this case, only the nurse manager responds (within minutes of the call). Even if the Code H turns out to be something very mild, families feel reassured to know that they will be heard.[22] Using RRT and Code H saves lives and improves nurses' job satisfaction, as nurses get help when they need it.[23]

Disease and Disability Management

Disease and disability management—a model of care that focuses on keeping people with chronic diseases and disabilities healthy—is an important part of the PPMP approach. We now *manage* chronic conditions over time, rather than waiting for episodes of relapse or crisis. For example, with asthma, we don't just keep *treating* asthma attacks. We *manage* the asthma by monitoring asthmatics *when healthy,* fine-tuning medications and inhalers to keep them symptom-free. In this way, we can ensure that they receive the most current, effective drugs with the least side effects.

We can expect nursing roles related to disease and disability management to grow. Studies find that using team-based, nurse-led care models significantly improves the condition and quality of life of patients with multiple chronic illnesses. Patients receiving this type of care achieve better control of chronic conditions such as depression, heart disease, and diabetes compared with those given standard care in a primary care setting.[24]

Box 3-5 (next page) summarizes additional trends that affect nurses' thinking.

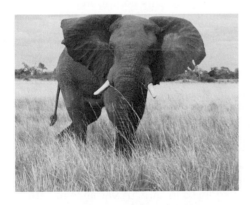

What does this elephant have to do with clinical judgment and the PPMP model? When we were in Africa, this elephant gave us a menacing look. As our guide quickly put the jeep into reverse, someone asked, "Do they teach you how to use that gun on the dashboard?" The guide replied, "Yes. But, even more important—they teach us how not to get in the position that we need it." Be proactive. Predict and prevent complications. Be ready to manage unavoidable complications. Promote health through patient teaching.

OUTCOME-FOCUSED, EVIDENCE-BASED CARE

From professional and economic perspectives, the care we give must focus on outcomes and be driven by the best available evidence. We must be able to answer questions like the following:

1. Exactly what does the patient, family, client, or group need to achieve?
2. Have the best-qualified professionals decided what, realistically—based on circumstances—can be achieved?

3. Have the key stakeholders—the people who will be most affected by care (e.g., patients and families) or from whom requirements will be drawn (e.g., caregivers, third-party payers, and health care organizations)—been included in decision-making?
4. What evidence indicates that the outcomes are likely to be achieved in this particular situation?

Evidence-based care is discussed in depth in Chapter 4. For now, just remember that it's important to evaluate the strength of the evidence that supports your plan of care.

Chapter 5 gives detailed information on the key clinical reasoning skill of *Determining Patient-Centered (Client-Centered) Outcomes*. For now, just remember the

---

BOX 3-5   TRENDS THAT AFFECT NURSES' THINKING

- **Nurses at all levels take on more responsibilities.** Licensed practical nurses, registered nurses, and advanced-practice nurses (APNs) continue to gain responsibilities, making it important to know how to decide whether you are qualified to accept new responsibilities.
- **New threats emerge.** Emergence of resistant bacteria such as methicillin-resistant *Staphylococcus aureus* (MRSA) point out the need for meticulous hand hygiene and management of invasive treatments and open wounds. International travel brings threats of pandemics (epidemics over a wide geographic area and affecting a large part of the population). Terrorism, including bioterrorism, is a constant threat, requiring new levels of preparedness and responsiveness.
- **Many people live longer with illnesses and disabilities.** An alarming number of people with obesity and diabetes are major health care concerns, as these problems contribute to many other health problems.
- **New diagnostic imaging and treatment modalities** such as vaccine use, stem cell use, and genetic manipulation emerge.
- **Ethical dilemmas grow.** Ethical issues (e.g., end-of-life care, assisted suicide, fertility issues, cloning, stem-cell research) require in-depth thinking that's clearly grounded in ethical principles (see Chapter 4).
- **Technology moves into homes.** Nurses must be able to give "high-tech" care in homes and must have excellent assessment and interpersonal skills. Being flexible, resourceful, and practical in homes is key.
- **Case management**—the use of collaborative approaches to ensure that the best available resources are used to reach outcomes efficiently—promotes quality. This approach is grounded in prevention and early intervention. Today all nurses are expected to be "case managers," closely monitoring progress toward outcomes to detect variances in care. (A variance in care is when a patient isn't progressing toward outcomes in the expected time frame—for example, if someone has surgery and is expected to get out of bed on the first day after surgery but is unable to do so, it's considered a variance in care, which requires further evaluation.)
- *Healthy People 2020* **initiatives** guide organizations, businesses, and communities to come together to achieve two major goals: (1) to help people of all ages improve life expectancy and quality of life, and (2) to eliminate health disparities among different segments of the population. (See www.healthypeople.gov/.)
- **Holistic and alternative therapies**—for example, diet, exercise, acupuncture, and stress reduction through meditation and aromatherapy—are recognized as key strategies for triggering the body's natural healing powers.

importance of identifying both goals and outcomes, as they address exactly *what you need the patient to be able to do* (outcome) and *what you need to do* (goal), as in the following example.

- **Example Outcome:** After completing the diabetic teaching module, Jim will be able to manage his diabetes independently at home, including blood glucose monitoring and medication, nutrition, and exercise management by Friday.
- **Example Goal:** Our goal is to work with Jim to help him review and complete the diabetic teaching module, teaching and supporting him as needed.

Sometimes goals and outcomes are very similar and only outcomes are needed. However, reflecting on whether you have really considered *both* goals and outcomes often brings to light flaws in thinking.

Clinical, Functional, and Other Outcomes

Because determining *overall* quality of care requires you to examine outcomes from *several* perspectives, this section explains clinical, functional, and other outcomes. Study the following types of outcomes listed in the context of a surgical repair of a fractured hip. Think about the importance of considering all the outcomes to determine overall care quality.

- **Clinical outcomes:** To what degree are the patient's health problems resolved? For example, is the hip healed?
- **Functional outcomes:** To what degree is the patient able to function independently, physically, cognitively, and socially? For example, is the person able to do required daily activities without help? Are there problems with cognitive function?
- **Symptom severity and quality of life outcomes:** To what degree is the patient free of symptoms and able to do desired, as well as required, activities? For example, is there any hip pain, and is the person able to meet physical work requirements and do favorite activities?
- **Risk reduction outcomes:** To what degree is the patient able to demonstrate ways to reduce health risks? For example, is he able to explain ways of improving safety, such as using a cane when fatigued? Does he keep his home free from hazards that may cause falls?
- **Protective factor outcomes:** To what degree does the patient's environment protect him from deteriorating health? For example, when bedridden, are bedrails up as needed and skin care protocols followed?
- **Therapeutic alliance outcomes:** To what degree does the patient express a positive relationship between himself and health care professionals? For example, when asked, does he state that he feels free to ask questions?
- **Satisfaction outcomes:** To what degree do the patient and family express satisfaction with care given? For example, when asked, do they state that they had competent, efficient treatment? Were services convenient?
- **Use of services outcomes:** To what degree were appropriate nursing services used? For example, was a case manager used, if needed?

> **RULE**
>
> **Outcome-focused thinking means more than "fixing the problems."** It means fixing the problems in ways that you get the *best results,* from a cost, time, and patient satisfaction perspective.

Dynamic Relationship of Problems and Outcomes

There's a close, dynamic relationship between problems and outcomes. Sometimes you'll find yourself focusing on *problems* and sometimes on *outcomes,* depending on the situation. Think about the following examples:

- You're working with a patient on a respirator, and the desired outcome is that the patient has *adequate ventilation.* You see that the patient seems to be struggling for air. You check the tubing and see a lot of water from condensation. You empty the water. If the patient is still struggling, you continue to look for other problems that might be interfering with the desired outcome of *adequate ventilation.* For example, you assess breath sounds and help the patient to get in a position to cough and clear mucus. You continue looking for problems until you reach your desired outcome.

- You're working with a group with many complex issues. Instead of getting bogged down in the problems, you say: "It's going to take us forever if we stay mired in long-standing, complicated issues. Let's focus on *results,* rather than *problems.* Let's decide together the major things we want to achieve and then get agreement on what we need to do to achieve them."

Critical Thinking Exercises

Example responses are on pages 267 to 268.

1. Study Box 3-3 on page 81 *(Speak Up),* and then decide how you would handle a drug addict who insists that he or she must have more medication.
2. Decide "what's wrong with the picture" in the following scenario.

Scenario
WHAT'S WRONG WITH THIS PICTURE?

Mr. Duncan, an elderly diabetic, is seen at home every other day by a nurse, who checks a healing incision. Mr. Duncan has been looking for an assistive device that he can attach to the toilet to help him get up and down. When he asks the visiting nurse if she knows where she can find such a device, the nurse replies, "I'm sorry. I know what you mean, but I don't know where you get them."

3. Using your own words and giving examples or drawing a map, explain how you use a PPMP approach to health care delivery.
4. Fill in the blanks in the following sentence: Critical thinking means more than fixing problems—it means fixing them in a way that gets the _____ _____ from a cost, time, and _____ _____ perspective.

Think, Pair, Share

1. Draw two columns on a piece of paper. On the left, list the key points of the applied critical thinking definition on page 71. On the right, write your own interpretation of what each key point implies about what you need to know and do to think critically in nursing. When you're done, swap papers with a partner and discuss your ideas.

2. Discuss where you stand in relation to the description in *Novice Thinking versus Expert Thinking* (see Table 3-1, page 77) and *How Novices Become Experts* (see Box 3-2, page 76).

3. Examine the relationship between the two boxes at the bottom of Figure 3-1 on page 74.

4. A healthy workplace forms the foundation for critical thinking. Share your thoughts and experiences in relation to the following.

> **Zero Tolerance for Bullying and Disrespect.** A key part of having a healthy workplace—which forms the foundation for critical thinking—is having "zero tolerance" for bullying and lateral violence. Lateral violence can be a variety of behaviors—from thoughtless acts to purposeful, intentional acts meant to harm, intimidate, or humiliate others. These types of behaviors create a hostile work environment. In its extreme form, lateral violence is bullying—a conscious, deliberate, hostile act intended to harm, demean, and induce fear. To read more on this topic, go to http://www.minurses.org/nursing-practice/lateral-violence.

5. **Pain-Free Hospitals?** Pain is a significant sign that may indicate deterioration in condition or a need for medication. Share the implications of the following: Utah nursing professor envisions pain-free hospitals. Retrieved January, 6, 2011, from http://www.sltrib.com/sltrib/home/50818890-76/pain-nursing-patients-hospitals.html.csp

6. Go to http://www.ipfcc.org/faq.html and discuss how the core concepts of patient- and family-centered care affect patient outcomes.

7. Draw a map of how to use a PPMP approach to health care delivery. Then swap maps with your partner and discuss them.

8. Think about people you know who are living with chronic diseases or disabilities. How does the PPMP model apply to keeping them healthy? Share their struggles and successes and the factors that help or hinder their ability to stay as well as possible.

9. Practice using the "Read Back" and "Repeat Back" rules (page 82) and the SBAR tool (page 83) with one another.

10. Go to http://www.ahrq.gov/questionsaretheanswer/ and discuss the following topics: Reducing Medical Mistakes, Talking with Your Clinician,

Getting Medical Tests, Planning for Surgery, Getting a Prescription, and Build Your Question List.

11. Critical thinking is guided by laws and standards. Discuss the following article: *Protect yourself: Know your nurse practice act* by Nancy Brent. Retrieved from http://ce.nurse.com/CE548/Protect-Yourself--Know-Your-Nurse-Practice-Act/.

NURSING PROCESS: A CLINICAL REASONING TOOL

As evidence-based approaches continue to evolve, you can expect that the nursing process won't be the *only* tool you will learn to promote critical thinking. Learning several models improves your ability to think critically for two reasons: (1) Each model brings new insights, and (2) some models work better in one context than another.

RULE

Nursing process principles form the basis for virtually all care models, and for nursing documentation. When something goes wrong, one of the first things that's examined is whether assessments, diagnoses, outcomes, interventions, and evaluation of progress has been recorded. Knowledge of nursing process is also key to passing NCLEX® and other certification tests.

The following section summarizes the purpose and process of each step of the nursing process. Keep in mind that it's important to remember the *purpose* of each phase, and that the phases are interrelated. What happens in one phase affects the others.

Applying the Nursing Process

NOTE: Remember that the following nursing process phases are dynamic, not linear. *Assessment* should ALWAYS be addressed first—never skip this step. An example of how the nursing process is dynamic is that if you get to the second phase (Diagnosis/Outcome Identification) and the problems are still not clear, you need to go back to check whether your assessment data is factual and complete. Chapter 5, *Practicing Clinical Reasoning Skills: Applying the Nursing Process*, gives opportunities to practice applying nursing process principles.

Assessment

Purpose: Collect and record data to provide the information needed to:

- Predict, prevent, detect, manage, and resolve problems, issues, and risks.
- Clarify expected outcomes—observable desired results and benefits—of care.

- Identify individualized interventions to achieve outcomes, promote health, and attain optimum function and independence.

Diagnosis/Outcome Identification

Purpose: Analyze data to (1) clarify realistic expected outcomes (benefits of care), and (2) identify the problems, risks, or issues that must be managed to achieve the outcomes. *Diagnosis* and *outcome identification* often happen almost simultaneously (a "chicken or egg" situation) with thinking going back and forth between questions like "What are the major problems, issues, and risks?" "What does the patient want to achieve?" "What, realistically, must be achieved?" During this phase, in addition to clarifying outcomes, you:

- Identify signs and symptoms that may indicate the need for referral to a more qualified professional (report these immediately).
- Rule in and rule out suspected problems.
- Decide what problems, issues, and risks must be managed in order to achieve the outcomes.
- Identify risk factors that must be managed.
- Determine the patient's resources, strengths, and use of healthy behaviors.
- Recognize health states that are satisfactory but could be improved.
- Reflect on thinking to determine whether (1) Patient participation in the process has been at an optimum level; (2) data are accurate and complete; (3) assumptions have been identified, and thinking tailored to individual patient and circumstances; (4) conclusions are based on facts (evidence), rather than guesswork; and (5) alternate conclusions, ideas, and solutions were considered. **(Reflecting on thinking applies to all the phases, but is placed here because it requires analysis, which is the focus of this phase.)**

Planning

Purpose: Ensure that there's a comprehensive, recorded, outcome-focused plan that's tailored to the individual patient and circumstances. The plan should be designed to do the following:

- Specify short-term and long-term outcomes.
- Monitor and manage *priority* problems, issues, and risks.
- Promote optimum comfort, function, independence, and health.
- Coordinate care and include patients as partners in decision-making and care.
- Identify what interventions must be managed by registered nurses and what may be delegated to other licensed and unlicensed workers
- Achieve the desired outcomes safely, efficiently, and cost-effectively

- Include teaching to help patients make informed decisions and become independent
- Provide a record that can be used to monitor progress and communicate care

Implementation
Purpose: Put the plan into action.
- Assess the patient to determine whether interventions are still appropriate and patient is ready.
- Prioritize, delegate, and coordinate care as indicated, including patients and other caregivers as partners in decision-making and care.
- Prepare the environment and equipment for safety, comfort, and convenience.
- Perform interventions, and then reassess to determine initial responses.
- Make immediate changes as needed; update the recorded plan if required.
- Record patient data and responses to monitor progress and communicate care.

Evaluation
Purpose: Determine where the patient stands in relation to desired outcomes; consider how the process can be improved.
- Assess patient status to determine whether expected outcomes have been met and what factors promoted or inhibited the success of the plan.
- Plan for ongoing assessment, improvement, and patient independence.
- Discharge the patient, or modify the plan as indicated.

*From: R. Alfaro-LeFevre handouts. Copyright 2011. www.AlfaroTeachSmart.com.

Proactive, Dynamic, and Outcome-Focused

Today we stress that the nursing process must be proactive and focused on outcomes, risk management, and health promotion—as well as dealing with problems. In the clinical setting, the nursing process is dynamic, unlike how it's described in books or classrooms. If you jump around in books or classrooms trying to explain how things happen in real life, you confuse people—you have to present content in a logical, step-by-step way.

In *real life*, the nursing process is fluid and changing. You apply principles of nursing process, but move back and forth within various phases. Think about the scenario on the next page, which shows the thinking that's likely to go on in a nurse's head as he applies the nursing process at the bedside.

In this scenario, Bob is experienced and comfortable in his role. If Bob were a novice, his thinking would be slower—hampered by lack of experience and lack of confidence. He would see a picture of the room, but he'd miss key details. He may also lose brainpower from dealing with his doubts about his own capabilities.

Scenario
**DYNAMIC
THINKING
AT THE
BEDSIDE**

Bob, a medical-surgical nurse, walks into a room. A picture flashes in his mind—his brain assesses the room in an instant. The picture he sees is that of bed linens in disarray, trash on the floor, and someone who is restless and has a distressed look. Bob's mind jumps to phase 2 of the nursing process (diagnosis), thinking, *there's a problem here*. Automatically, he goes back to basics—phase 1 (assessment)—and assesses closely to find out exactly what's going on. He may start thinking, "Something bad is happening here, and I need to get help," or he may simply intervene with a lot of little things, which resolves the *overall problem*. Either way, he is so busy *doing* that he's unaware that his brain is assessing, correlating, and forming opinions as he goes along.

RULE

Experts use the nursing process in dynamic ways because they quickly assess situations and correlate information in their heads. They know what steps can be safely skipped, combined, or delayed. They also know when situations warrant a rigorous, comprehensive, step-by-step approach. If you're inexperienced, you need to follow the steps more rigidly, carefully reflecting on each step. You take risks when you skip or delay steps.

Interplay of Intuition and Logic

Much has been written about the role of intuition in nursing. This section addresses the question: What roles do *both* intuition (knowing without evidence) and logic (rational thinking that's based on evidence) play in clinical judgment?

Most agree that intuition—an important part of thinking—is often seen in experts, as a result of years of experience and in-depth knowledge of patients. However, there's a concern that encouraging the use of intuition sends the message that it's okay to act on gut feelings without evidence, which is *risky*. To clarify the use of intuition and logic in clinical judgment, it's important to answer two questions:

1. Is the rapid thinking that goes on in experts' heads simply the use of intuition—what many describe as "knowing in your gut"?
2. If you can't explain your thinking, does it mean that you're thinking intuitively?

To the outsider, many experts' actions seem to be based on intuition alone. But, as in the example of Bob's thinking in the above scenario, this rapid thinking is usually the result of "thinking in pictures"—like watching a video—and using intuition and logic *together*. In experts' minds, there's a dynamic interplay between intuition and logic. Experts make leaps in thinking with intuitive hunches, then almost at the same time draw on logic and past experience to make well-reasoned conclusions.

Experts who juggle several priorities at once often have trouble explaining their thinking at the very moment it's happening. But, if it's really important—for example, if decisions are later challenged in court—they can readily reconstruct the logic of their thinking (and if they can't, they're in trouble). Remember the following rule:

RULE

Intuitive thinking is fostered by two things: (1) In-depth knowledge and experience related to the clinical situations at hand, and (2) deep understanding of the patient's normal patterns, circumstances, needs, and desires.

Clinical judgment requires using your whole brain—both the intuitive-right and logical-left sides. Use intuitive hunches as guides to search for evidence. Use logic to formulate and double-check your thinking, ensuring that your conclusions are based on the best available facts. In important situations, be careful about acting on intuition alone. Ask questions like "Does this make logical sense?" "How do I know I'm right?" "Could this situation actually be counterintuitive?" and "What could go wrong if I act on intuition alone?"

Thinking Things Through

In today's fast-paced world, we must remember the importance of thinking things through and not jumping to conclusions. In fact, this has become such a problem that there's a phrase to describe it: "Ready, fire, aim" (instead of "ready, aim, fire"). This phrase refers to what happens with poor assessment and planning. Critical thinking means not jumping to conclusions or acting on impulse. Time constraints today sometimes push you to make diagnoses before you have all the data. If you're not *sure* of the diagnosis or problem, however, it's best to say something like "there seems to be some issue with (whatever), but we don't know enough yet to completely understand what's going on." Remember that American Nurses Association (ANA) standards support this approach by saying that nurses deal with "diagnoses or *issues*."[25] *Issues* are problems that are still muddy and not clearly defined. Always ask yourself, "How complex is this situation, and have we really thought things through?"

Throughout this book, there are many guides to help you think through complex decisions. In Chapter 5, where we discuss the clinical reasoning skill *Evaluating and Correcting Thinking* (page 210), you will find a summary of questions to apply the nursing process to determine whether the depth and breadth of your thinking is sufficient. In the clinical setting, when faced with complex issues, ask whether there are electronic or print decision-support tools that you can use. These help your "human brain" be focused, organized, and prioritized when thinking complex situation through.

What about Creativity?

Every so often, I'm asked whether using creativity is acceptable in clinical judgment. This question surprised me at first. I wondered, Why not? Then nurses gave me two examples of dangerous or problematic creativity. The first example was of a nurse who was going to administer blood, but found that the blood warmer was broken. She used a "creative" (and dangerous) approach: she heated the blood in the microwave. The other example is that of nurses who continually reinvent the wheel, creating new approaches that aren't really better, or coming up with ideas that aren't practical or user-friendly. Creativity has an important place in clinical nursing. Be sure to use *principle-centered* creativity, and be sure that your ideas are useful to end users.

Don't be happy with the status quo. Think outside the box. Ask questions like "Are there new evidence-based approaches we should be using?" "Is there something creative we can do?" "How can technology help?" "What human resources might be willing to give their time?" and "How can we involve patients and families to get better results?"

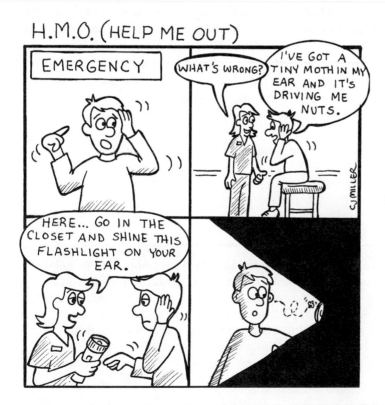

Using principle-centered creativity.

Collecting Versus Analyzing Data

It's important to remember that *collecting and recording information* isn't the same as *analyzing* it. After you *record* the data, you have to do a lot of *analysis* to clarify priority problems and risks. Patients rarely have just *one* problem. They usually have several problems that contribute to one another, requiring you to decide which problems must be dealt with *first*. (Chapter 5 gives detailed instructions and practice for *setting priorities*.)

Is the Care Plan Dead?

As we continue to use standard plans and EHR, some nurses wonder, "Is the care plan dead?" The answer is that the care plan is alive and well—it's just changed. Standards mandate that patients have an individualized recorded plan of care that demonstrates that specific needs and problems are being addressed.

You may not find the care plan all in one place. Rather, parts of the plan may be addressed in different places of the health record (e.g., the nursing assessment may be in one place, routine interventions may be covered in critical paths or protocols and an individual plan covered in another, and so on).

Why Learn Care Planning When We Use Computers?

Just as using a calculator doesn't replace having mathematical and problem-solving principles "in your head," using HIT and EHR doesn't replace the need to have basic principles of nursing process and care planning in your head. You need a deep understanding of these principles to apply them to your daily work at the bedside, to discuss patient care with others, and to determine whether the plan of care is sufficiently documented. The memory-jog **EASE** can help you remember the major care plan components.

Expected outcomes
Actual/potential problems that must be addressed to reach overall outcomes
Specific interventions designed to achieve the outcomes
Evaluation statements (charting/progress notes)

RULE

Gaining a deep understanding of nursing process and care planning principles is crucial to clinical reasoning. Gaining this type of understanding requires strategies that promote deep personal learning. For example, students learn nursing process principles and care planning in a step-by-step way, completing detailed maps and papers. These assignments not only promote deep personal learning, they help develop clinical reasoning skills by forcing learners to "think out loud," explain their reasoning, identify relationships, and apply *principles.*

EXPANDING ROLES RELATED TO DIAGNOSIS AND MANAGEMENT

Nurses now have greater accountability for various aspects of diagnosis and care management. We have moved from "nurses diagnose and treat only nursing diagnoses" to "nurses diagnose and manage various issues and problems, depending on their knowledge, expertise, and qualifications." For example, advanced-practice nurses (APNs) diagnose or manage problems that used to be managed only by physicians (e.g., stable hypertension and common infections).

Growing Responsibilities

Nursing responsibilities for all aspects of care continue to grow, requiring you to a gain strong sense of what nurses *do* in relation to managing medical and nursing problems. Think about the following quotes.

> *"Your doctor's job is to diagnose your medical problem and prescribe the necessary treatment. My job, as your nurse, is to monitor your body's response to treatment, help prevent complications before they begin, keep you comfortable, and help you be as independent as possible."*[26]
>
> *—Phyllis G. Cooper, MN, RN*

> *"The public needs to know that nurses—regular, ordinary bedside nurses, not just nurse practitioners or advanced practice nurses—are constantly participating in the act of medical diagnosis, prescription, and treatment and thus make a real difference in medical outcomes. Nurses can help the public understand that nursing is a package of medical, technical, caring, nursing know-how—that nurses save lives, prevent suffering, and save money. If nurses wear not only their hearts, but also their brains on their sleeves, perhaps the public ... will finally understand what nurses know and do."*[27]
>
> *—Journalist Susan Gordon*

The following blog also gives insight into the complexity of nursing today.

ICU Blog. Last night I took care of a man who was hypoxic and needed oxygen via mask. Most people tolerate masks fine, but there are a few that just can't handle having something on their face. He was one of those few. Even though the nasal prongs were doing the trick, the pulmonologist wanted us to use a mask because "he will probably take a turn for the worse eventually." (Side rant: This is the same pulmonologist who, upon walking onto the unit, said, "Geena, when you have a critically ill patient, wouldn't it be at the forefront of your mind to have the chart available?" I replied, "Dr. B, the very fact that I have a critically ill patient who is hypoxemic and trying to climb out of bed actually explains why I don't have the faintest idea where the chart is.") Anyway, owing to other circumstances, I didn't immediately connect that the patient became severely agitated when we applied the oxygen mask. I had to give him an antipsychotic shot and spent as much time as I could at his bedside to avoid having to restrain his arms (which I correctly assumed would make him worse and wouldn't work anyway ... when another nurse watching him for me went ahead and restrained him, he just bent over and put his face to his hand to take the mask off). I tried to chat with him about other things to help take his mind off the bothersome mask, and he finally stopped struggling against the restraints and lay back on the pillow. After a few moments, he looked at me and asked, "How long have you been working here?"

Continued

"Three years," I replied. "Before that, did you get your bachelor's, or your master's …?" Before I could answer him, he finished, *"IN TORTURE???"*

I'm sure it's not good nursing etiquette, but I laughed quite hard at that—which made him laugh. I eventually decided that the amount of energy he was exerting to remove the mask far outweighed the benefits of it, so I switched him to the nasal prongs again. After a few minutes of low oxygen saturation (O_2 sats) readings, he calmed down considerably and actually drifted off to sleep. His O_2 sats came up perfectly, and the rest of the night was fabulous.

Adapted with permission from www.codeblog.com.

Legal Implications of Diagnosis

As nursing responsibilities continue to grow, remember the following rule.

> **RULE**
>
> **The terms *diagnose* and *diagnosis* have legal implications.** They imply that there's a specific problem that requires management *by a qualified professional*. If you make a diagnosis, it means that you accept accountability for accurately naming and managing it. If you treat a problem or allow a problem to persist without ensuring that the *definitive diagnosis—the most specific, correct diagnosis—has been made*, you may cause harm and be accused of negligence. For example, if you deal with the problem of *chronic constipation* without determining whether the constipation has been evaluated by a physician, you may be missing a *major symptom* of *colon or ovarian cancer*.

Because of the importance of keeping patients safe and remembering the legal implications associated with diagnosis, when treating patient signs and symptoms or starting people on diet or exercise routines, always ask: "Have this patient's signs and symptoms been evaluated by a primary care provider (e.g., medical doctor, advanced practice nurse)?" "Does this diet or exercise routine need approval?" Let the caution to *see your doctor first* resonate in your head.

SCOPE OF PRACTICE AND CLINICAL DECISION-MAKING

With nursing roles and responsibilities constantly growing, how do you know when you are the one who is allowed—who is accountable—for diagnosing and managing specific problems? How do you determine your scope of practice? This question is especially difficult for beginners.

Scope of nursing practice varies from state to state and setting to setting depending on: (1) laws outlined in your state nursing practice act; (2) rules and regulations defined by your state board of nursing (SBN), which is in charge of enforcing the state laws and specifying what nurses may and may not do; and (3) professional standards, policies, procedures, competencies, and job descriptions.[28]

Figure 3-2 (next page) shows the questions you need to answer to make decisions about your scope of nursing practice.

USING STANDARD OR RECOGNIZED TERMS

Many organizations have addressed the need to improve communication and documentation by using standard terms and abbreviations. The ANA supports the use of twelve terminologies that support nursing practice.*

Deciding what terms to use can be a challenge, as terminology development is a lengthy process that is still evolving. Use of terms has shifted from "We use a specific taxonomy of terms" to "We use terms that are best understood by the multidisciplinary health team (terms may be derived from any accepted taxonomy and are usually chosen by experts as documentation systems are developed). Usually, you will use the terms that have the best evidence to support them. For example, you are more likely to use the term *dehydration* than *fluid volume deficit*.

You'll readily learn what terms to use as you work with EHR and standard tools.

RULE

When deciding what terms to use, remember: Use the terms that are required by the school you attend or the place where you work. Also remember that almost all organizations have Do No Use Lists that address abbreviations and acronyms that shouldn't be used because they are error-prone.[29]

UNIQUE NURSING ROLE

Your understanding of the unique role of nurses in health care is key to critical thinking. You'll deal with many aspects of managing health problems. However, as you read through this section, keep the following rule in mind.

RULE

Nurses' unique role is to identify and manage problems or issues related to *human responses* (how health problems influence each person's sense of well-being and ability to function independently as a bio-psychosocial human being).[25]

---

*Download a list of approved terminologies from http://www.nursingworld.org/Terminologies.

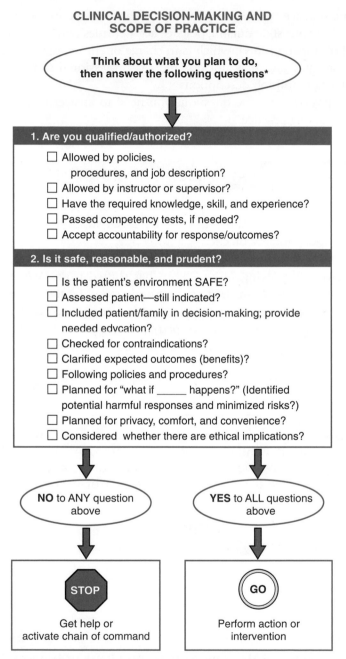

FIGURE 3-2 Clinical decision-making. Source: Alfaro-LeFevre (2011). *Critical thinking tool #1: Scope of practice and clinical decision-making.* Copyright 2011 by R. Alfaro-LeFevre. www. AlfaroTeachSmart.com.

NURSING SURVEILLANCE: MONITORING CLOSELY

As a nurse, you have specific accountability for surveillance—close monitoring of both human responses and medical problems.

For example, suppose that you're caring for Mrs. Hernandez, who has the medical problem of congestive heart failure. Her *response* to the heart problem is *activity intolerance.* As a nurse, you're accountable for monitoring and managing the nursing problem of *activity intolerance.* But you must assess the status of the *cardiac problem* before dealing with the *activity intolerance.* If her vital signs are *unstable,* you're accountable for notifying the physician or APN before dealing with the *activity intolerance.*

You're accountable for detecting signs and symptoms of problems that are within your expertise to manage independently. To gain an understanding of the types of problems and complications that nurses frequently encounter, study Boxes 3-6, 3-7, and 3-8.

With common medical diagnoses and complications, you're accountable for certain aspects of care management. For example, as a nurse, you are *not* qualified to diagnose and treat medical diagnoses independently. But, you *are* accountable for the following aspects of care related to medical diagnoses.

- **Monitoring patients closely to detect and report signs and symptoms that may suggest a medical diagnosis or complication** (e.g., notify the physician if a patient has fever, productive cough, fatigue, and malaise—all symptoms of *pneumonia*)

BOX 3-6   COMMON PRIORITY NURSING PROBLEMS IN ACUTE CARE*

- Risk for infection or infection transmission
- Airway and breathing problems
- Impaired swallowing—risk for aspiration
- Safety risks—fall risks
- Impaired circulation
- Altered mental status—confusion
- Impaired communication
- Pain, nausea, discomfort
- Anxiety, mental stress
- Risk for violence or self-harm
- Poor oral hygiene**
- Risk for pressure ulcer or impaired skin integrity
- Immobility
- Activity intolerance
- Self-care deficits (feeding, bathing, dressing, toileting, activities of daily living)
- Altered nutrition
- Altered bowel elimination
- Altered urinary elimination
- Constipation
- Diarrhea
- Dehydration
- Insomnia—sleep deficits
- Patient education (safety and infection risks, illness, disability management, immobility hazards, health promotion, risk management)
- Medication and other treatment management problems
- Smoking cessation, weight management
- Spiritual distress

*Partial list. Problems are summarized, rather than given specific labels.
**Linked with incidence of pneumonia

BOX 3-7 COMMON MEDICAL PROBLEMS AND THEIR POTENTIAL COMPLICATIONS

Angina/Myocardial Infarction
Dysrhythmias
Congestive heart failure/pulmonary edema
Shock (cardiogenic, hypovolemic)
Infarction, infarction extension
Thrombi/emboli formation (pulmonary emboli, stroke)
Hypoxemia
Electrolyte imbalance
Acid-base imbalance
Pericarditis
Cardiac tamponade
Cardiac arrest
See also Kidney Disease

Lung Diseases (e.g., Asthma, COPD)
Hypoxemia
Acid-base and electrolyte imbalance
Respiratory failure
Infection
See also Pneumonia and Angina/Myocardial
    Infarction

Pneumonia
Respiratory failure
Dehydration
Sepsis/septic shock
Pulmonary embolus
Pulmonary hypertension
See also Angina/Myocardial Infarction

Diabetes
Hypoglycemia (diabetic shock)
Hyperglycemia (diabetic coma)
Compromised circulation—pressure and leg ulcers
Delayed wound healing
Hypertension
Eye problems (retinal hemorrhage)
Infection
Dehydration
See also Angina/Myocardial Infarction and Kidney
    Failure

Hypertension
Stroke (cerebrovascular accident [CVA])
Transient ischemic attacks (TIAs)
Hypertensive crisis
See also Angina/Myocardial Infarction and Kidney
    Failure

Kidney Disease
Congestive heart failure
Kidney failure

Edema
Hyperkalemia
Electrolyte/acid-base imbalance
Anemia
See also Hypertension and Urinary Tract Infection

Urinary Tract Infection (UTI)
Septic shock
Kidney failure

HIV and Immunosuppression
Opportunistic infections (e.g., tuberculosis, herpes,
    intestinal organisms)
Severe diarrhea
See also Lung Diseases and Pneumonia

Fractures
Bleeding (internal or external)
Bone fragment displacement
Edema/pressure points
Compromised circulation
Nerve compression
Compartment syndrome
Thrombus/embolus formation
Infection

Head Trauma
Respiratory depression
Airway occlusion
Aspiration
Bleeding (internal or external)
Shock
Brain swelling
Increased intracranial pressure
Seizures, coma
Hyperthermia/hypothermia
Infection

Other Trauma
See Anesthesia/Surgical Invasive Procedures in
    Box 3-8.

Depression/Psychiatric Disorders
Reality distortion
Dehydration, malnutrition
Suicide
Violence (against self or others)
Self-protection problems
Trauma, death
Medication side effects

BOX 3-8 COMMON COMPLICATIONS RELATED TO TREATMENTS AND INVASIVE PROCEDURES

Anesthesia—Surgical Procedures
Respiratory depression
Airway management problems
Aspiration
Atelectasis, pneumonia
Bleeding (internal or external)
Hypovolemia/shock
Infection/septic shock
Fluid/electrolyte imbalance
Thrombus/embolus
Paralytic ileus
Urinary retention
Incision complications (infection, poor healing, dehiscence/evisceration)
See also Angina/Myocardial Infarction (Box 3-7).

Cardiac Catheterization—Invasive Monitoring
Bleeding (internal or at insertion site)
Hemopneumothorax
Thrombus/embolus formation
Stroke
Infection/sepsis
See also Angina/Myocardial Infarction (Box 3-7).

Chest Tubes—Thoracentesis
Bleeding (internal or at insertion site)
Hemopneumothorax
Atelectasis
Chest tube malfunction/blockage
Infection/sepsis

Foley Catheter
Infection/sepsis
Catheter malfunction/blockage
Bladder spasms

IV Therapy
Bleeding (internal or at insertion site)
Air embolus
Phlebitis/thrombophlebitis
Infiltration/extravasation/tissue necrosis
Fluid overload
Infection/sepsis

Medications
Adverse reactions (allergic response, exaggerated response, side effects)
Drug interactions
Overdose/toxicity

Nasogastric Suction
Electrolyte imbalance
Tube malfunction/blockage
Aspiration
Bleeding

Paracentesis
Bleeding (internal or at insertion site)
Paralytic ileus
Infection/sepsis

Skeletal Traction/Casts
See fractures (Box 3-7)

Source: Copyright 2011. www.AlfaroTeachSmart.com.

- **Ensuring that medical problems are monitored and treated** according to the treatment plan (e.g., with *pneumonia*, monitor lung sounds, oxygen administration, IV management, and vital signs).
- **Preventing common complications** by recognizing when your patient is at risk, monitoring closely, and performing preventative nursing interventions (e.g., elderly postoperative patients are at risk for *pneumonia*—a key priority is to monitor respiratory and hydration status and help them cough and breathe deeply)

- **Identifying and managing *human responses* to health problems** (e.g., humans often respond to having pneumonia by experiencing fatigue, lack of appetite, dehydration, and difficulty clearing mucus)
- **Identifying and managing problems with independence** (e.g., if the person with pneumonia lives alone, he or she is likely to need assistance with shopping and preparing meals)
- **Monitoring treatment and medication regimens for adverse reactions,** as well as individualizing the regimens within prescribed parameters. Nurses are very involved in ensuring that overall regimens are as safe, effective, cost-effective, and convenient as possible, considering the age, culture, religion, roles, occupation, and lifestyles of those involved. For example, with *pneumonia*, ask whether prescribed antibiotics are the best available, considering cost, convenience, and results. The shaded section after the following rule gives a memory jog for monitoring medication and treatment regimens.

RULE

Nurses play key roles in monitoring for complications related to medication and treatment regimens. Medication reconciliation—checking to ensure that the patient's medication orders are up-to-date and complete—is the first step to reducing complications.[30]

Use **TACIT** to remember the key things you must monitor when caring for patients on various medication and treatment regimens:

Therapeutic effect—Is there a therapeutic effect?

Allergic or Adverse reactions—Are there allergic or adverse reaction signs?

Contraindications—Are there contraindications to giving this drug?

Interactions?—Are there possible drug interactions?

Toxicity or overdose—Are there signs of toxicity or overdose?

Activating the Chain of Command

When a patient's status indicates the need for more qualified help, you are responsible for *activating the chain of command*. Activating the chain of command means following communication policies and *staying with the problem* until the appropriate qualified professional has responded. Think about the following example.

Example: Activating the Chain of Command. You give medication for incisional pain, but the patient has no relief. You try repositioning and other holistic measures, but the person still has no relief. You leave two messages for the doctor to call you about this problem. One hour later, you haven't heard from the doctor, and the patient is still in distress. You are accountable for activating the chain of command and notifying your supervisor about this problem and finding out what to do next.

RULE

Using sound clinical judgment means *drawing valid conclusions and acting appropriately* **based on those conclusions** (e.g., monitoring closely, initiating treatment, or contacting a more experienced professional to activate the chain of command).

Monitoring for Dangerous Situations

While preventing errors is addressed in detail in Chapter 6, it's worthwhile to address the importance of monitoring for dangerous situations as part of nursing surveillance. Front-line nurses play an important part in identifying, interrupting, and correcting mistakes. Think about the following, which gives strategies that research shows nurses use to prevent and correct mistakes.

Strategies Nurses Use to Identify, Interrupt, and Correct Errors

- **Error identification strategies:** knowing the patient, knowing the "players," knowing the plan of care, surveillance, knowing policy/procedure, double-checking, using systematic processes, and questioning.
- **Error interruption strategies:** offering help, clarifying, and verbally interrupting.
- **Error correction strategies:** persevering, being physically present, reviewing or confirming the plan of care, offering options, referencing standards or experts, and involving another nurse or physician.

Source: Summarized from Henneman, E., Gawlinski, A, Blank, F., et al. (2010). Strategies used by critical care nurses to identify, interrupt, and correct medical errors. *American Journal of Critical Care*, 19(6), 500-509.

Study Figure 3-3 (next page), which shows how nursing surveillance for dangerous situations can promote early intervention and keep patients safe.

Failure to Rescue

Let's finish this section on surveillance by addressing an issue identified by researchers Clarke and Aiken at the University of Pennsylvania: Failure to Rescue.[31,32] Failure to Rescue is defined as a clinician's inability to save a hospitalized patient's life when he or she experiences a complication (a condition not present on admission).[32] This research, and subsequent work by others, has significantly improved our ability to identify and correct issues related to problems with nursing surveillance. A Google search will give you many articles on this topic, most addressing the need for nurses to identify and manage potential complications. The following articles give excellent information and case examples for failure to rescue.

■ Friese, C., and Aiken, L. (2008). Failure to rescue in the surgical oncology population. *Oncology Nursing Forum*, 35(5), 779-785. Retrieved January 4, 2011, from http://www.medscape.com/viewarticle/583103.

■ McGee, E. (2010). Failure to rescue. Retrieved January 4, 2011, from http://nursing.advanceweb.com/Article/Failure-to-Rescue.aspx.

POTENTIAL DANGEROUS SITUATIONS

TECHNICAL ISSUES

Examples: alarms not working, broken equipment, computer issues

HUMAN ISSUES

Examples: poor attention, knowledge, or skill; fatigue; failure to follow policies and procedures

SYSTEM FAILURE ISSUES

Examples: poor staffing; poor training; room design that makes it difficult for nurses to maintain infection control; poorly designed workflow. Technical and human issues on left may also be the result of system failure issues.

NURSING SURVEILLANCE AND SAFETY NETS: Monitoring for the above dangerous situations; interrupting and correcting error-prone situations; early correction of mistakes.

☐ Early detection, prevention, and correction of errors.
☐ Reporting organizational failure issues.

☐ **No adverse patient outcome (or reduction in severity of adverse patient outcome)**
☐ **Correction of system failure issues—improved organization safety measures**

FIGURE 3-3 Nursing surveillance: monitoring for dangerous situations and keeping patients safe. Source: Copyright 2011 by R. Alfaro-LeFevre. www.AlfaroTeachSmart.com. Recommended: Henneman, E., Gawlinski, A, Blank, F., et al. (2010). Strategies used by critical care nurses to identify, interrupt, and correct medical errors. *American Journal of Critical Care,* 19(6), 500-509.

ADDITIONAL NURSING RESPONSIBILITIES

The following are additional key nursing responsibilities related to managing various health problems. While we have already addressed the importance of safety, infection prevention, and managing risks, this point is placed once again at the top of the following list because it should be foremost in your mind *in all nursing situations.*

- **Promoting safety and preventing infection; detecting and managing risks:** At every patient encounter, you're accountable for keeping patients safe and preventing injury and complications. For example, you must detect, record, and manage patients at risk for falls, skin breakdown, infection, violence, or self-harm. Be vigilant in observing for problems within health care systems that may put patients at risk (e.g., if a new drug is ordered and no one seems to be very informed about it, you would report this to your manager).
- **Monitoring for changes in health status:** Because nurses spend the most time with patients—the ones in the "front line"—they are responsible for detecting signs and symptoms of possible problems requiring medical (or other multidisciplinary) management. For example, in the case of surgery, nurses are accountable for monitoring for signs of potential complications, such as bleeding.
- **Managing emotional and physical discomfort,** through both prescribed and holistic strategies (e.g., managing pain medications, using therapeutic communication, and repositioning patients).
- **Identifying and meeting learning needs:** Nurses must ensure that patients and caregivers have the knowledge and ability to manage their own health; for example, ensuring that parents know how to care for their newborn at home.
- **Promoting optimum health, sense of well-being, and quality of life:** Nurses promote health by teaching about healthy behaviors. They "raise the bar" of care by focusing on *what each individual patient wants to do in life* (e.g., horseback riding may be important to one patient, and sewing may be important to another).

The following is a summary of what you must know about common problems and potential complications.

What You Must Know about Common Health Problems

- What are the signs, symptoms, and risk factors of each problem or complication?
- What is the related pathophysiology?
- What are the common issues with independence and quality of life related to these problems?
- How do you monitor for the status or onset of each problem?
- What interventions are commonly used to prevent and manage each problem?
- What are the common complications of each problem?
- Who is ultimately accountable for developing and recording a plan to monitor, prevent, and manage each problem? (Accountability changes, depending on setting and complexity of the problem.)
- How do you find out what your responsibilities are in relation to each problem?

As you can see, depending on your education, qualifications, and clinical setting, you may be accountable for managing a *variety* of issues. What's most important is that you determine your responsibilities related to risk management, diagnosis, interventions, and outcomes *in each particular clinical setting.*

DEVELOPING CLINICAL JUDGMENT

Developing clinical judgment is one of the most important and challenging aspects of becoming a nurse. It's important because people's lives depend on it. It's challenging because thinking in the clinical setting is often fraught with more anxiety and risks than other situations.

Clinical judgment entails things like knowing how to recognize when a patient's status is changing, and what to do about it. For beginners, this is particularly taxing because it requires an ability to recall facts, put them together into a meaningful whole, and apply the information to a current clinical situation (a situation that is often fluid and changing). For example, you note that someone is pale and sweaty and has a rapid pulse. To use good clinical judgment, you must be able to *recall* that these are symptoms of shock and that an immediate priority is to take a complete set of vital signs to further evaluate the patient's condition.

DECISION-MAKING AND STANDARDS AND GUIDELINES

Critical thinking and clinical reasoning is guided by professional standards. Think about the following descriptions of *standards.*

Standards[33]
- Authoritative statements by which the nursing profession describes the responsibilities for which its practitioners are accountable.
- Reflect the values and priorities of the profession, and provide direction for professional nursing practice and a framework for the evaluation of this practice.
- Define the nursing profession's accountability to the public and the outcomes for which registered nurses are responsible.

National practice standards give broad standards that address how nurses are expected to plan and give care. ANA practice standards apply to all nursing care (see Appendix D). Each specialty organization (e.g., American Association of Critical Care Nurses, Association of Rehabilitation Nurses) develops its own unique standards. The Joint Commission sets many standards for health care organizations. These standards are often tailored to each organization. Each health care organization usually develops standards to guide decision making in specific situations (e.g., standards of care, policies, protocols, procedures, care plans, critical paths).

When determining care management, there are three main questions to answer related to standards:

1. Has this facility developed specific standards, guidelines, or policies for the care of this specific situation? For example, if you're caring for someone with a mastectomy, ask, "Has this facility developed guidelines or pathways for someone undergoing a mastectomy?"

2. Are there national or local evidenced-based practice guidelines relating to this particular problem?

3. To what degree do these standards and guidelines apply to my patient's particular situation?Practice standards and guidelines are crucial tools to help you make care decisions. However, don't follow guidelines blindly. Decide whether they are appropriate by carefully comparing your patient's situation with the information in the guidelines. For example, suppose that you're looking after an elderly man after prostate surgery, and the critical path for this problem states that on the first postoperative day, the patient gets out of bed twice. On the first postoperative day, you assess the man and find he has chest pain. This finding is significant enough for you to question whether he should indeed get out of bed. Could this man be suffering a complication such as myocardial infarction or pulmonary embolus? In this case, it's your responsibility to report the symptoms and keep the man in bed until a physician or more qualified nurse evaluates him.

DELEGATING SAFELY AND EFFECTIVELY

As staffing patterns change, delegation—authorizing someone to perform a selected task in a selected situation, while retaining accountability for results[33]—is an important part of managing time and resources. It's also important for passing the NCLEX®, since the exam tests knowledge of delegation principles. When you delegate tasks, you're accountable for decisions made, actions taken, and patient responses during the course of that delegation). Delegating effectively—a skill that's developed over time with experience—takes significant critical thinking and judgment. It requires you to understand both patients' needs and workers' needs and capabilities. The following section addresses when it's safe to delegate, the four steps of delegation, and the five "rights" of delegation.[34]

When Is It Safe to Delegate?

Delegate When:

- The patient is stable.
- The task is within the worker's job description and capabilities.
- You're able to do the teaching and supervision the worker needs.
- You've planned how to monitor patient results yourself.

Don't Delegate When:

- Complex assessment, thinking, and judgment are required.
- The outcome of the task is unpredictable.

Continued

- There's increased risk of harm (e.g., arterial puncture can cause more severe complications than venous puncture).
- Problem solving and creativity are required.

Four Steps of Delegation

1. **Assess and Plan:** Consider the patient, the task, and worker competencies to make a plan for what tasks you will assign to whom.
2. **Communicate:** Give clear, concise, complete directions about what must done, how it must be done, what needs reporting, and when to touch base with you (verify that worker understands directions).
3. **Ensure Surveillance and Supervision:** Monitor the patient and worker performance as frequently as needed based on the above.
4. **Evaluate and Give Feedback:** Evaluate the effectiveness of the delegation by assessing patient response yourself. Decide whether you need to make changes in the patient's plan of care or how the worker is completing the task. Evaluate the worker's performance, and give teaching and feedback as needed (this helps the worker improve skills and ultimately frees you for other important work).

Five "Rights" of Delegation

Delegate: (1) the *right task*, (2) in the *right situation*, (3) to the *right worker*, (4) with the *right direction and communication*, and (5) the *right teaching, supervision, and evaluation*.

RULE

You are accountable for the outcomes of your decision to delegate. When you delegate tasks, teach and supervise as needed. Follow up after tasks are done by *assessing patient responses yourself.* This does two things: (1) you have firsthand knowledge of how the patient responded to care, and (2) when workers know that you check results *directly with the patient,* they're more likely to do a good job.

---

10 STRATEGIES FOR DEVELOPING CLINICAL JUDGMENT

Developing clinical judgment comes with *clinical experience.* It requires a commitment to study common health problems, seek out clinical experiences, and come prepared to the clinical setting. The following strategies help you plan ahead and make the most of clinical learning opportunities.

1. **Keep references—texts, handheld computers, pocket guides, and personal "cheat sheets"—handy,** and be sure that you:

- **Learn terminology and concepts.** If you encounter words like *embolus, thrombus,* or *phlebitis* and you don't know what they mean, look them up as you encounter them, so that they become part of your long-term memory. Learning terms *in context* helps your brain to store information in related groups, rather than as isolated facts.
- **Become familiar with normal findings** (e.g., normal lab values, assessment findings, disease progression, growth and development) before being concerned with abnormal findings. Once you know what's normal, you'll readily recognize when you encounter information that's *outside the norm* (abnormal).
- **Ask why?** Find out why normal and abnormal findings occur (e.g., Why is there edema in heart failure, yet none when the heart is functioning normally?)
- **Learn problem-specific facts.** You need to know how problems usually present themselves (their signs and symptoms), what usually causes them, and how they're managed. The following gives questions you need to answer to be prepared for going to the clinical setting:

QUESTIONS TO ANSWER BEFORE GOING TO THE CLINICAL AREA
- What common problems are seen in this particular setting?
- What are the signs and symptoms of these problems?
- What risk factors do I know or suspect patients in this setting have?
- What do I assess to determine the status of these signs, symptoms, and risk factors?
- What are the usual causes of these problems?
- What do I assess to determine the status of the causes of the problems?
- How do these problems usually progress, and how are they managed?
- How can these problems be prevented?
- What are the signs and symptoms of potential complications of these problems, and how will I monitor for them?
- How can I be prepared to manage potential complications?
- What medications and treatments are likely to be used, and why?
- What medication-related or treatment-related problems might I encounter, how will I monitor to detect them, and how are they usually managed?
- What population-based factors (e.g., age group, lifestyle, culture, beliefs, language needs) might have bearing on health practices related to these health problems?
- What are the key things people need to know to manage these problems independently, and what will I do to ensure that this knowledge is gained?

2. **Apply principles of the nursing process.** For example, assess before acting, anticipate, and change approaches as needed. Make judgments based on evidence rather than guesswork.

RULE

Always consider your *direct assessment* of the patient to be the *primary source* of information (e.g., if someone tells you a patient has pain, assess the pain *yourself* before giving a medication). **Always ask yourself whether your patient's signs and symptoms could be related to medical problems, medication problems, or possible allergies.** Use the memory jog "MMA" to remember "medication problems, medical problems, allergies."

- Ask your mentor, teacher, or manager whether there are printed or electronic standard tools to guide thinking and documentation in various situations. You'll find *comprehensive assessment tools* and *focused assessment tools.* Comprehensive tools are usually used for patient admissions (see Appendix E). Focus assessment tools are usually used to monitor a specific problem (see example on page 172).
- Be sure you understand the reasoning behind the tools you use. Finding out *why* you collect each piece of data on the tool helps you learn what's *relevant* to each situation.
- Don't just record the data. Reflect on what you recorded, looking for patterns and omissions.
- Realize that the tool you use affects how you think about the data. For example, Box 3-9 shows *Gordon's Functional Health Patterns*, a framework that's often used to organize data to identify problems with *human functioning*. Figure 3-4 shows the *Body Systems* approach to collecting data, which helps identify medical problems. Realize that using both ways of organizing data—*Functional Health Patterns* and *Body Systems*—helps you to identify nursing problems (e.g., human responses or problems with independence and well-being) and signs and symptoms of medical issues that should be reported to the primary care provider.

3. **Learn to think ahead, think-in-action, and think back** (reflect on your thinking).
4. **Follow policies, procedures, and standards of care carefully, with a good understanding of the reasons behind them.** Policies, procedures, and standards of care are designed to help you use good judgment, but you must know the *reasons behind them* to know when and how they apply.
5. **Determine a system that helps you make decisions about what must be done now and what can wait until later** (see *Setting Priorities* in Chapter 5).
6. **Never perform actions (interventions) if you don't know why** they're indicated, why they work (the rationale), and what the risks of harm are in the context of the current patient situation.
7. **Learn from human resources** (e.g., educators, preceptors, classmates, other nurses). When in doubt, activate the chain of command—get help from a qualified

BOX 3-9 GORDON'S FUNCTIONAL HEALTH PATTERNS

1. **Health perception–health management pattern:** Perception of health and well-being; knowledge of and adherence to health promotion regimens
2. **Nutritional-metabolic pattern:** Usual food and fluid intake; height, weight, age
3. **Elimination pattern:** Usual bowel and bladder elimination patterns
4. **Activity-exercise pattern:** Usual activity and exercise tolerance
5. **Sleep-rest pattern:** Usual hours' sleep and rest.
6. **Cognitive-perception pattern:** Ability to use all senses to perceive environment; usual way of perceiving environment
7. **Self-perception or self-concept pattern:** Perception of capabilities and self-worth
8. **Role-relationship pattern:** Usual responsibilities and ways of relating to others
9. **Sexuality-reproductive pattern:** Knowledge and perception of sex and reproduction
10. **Coping-stress tolerance pattern:** Ability to manage and tolerate stress
11. **Value-belief pattern:** Values, beliefs, and goals in life; spiritual practices

Source: Summarized from Gordon, M. (2010). *Manual of nursing diagnosis* (12th ed.). Sudbury, MA: Jones & Bartlett.

BODY SYSTEMS ASSESSMENT

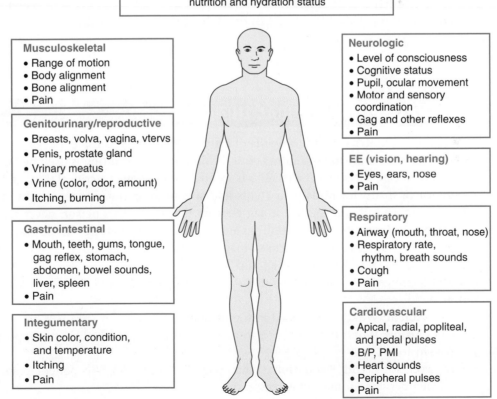

General appearance, age, height, weight, allergies, current medications, medical problems and treatments, nutrition and hydration status

Musculoskeletal
- Range of motion
- Body alignment
- Bone alignment
- Pain

Genitourinary/reproductive
- Breasts, volva, vagina, vtervs
- Penis, prostate gland
- Vrinary meatus
- Vrine (color, odor, amount)
- Itching, burning

Gastrointestinal
- Mouth, teeth, gums, tongue, gag reflex, stomach, abdomen, bowel sounds, liver, spleen
- Pain

Integumentary
- Skin color, condition, and temperature
- Itching
- Pain

Neurologic
- Level of consciousness
- Cognitive status
- Pupil, ocular movement
- Motor and sensory coordination
- Gag and other reflexes
- Pain

EE (vision, hearing)
- Eyes, ears, nose
- Pain

Respiratory
- Airway (mouth, throat, nose)
- Respiratory rate, rhythm, breath sounds
- Cough
- Pain

Cardiovascular
- Apical, radial, popliteal, and pedal pulses
- B/P, PMI
- Heart sounds
- Peripheral pulses
- Pain

FIGURE 3-4 Body systems assessment. To prioritize, go clockwise, starting at "12 o'clock."

professional. Your patients' right to timely care takes precedence over your need to learn independently. Other professionals can help you decide whether you have time to look up your concerns in a reference. Also learn from your peers' experiences. Collaborating with classmates is a win-win situation: Asking questions like "What did you look for in that patient?" "How did you know?" and "What was the biggest thing you learned?" helps your classmates clarify their knowledge and helps you learn from being involved in real situations. However, don't use names or talk about patients in public places where others might overhear (e.g., cafeteria, elevators)—you may be violating HIPAA privacy laws.

8. **Seek out simulated experiences.** Become familiar with the technology you'll use (e.g., IV pumps, computers, heart monitors) and the types of problems you'll encounter before you go to the clinical setting.

9. **Remember the importance of caring.** Patients describe caring as *vigilance* (attentiveness, highly skilled practice, basic care, nurturing, and going the extra mile); *mutuality* (building relationships among nurses, patients, and families); and *healing* (lifesaving behaviors and freeing the patient from anxiety and concerns).

10. **When planning time for nursing care**, consider the time required for (a) direct care interventions (things you do directly for or with the patient, such as helping someone walk), and (b) indirect care interventions (things you do away from the patient, such as consulting with the pharmacist or analyzing lab study results).

CHARTING THAT SHOWS CRITICAL THINKING

Let's end this chapter with a few words of caution: Whether you use paper or electronic charting, be sure your charting shows critical thinking. Your charting is used by others to make patient care decisions. It also reflects whether or not you're a critical thinker. If your supervisor or instructor reads your charts and sees nothing but rote repetition of what the person ahead of you charted, a flag goes up that says, "This person never seems to have an original thought." Follow policies and procedures for charting—these may include using a system of flowcharts and check marks—but always ask yourself whether there is something *different* today that you should add.

Make sure your charting reflects use of the nursing process and a strong focus on the following:

1. **Assessment:** What you assessed in the patient
2. **Conclusion:** What you concluded about your patient—state the facts to support your conclusions
3. **Interventions and Evaluation:** What you did, and how the patient responded (remember: assess, intervene, reassess)
4. **Safety Measures:** Anything you did to correct or prevent adverse responses

Example: Rates incisional pain at 7. Dressing clean and dry. Vital signs normal. Appears stable. Pain med given. Bedrails raised. Call bell given and told to call for help if needed. Reassessed 30 min later and rates pain at 2.

RULE

Timely charting not only improves accuracy, it helps you to pick up patient problems, and recognize things you forgot to do. Chart *as soon as you can.* If you can't get to the chart or computer right away, jot important data down on a personal worksheet. *Think* about what you record. When using computers, don't just dump data in—find ways to *reflect* on your charting and patient care (using printouts or summary screens).

CRITICAL MOMENTS

REFLECTING ON THINKING IMPROVES PERFORMANCE

Learning how to reflect your thinking in an objective, honest way is one of the most powerful tools you have to improve clinical reasoning. When you deconstruct your thinking—reflect on it and break it down into what was going on in your head at certain points in time—you can identify "pieces of thinking" that you're doing well and "pieces" you need to correct. You can also identify system things that need correcting. For example, one nurse deconstructed her thinking like this: "I came to work very tired because I had been up with a sick child. We were very busy and I was handling several priorities. The computer froze again and I had to deal with that. I totally know our protocols and time frames for this problem, but I simply couldn't get the patient to x-ray within the one-hour time frame. I probably should have gotten help. The thing that bothers me the most though, is that I made some assumptions that I shouldn't have. I know we all make assumptions, but I'll assess more carefully next time, even when it seems to be a straight-forward problem."

COMPUTERS BELIEVE WHAT YOU TELL THEM

Have you heard anyone say *you have to tell the computer that ...?* While we have some safeguards in place that prevent you from entering totally incorrect information, don't let your brain slip into neutral simply because you're entering data into a computer. You need an active mind that considers both the data and the patient's circumstances to make sure the computer does what you mean for it to do.

STANDARD TOOLS IMPROVE HUMAN PERFORMANCE

To grasp the importance of helping our brains to remember by using computers and standard tools, answer this question: The next time you're on an airplane, do you want the pilot to rely on his or her memory to check that "all systems are go"? Do you want him to use his own tool? Or, do you want him to use a tool designed by the Federal Aviation Administration (FAA)? Consider this in relation to thinking in the clinical setting.

ELDERLY AND CHRONICALLY ILL: DON'T ASSUME

When dealing with elderly and chronically ill clients, be especially careful of the human tendency to make assumptions. The complexity of their health status often hides problems that might otherwise be quite obvious. For example, we had a 70-year-old man with chronic back pain. He complained of increasing pain for weeks before someone said, "Maybe it's not his back. Has anyone checked his kidneys?" Only then were kidney stones diagnosed. Getting results requires you to examine alternative explanations, problems, or solutions. The more alternative solutions, explanations, and problems you consider, the more likely it is that you're thinking critically.

"NO PAIN, NO GAIN" CAN DAMAGE

While the "No pain, no gain" rule may be true during physical therapy, it can backfire on you. For example, I started lifting weights to strengthen my arm muscles. I began to have shoulder pain and told myself to "work through the pain." The result was a damaged shoulder joint. Never work through pain (or allow a patient to do it) without checking with a doctor or physical therapist.

CRITICAL PATHWAYS: NOT LIKE OZ

Critical pathways, protocols, and other standard plans aren't meant to be like the yellow brick road in the land of Oz, which allowed Dorothy to find the wizard without much thought. Use critical pathways as maps, carefully considering how they apply to your particular patient situation. Think about this analogy: Imagine you're driving down the road, and you come to a temporary roadblock. Even though the map says you have to go straight, you clearly have to figure out another way. Whether talking about care maps or road maps, you are the one who has to "assess the actual road conditions, change speed, and make detours" as needed. When using standard plans, don't be a task-oriented thinker. Think about the difference between the approaches at the top of the next page:

Task-Oriented Thinking: "I have a critical path for this patient's problem. This will be easy and straightforward because I already know what the problems are going to be."

Critical Thinking: "I'm familiar with the critical path for my patient's problem. I wonder how he's doing in relation to the predicted care on the path."

OTHER PERSPECTIVES

CARING NO SUBSTITUTE FOR COMPETENCE

"Compassion is no substitute for competence. In superficial, short-term medical encounters, a smiling face and a gentle hand impress. In the long term, it's competence that you begin to value. You find that kindness is a relatively abundant commodity. It's confidence, borne of knowing, that's too often in short supply. Does this mean I found myself disinterested in compassion? Not at all. But I also found it didn't count for much unless it was bundled with competence."[35]

—*Daniel Beckman, parent of an acutely ill child*

WHAT GOOD NURSING LOOKS LIKE

When my father almost died, he had a seamless hospital experience, marked by a world-class nursing staff that was ranked as Magnet by the American Nurses Credentialing Center. Throughout a long weekend the nurses kept my family involved with Dad's progress through flexible visiting hours, countless phone calls, and e-mails—even in the middle of the night. And my family of lawyers, physicians and nurses can be fussy.[36]

—*Robert Hess, RN, PhD, FAAN, Founder of* Forum for Shared Governance
(info@sharedgovernance.org)

CRITICAL THINKING: A SIXTH SENSE?

"Critical thinking is a 'sixth sense' that's developed over time from an accumulation of years of knowledge and experience—both personal and what you've learned from others. When you do a job for years, you learn what to look for and what to do. In almost a split second, you evaluate what you see, correlate it with what you've learned, and take appropriate action."

—*Doris Alfaro, SRN, class of 1944, Chesterfield Royal Hospital*

HOW NOVICES AND EXPERTS DIFFER

"The main difference between expert clinicians and students is that experts generate better hypotheses (from the beginning, they have better hunches about what the problems may be)."[37]

—*Dr. Geoffrey Norman*

HOW TO KEEP PATIENTS SAFE

There is something to be said for reporting system issues and organizational failure. This includes alarms not working, broken equipment, incompetent colleagues (knowledge or skill deficit). I think individual accountability by the nurse is also key ... what are YOU the staff nurse doing to keep the patient safe? What about monitoring the patient? Keeping patients safe involves always following standard procedures (keeping the alarms on, washing those hands and other infection control activities) and identifying patient needs accurately and doing something about them (implementing falls precautions or measures to prevent pressure ulcers). Also identifying complications or problems the patient may be having and intervening appropriately to avoid failure to rescue situations.[38]

—*Nancy Konzelmann, MS, RN-BC, CPHQ, Nursing
Professional Development Specialist*

DELEGATING: LET GO OF GUILT AND MICROMANAGEMENT

"As a novice delegator, I was often unable to let go of tasks. Therefore, I micromanaged, duplicated duties and did not plan ahead. In this new leadership role I lacked the skills necessary to effectively guide patient care, accomplish goals and lead staff. One of my first struggles as a delegator was a terrible sense of guilt I felt when it came to delegating to CNAs. I identified with the difficulty of their job, feared being disliked and was very insecure. This caused me to take back delegated tasks and undermine my own leadership capabilities."[39]

USING INTUITION AND LOGIC: DO A LITTLE DANCE

"I use both intuition and logic. I'm told I 'do a dance' when my gut tells me something's wrong with my patient but I'm not sure what. First, I get quiet. Second, I gather all my information—the progress notes, medication record, etc. I take more vital signs. Then, I sort of pace back and forth, thinking about what's going on. I reassess the patient and review the trends for the day. I check lab results, urine output, etc. Then, when I 'get it,' I get verbal again. I page the doctor or consult a more experienced nurse. My group calls it my 'intuitive dance.' Once I get the hunch something's up, I keep going until it makes sense."[40]

—*Elizabeth E. Hand, MS, CCRN*

DEALING WITH HIPAA PRIVACY LAWS

"Maintaining patient privacy is important. But, sometimes patients' families need information before it's officially released. In this case, I use my judgment and say something like, 'Because of privacy laws, I can't tell you what's going on with your family member. I can tell you what typically happens in situations like this is, but I can't be sure that this is what will happen now.'"[41]

—*Matthew Riley*

DECISION MAKING: A LEARNED SKILL

Nurses aren't born good decision makers. They develop their skills through constant reflection on their practice. One thing you can do to develop your skills is to ask yourself, What could happen next? or What if _____ happens? Thinking ahead helps you consider solutions in advance. This 'what if' mentality is a characteristic of expert decision-makers."[42]

—*Bernie Garrett, Author of* Student Nurses' Perceptions of Clinical Decision-Making in Their Final Year of Adult Nursing Studies[43]

GETTING LEARNERS AND MENTORS ON THE SAME PAGE

"Paying attention to personality and learning style differences, and getting 'on the same page' about what behaviors promote critical thinking is key to mentor-learner success. For example, when mentors and learners use CTIs in the form of a checklist, they have a 'language' to talk about critical thinking. They can reflect on the ideal behaviors, compare them with current status, and develop a plan to improve."[44]

—*Kathie Kulikowski, MSN, RN, BC*

THANK GOD I'M A NURSE

"I thank God for every day that I was a nurse because I had so many wonderful experiences and learned so much."

—*Actress Bonnie Hunt, as heard on television*

MISCOMMUNICATION

Overheard in the emergency department: "Why do you think you passed out?" "Because when I woke up I was on the floor."

Critical Thinking Exercises

Example responses are on pages 268 to 269.

1. Explain the how the situations in *a* and *b* relate to *novice* and *expert thinking* as described in this chapter.
   a. Compare how your brain thinks when encountering familiar situations with what happens when you encounter unfamiliar situations: For

example, think of the difference between what you see and understand the minute you walk into your own home, compared to what it's like when you are a first-time visitor in someone's home.

b. Think about the following analogy: When you go to a new clinical setting or have a patient for the first time, it's like watching a movie for the first time. Each time you see the same movie over and over, you understand it better and see new things. The same thing happens when you are familiar with patients, staff, and routines in a particular clinical setting.

c. What are some things you can do to increase your ability to function in unfamiliar situations?

2. Using the clinical decision guide on page 102, decide whether you're allowed to irrigate a nasogastric tube in the clinical setting where you are currently working.

3. An important aspect of developing clinical judgment is being willing to focus on wants and needs of patients and families. Keeping this in mind, how would you interpret the statements made by the off-going nurse below?

On-coming nurse: "How is the family doing?"

Off-going nurse: "They seem to be fine. They don't say much, but they're sticking to visiting hours and have been here 15 minutes this morning and 15 minutes this afternoon."

4. How do you use the memory jogs MMA and EASE?

5. Imagine that you have a postoperative patient whose blood pressure is alarmingly high. You call the doctor twice, but there is no response. How will you know what to do to activate the chain of command?

6. Suppose your neighbor asks you whether it's okay to give an aspirin to her normally healthy 5-year-old who is alert, but has a fever of 100° F, orally. Apply the 10 critical thinking questions on the inside back cover to this situation, and decide how you will respond.

 Think, Pair, Share

1. Discuss the following in relation to the blog on page 99.
   a. Risks of applying restraints
   b. Independent thinking on the part of the nurse
   c. The value of the human relationship between the nurse and the patient
   d. The many things that influence hypoxia

2. Take the stress scale test at www.teachhealth.com. Identify the stressful things in your life. How are you handling them? What healthy behaviors might help?

3. Control over practice means being "allowed" to exercise nursing judgment for patient care is a key factor in patient outcomes. Learn the main issues

by reading Hess, R. *From bedside to boardroom—Nursing shared governance: definition and history: Who's the Boss?* Retrieved January 7, 2011, from http://www.medscape.com/viewarticle/490757_2.

4. Discuss the implications of what's new in *Medication Reconciliation*. Read the Patient Safety Primer at http://www.psnet.ahrq.gov/primer.aspx?primerID=1#extra.

5. Address some of the issues raised in Chizek, M. (2010). Documentation: Getting it right. Retrieved January 7, 2011, from http://nursing.advanceweb.com/Continuing-Education/CE-Articles/Documentation-Getting-It-Right.aspx.

6. Share your thoughts on *Advancing effective communication, cultural competence and patient- and family-centered care: A road map for hospitals* (available at http://www.jointcommission.org/assets/1/6/ARoadmapforHospitalsfinalversion727.pdf.

7. Discuss the challenges of delegating effectively as addressed in the following document: ANA and NCSBN (2006). Joint Statement on Delegation, Retrieved January 7, 2011, from https://www.ncsbn.org/Joint_statement.pdf.

8. Discuss the implications of the *Critical Moments* and *Other Perspectives* in this chapter.

9. Decide where you stand in relation to achieving the outcomes on pages 67 to 68.

KEY POINTS/SUMMARY

- Figure 3-1 (page 74) maps key features of critical thinking that are integrated throughout this book.
- The applied definition of critical thinking, clinical reasoning, and clinical judgment on page 70 gives key information on thinking in the clinical setting.
- Problem-solving skills are crucial to critical thinking—but critical thinking requires more than problem solving. It requires creativity, risk management skills, and constantly striving to improve.
- Being familiar with CTIs—short descriptions of behaviors that demonstrate the knowledge, characteristics, and skills that promote critical thinking—is central to learning to think critically.
- The 4-circle CT model on the inside *front* cover helps you assess your ability to think critically and target areas to develop.
- The questions on the inside *back* cover can be used as a guide to critical thinking.
- Pages 75 to 77 address how novice thinking differs from expert thinking.
- IOM and QSEN competencies require nurses to be able to provide patient-centered care, work in interdisciplinary teams, employ evidence-based practice, apply quality improvement methods, and use informatics.

- The concept of *stewardship* stresses that your job is to protect patients and *empower them* to navigate safely through the health care system.
- Care has shifted from a *diagnose and treat* (DT) approach—which implies that we wait for evidence of problems to start treatment—to a *predict, prevent, manage and promote* (PPMP) approach, which focuses on early detection and treatment.
- Nursing surveillance—monitoring patient status and paying attention to dangerous situations—is a key nursing role today. A clinician's inability to save a hospitalized patient's life when he or she experiences complications is called Failure to Rescue.
- *Disease and disability management* is a model of care that focuses on keeping those with chronic diseases as healthy as possible by managing risks and illnesses, even when symptoms aren't obvious (e.g., determining whether an asthmatic who has no asthma attacks is on the best prevention regimen with the lowest side effects).
- From professional and economic perspectives, the care we give must be driven by the best available evidence.
- Page 89 explains the importance of looking at clinical, functional, and other outcomes.
- Outcome-focused thinking requires fixing problems in ways that you get the *best results*, from cost, time, and patient satisfaction perspectives.
- Understanding nursing process *principles* is the key to learning other CT models and also to think your way through NCLEX and other certification tests.
- Pages 92 to 94 summarize the phases of the nursing process, a tool that the ANA states serves as a CT model to give competent care.
- Experts use the nursing process in dynamic ways because they quickly assess situations and correlate information in their heads.

Novices need to learn nursing process principles through deep personal learning (doing detailed maps and papers).
- *Ready, fire, aim* is a phrase that describes the risks of working in today's fast-paced world—critical thinking means not jumping to conclusions or acting on impulse.
- Intuitive thinking is fostered by (1) in-depth knowledge and experience related to the clinical situations at hand, and (2) deep understanding of the patient's normal patterns, circumstances, needs, and desires.
- Use intuitive hunches to search for evidence. Use logic to formulate and double-check your thinking.
- Remember three things about electronic and printed tools: (1) Recording data *in a standard way* reduces omission errors and promotes safety, consistency, and efficiency. (2) Tools must be designed for specific purposes: One size doesn't fit all. (3) Tools don't *think* for you—*you* are accountable for making independent judgments.
- While standards mandate that patients have individualized plans of care, care plans may not be all in one place. Use the memory-jog **EASE** (page 98) to remember the major care plan components.
- Using sound clinical judgment means *drawing valid conclusions* and *acting appropriately* on those conclusions (e.g., monitor closely, begin independent treatment, or activate the chain of command).
- National practice standards provide broad standards that address how nurses are expected to plan and give care. The facility where you work has detailed standards, policies, and procedures—become familiar with them.
- Knowing how to delegate effectively (page 111) is an important part of managing time and resources. It's also important for passing

the NCLEX® exam. You're accountable for the outcomes of your decision to delegate. After you delegate a task, follow up *with your direct assessment* of the patient.

- Developing clinical judgment comes with *clinical experience*. It requires a commitment to study common health problems, seek out clinical experiences, and come prepared to the clinical setting.
- Thinking ahead, thinking-in-action, and thinking back (reflecting on thinking) are important parts of using sound clinical judgment.

- Documentation tools influence how you *think* about data. *Gordon's Functional Health Patterns* (p. 115) *is* a framework that's often used to organize data to identify problems with *human functioning*. Page 115 shows the *Body Systems* approach to organizing data, which helps identify *medical problems*. Using *both* ways of organizing data—*Functional Health Patterns* and *Body Systems*—helps to identify both nursing and medical problems.
- Scan this chapter to review all highlighted rules.

REFERENCES

1. Gallup. Nurses top honesty and ethics list for 11th year. Retrieved January 6, 2011, from: http://www.gallup.com/poll/145043/Nurses-Top-Honesty-Ethics-List-11-Year.aspx.
2. Tanner, C. A. (2006). Thinking like a nurse: A research based model of clinical judgment. *Journal of Nursing Education*, 45(6), 204-211.
3. Hansten, R. (January 2011). E-mail communication.
4. Ignatavicius. D. (January 2011). E-mail communication.
5. Valiga, T. (January 2011). E-mail communication.
6. Elechko, K. (January 2011). E-mail communication.
7. McGuire, M. (January 2011). E-mail communication.
8. Institute of Medicine. (2000). *To err is human: Building a safer health system*. Washington, DC: National Academies Press.
9. Institute of Medicine. (2001). *Crossing the quality chasm: A new health system for the 21st century*. Washington, DC: National Academies Press.
10. Institute of Medicine. (2004). *Keeping patients safe: Transforming the work environment of nurses*. Washington, DC: National Academies Press.
11. Quality and Safety Education for Nurses (QSEN) goal statement. Retrieved January 2, 2011, from www.QSEN.org.
12. The Joint Commission. (2010). 2010 National patient safety goals. Retrieved January 3, 2011, from http://www.jointcommission.org/PatientSafety/NationalPatientSafetyGoals/.
13. Understanding patient safety confidentiality. Retrieved January 2, 2011, from http://www.hhs.gov/ocr/privacy/psa/understanding/index.html.
14. Institute for Patient- and Family-Centered Health Care. (Web page). Retrieved January 6, 2011, from http://www.ipfcc.org/.
15. Prion, S. (January 2011). E-mail communication.

16. Singer, S. (June 6, 2010). Electronic medical records may cause patient care errors, Florida medical board says. The Palm Beach Post. Retrieved January 10, 2011, from www.palmbeachpost.com/news/electronic-medical-records-may-cause-patient-care-errors-729288.html?cxtype=rss_news.

17. Freeman, S. (2010). The challenge of hospital safety: A success story. Retrieved January 3, 2011, from http://www.huffingtonpost.com/seth-freeman/the-challenge-of-hospital_b_651375.html.

18. The North American Thrombosis Forum. (Web page). Retrieved January 3, 2011, from http://www.natfonline.org/.

19. Carpenito-Moyet, L. (2009). *Nursing diagnosis: Application to clinical practice* (13th ed.). Philadelphia: Lippincott Williams & Wilkins.

20. Shever, L., Titler, M., Kerr, P., et al. (2008). The effect of high nursing surveillance on hospital cost. *Journal of Nursing Scholarship*, 40(2), 161-169.

21. Josey King Foundation. (Web page). Retrieved January 6, 2010, from http://www.josieking.org/.

22. Hilton, L. (2007). Nyack Hospital's code H spells safety and satisfaction. Retrieved January 3, 2011, from http://news.nurse.com/apps/pbcs.dll/article?AID=/20071203/NJ02/712030311.

23. Metcalf, R., Scott, S., Ridgway, M., et al. (2008). Rapid response team approach to staff satisfaction. *Orthopaedic Nursing*, 27(5), 266-271.

24. Nurse leadership helps treatment of patients with multiple conditions. (2010). Retrieved January 11, 2011, from http://news.nurse.com/article/20101230/ALL01/101030003/-1/frontpage.

25. American Nurses Association. (2010). *Nursing scope and standards of performance and standards of clinical practice* (2nd ed.). Silver Spring, MD: nursesbooks.org.

26. Cooper, P. G. (2007). Professionalism means clarity about what we do. *Nursing Forum*, 39(1), 3.

27. Gordon, S. (2006). What do nurses really do? *Topics in Advanced Nursing Journal*, 6(1). Retrieved June 1, 2011, from http://www.medscape.com/viewarticle/520714.

28. Chitty, K., & Black, B. (2011). *Professional nursing: Concepts & challenges* (6th ed.). Maryland Heights, MO: Saunders.

29. The Joint Commission. The official "do not use" list of abbreviations. Retrieved January 6, 2011, from http://www.jointcommission.org/Do_Not_Use_List_of_Abbreviations/.

30. AHRQ. (2011). Medication reconciliation. Retrieved January 6 from http://www.psnet.ahrq.gov/primer.aspx?primerID=1#extra.

31. Friese, C., Aiken, L. (2008). Failure to rescue in the surgical oncology population. *Oncology Nursing Forum*, 35(5), 779-785. Retrieved January 4, 2011, from http://www.medscape.com/viewarticle/583103.

32. McGee, E. (2010). Failure to rescue. Retrieved January 4, 2011, from http://nursing.advanceweb.com/Article/Failure-to-Rescue.aspx.

33. American Nurses Association. (Web page). Retrieved January 6, 2011, from http://www.nursingworld.org/MainMenuCategories/ThePracticeofProfessionalNursing/NursingStandards.aspx.

34. American Nurses Association & National Council of State Boards of Nursing. (2006). Joint statement on delegation. Retrieved January 7, 2011, from https://www.ncsbn.org/Joint_statement.pdf.

35. Beckman, D. (1993). Andrew's not-so-excellent adventure. *Healthcare Forum Journal*, May/June, 90-96.

36. Hess, R. (October 2010). E-mail communication.

37. Norman, G. (1988). Problem-solving skills, solving problems and problem-based learning. *Medical Education, 22*(4), 279-286.
38. Konzelmann, N. (January 2011). E-mail communication.
39. Goldwire, R. (2010). Nurse delegation. *Advance for Nurses*. Retrieved January 10, 2011, from http://nursing.advanceweb.com/Features/Articles/Nurse-Delegation.aspx.
40. Hand, E. (January 2011). E-mail communication.
41. Riley, M. (January 2011). E-mail communication.
42. Garrett, B. (January 2007). E-mail communication.
43. Garrett, B. (2005). Student nurses' perceptions of clinical decision-making in their final year of adult nursing studies. *Nurse Education in Practice, 5*(1), 30-39.
44. Kulikowski, K. (January 2011). E-mail communication.

Ethical Reasoning, Evidence-Based Practice, Teaching Others, Teaching Ourselves, and Test-Taking

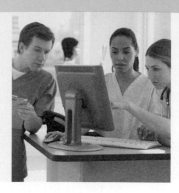

This chapter at a glance ...

Decide where you stand in relation to the following learning outcomes.

Learning Outcomes

After completing this chapter, you should be able to:

1. Develop or adopt a personal code of conduct based on your personal values and content in this chapter.
2. Compare and contrast the terms *moral reasoning* and *ethical reasoning*.
3. Make prudent decisions based on ethical principles, codes, and practice standards.
4. Explain (or map) the relationship between nursing research and evidence-based practice (EBP).
5. Describe your responsibilities for research, EBP, surveillance, and quality improvement (QI).
6. Choose refereed (peer-reviewed) journals and reliable websites to learn more about up-to-date EBP on specific topics.
7. Use critical thinking to create individualized patient teaching plans.
8. Address the roles of memorizing and reasoning in teaching ourselves.
9. Identify strategies that help you learn deeply and efficiently.
10. Describe five strategies that help you improve your test scores and pass the NCLEX® on the first try.

REASONING IN FIVE MAJOR NURSING CONTEXTS

Having examined clinical reasoning and clinical judgment in Chapter 3, let's go on to consider reasoning in five other major nursing contexts: (1) moral and ethical reasoning, (2) research and evidence-based practice, (3) teaching others, (4) teaching ourselves, and (5) test-taking. Learning to think critically in each of these situations is central to your success as a nurse. In the clinical setting, you must be able to reason about ethical issues, apply evidence-based practice, and teach others and yourself. Test-taking skills—your ability to reason your way through tests such as the NCLEX®, competency exams, and advanced certification exams—can make the difference between passing on the first try and having to retake the test or failing completely.

This chapter helps you gain the knowledge and skills you need to succeed in context of all the above situations. Let's start with moral and ethical reasoning, a process that is integral to everyday nursing practice. In this complex, multicultural world, how can you learn to make ethical decisions that are in *your patients' best interests?*

MORAL AND ETHICAL REASONING

Treatment advances, longer life spans, and more emphasis on partnering with patients to improve outcomes continue to create new challenges. Questions related to end-of-life care, genetic advances, quality of life, and the distribution of resources are common. On a daily basis, nurses are involved in many aspects of the ethics of caregiving. Knowing how to reason your way through moral and ethical issues and help your patients do the same is a cornerstone of competent nursing practice.

Clarifying Values

Your values and beliefs affect your thinking at a subconscious level. Unless you spend considerable time getting in touch with your deep personal beliefs—and the implications of these beliefs—you're making "gut," not ethical, decisions. For this reason, *clarifying values* is a major starting point for moral and ethical reasoning.

There are two main ways of looking at values:

■ **Personal values:** These are the beliefs, qualities, and standards that you're passionate about—things you hold "near and dear," for example, your sense of right and wrong. We all have significant emotional investment in our personal values. Yet, it often takes "serious thinking" to get in touch with them. Once you clarify what you believe, why you believe it, and how it affects your ability to be objective in various situations, you improve your ability to deal with moral and ethical issues.

■ **Organizational values:** These are deeply held beliefs within an organization (e.g., a school or hospital). These values are expected to be demonstrated through the day-to-day behaviors of all organizational members. Examples of common organizational values are leadership, collaboration, honesty, integrity, dedication to customer service, and respect for diversity.

Think about what's important to you as a person and nurse. For example, what are your beliefs about how terminal illnesses should be managed, how people should treat one another, and how much autonomy and responsibility students and patients should have? Reflect on the values of your school or hospital. Are they compatible with your own values? Think about where you stand in relation to the following quotes.

> *"An ethic of care respects individual uniqueness, personal relationships, and the dynamic nature of life. Essential to an ethic of care are compassion, collaboration, accountability, and trust."*[1]
>
> **—American Association of Critical Care Nurses**

> *"Everyone has an ethical framework—the question is how aware of it are they? We all need to clarify our ethical frameworks before we're faced with dilemmas. Just as we're too late if we're flipping through our advanced life support book during a code, we can make some regrettable decisions if we haven't given thought to how we'll respond to difficult situations."*[2]
>
> **—Michael Riley, LMSW, LPC, EMT, Paramedic**

Moral Versus Ethical Reasoning

The terms *moral reasoning* and *ethical reasoning* are often used interchangeably. There is, however, a difference between these two terms:

- **Moral reasoning:** Refers to judgments made based *on personal standards of right and wrong* (e.g., I personally believe it's okay to tell little white lies now and then).
- **Ethical reasoning:** Refers to professional judgments made based *on standards derived from the formal study of what criteria should to be used to determine whether actions are justified and therefore ethically right or wrong* (e.g., I personally don't think that there's anything wrong with little white lies, but the ANA's Code of Ethics stresses the importance of being honest and telling the truth).[3]

To better grasp the difference between *moral* and *ethical reasoning*, imagine that you're caring for a woman who is freely and knowledgeably asking for her tubes to be tied to prevent pregnancy. *Morally* (according to your personal standards), you believe sterilization is wrong. However, you know that professional standards and ethics codes stress that people have the right to make their *own choices*, based on their own beliefs. It's *unethical* for you, as a nurse, to tell her that sterilization is wrong.

How Do You Decide?

So how do you make decisions about moral and ethical issues? The answer is: It's not easy. These types of issues are rarely simple. Let's look at how to handle situations that have no clear "right" answers—when each answer has its own merits and drawbacks, and it's hard to say that one is better than another.

Moral and ethical problems may be divided into three categories:

■ **Moral uncertainty:** You aren't sure which moral or ethical principles apply. Example: A patient asks you whether you think his doctor is a good doctor. You don't think the doctor is very competent. Do you tell him?

■ **Moral dilemma:** You're faced with a situation in which you have two (or more) choices available, but neither (or none) of them seems satisfactory. Example: A doctor takes you aside and tells you she's sure your friend Susan has cancer, but she tells Susan, "I won't know anything until the diagnosis is made by the lab next week." When Susan begs you to tell her what the doctor knows, what do you do? If you tell her you don't know, you're lying. If you tell her what the doctor told you, you risk breaking Susan's trust in her doctor.

■ **Moral distress:** You know the right thing to do, but institutional constraints make it nearly impossible to do what is right. Example: You think a patient isn't ready for discharge because his wife is unprepared to care for him. When you report this problem to the physician, you're told the hospital has "no choice" but to discharge him. What do you do?

Did you know what to do in the above examples? If so, on what did you base your decisions? Gut feelings? Personal values? Professional standards? Making moral and ethical decisions requires knowledge of personal values, ethical principles, and codes, as discussed in the next section. As a nurse, you must know the standards and principles that guide moral and ethical reasoning—and be able to justify your actions to others in a professional way.

Seven Ethical Principles

There are seven ethical principles you should apply when making ethical decisions.

1. **Autonomy.** People have the right to self-determination and to make legally acceptable decisions based on (a) their own values and beliefs, (b) adequate information that is given free from coercion, and (c) sound reasoning that considers all the alternatives.
2. **Beneficence.** Aim to benefit others and avoid harm.
3. **Justice.** Treat all people fairly, and give what is due or owed.
4. **Fidelity.** Keep promises, and don't make promises you can't keep.
5. **Veracity (truth telling).** Be honest and tell the truth.
6. **Confidentiality.** Keep information private. This is now law according to Health Insurance Portability and Accountability Act (HIPAA) privacy rules.
7. **Accountability.** Accept responsibility for the consequences of your actions.

Standards, Ethics Codes, and Patients' Rights

Standards, ethics codes, and statements of patients' rights also influence how you conduct yourself as a nurse. For example, the American Nurses Association's (ANA's) *Code of Ethics* stresses that nurses must:[3]

■ **Practice with compassion and respect for each person's dignity, worth, and unique individuality.** This applies to co-workers, families, and patients, regardless of the nature of health problems present, socio-economic status, or culture.

- **Keep your primary commitment to consumers (patients, families, and communities).** It's your responsibility to promote, advocate, and protect the health, safety, privacy, and rights of consumers.
- **Maintain professional relationships.** Although nursing is inherently personal—often requiring a friendly attitude—maintain professional boundaries. You're the professional. The patient isn't your friend.
- **Ensure safe, effective, efficient, ethical care by collaborating with others, seeking professional opinions, and delegating tasks appropriately, when needed.** Involve consumers and care providers to make shared decisions and goals. Recognize when you have an ethical dilemma that requires input from qualified ethicists. Get informed consent from patients involved in research studies.
- **Respect your own worth and dignity.** Maintain a healthy lifestyle. Strive to grow personally and professionally. Broaden your knowledge, and seek out learning experiences. Help advance the profession by contributing to practice, education, administration, and knowledge development (this improves patient care and your own worth and employability).
- **Participate in establishing, maintaining, and improving the health care environment.** Work to ensure that the physical environment and conditions of employment are conducive to providing quality health care.
- **Get involved in professional organizations.** Help clarify nursing values, shape policies, and maintain and improve the integrity of the profession and its practice.

Appendix C (page 283) gives an example of a *patients' bill of rights*. Bills of rights (e.g., a pregnant patient's bill of rights and a nursing home resident's bill of rights) also guide how you respond to ethical issues.[4] Advance Directives (Box 4-1 on the next page) help us make decisions about cardiac resuscitation and other end-of-life treatments.

Steps for Moral and Ethical Reasoning

The following steps help you develop an in-depth approach to moral and ethical reasoning.*

1. **Clearly identify the ethical issues** based on the perspectives of the *main stakeholders*—the people who will be most affected by care (patients and families) or from whom requirements will be drawn (caregivers, insurance companies, third-party payers, health care organizations.) The patient's perspectives should be considered first, but families and caregivers must also be considered. For example, Mrs. Morris, an elderly woman who lives alone, tells you she doesn't want her leg amputated and that she'd rather die than live as an amputee. Mrs. Morris's daughter tells you her mother is incompetent to make this decision. Who has the right to make this decision? Is Mrs. Morris competent? Does she have the right to refuse surgery? Does the daughter have the right to overrule her mother?

---

*The author acknowledges the help of Carol Taylor, RN, PhD, Director, Center for Clinical Bioethics, Georgetown University, Washington, DC.

BOX 4-1   WHAT ARE ADVANCE DIRECTIVES?

Advance directives include two documents*:
1. **Living will:** Designates the types of medical treatments you would or wouldn't want in specific instances (e.g., whether you want to continue ventilator support if you become permanently unconscious).
2. **Durable power of attorney for health care (DPAHC):** Identifies who you want to make treatment decisions if there comes a time when you aren't able to do so for yourself.
   Don't wait too late: Too many people wait until it's too late to address advance directives. Encourage people to talk with loved ones about what they would want if they were unable to speak for themselves. This eases the burden of making tough decisions about whether to refuse aggressive treatment that merely prolongs dying.

---

*These two documents may be combined into one document called a *combination directive*.

2. **Clarify your personal values and how they influence your ability to participate in decision-making.** For example, in Mrs. Morris's case, do you believe that no one has the right to refuse lifesaving surgery? If so, how would this affect your ability to help Mrs. Morris with this decision? If you can't be objective, let your supervisor know so that another caregiver can assist with decision-making.

3. **Decide what your role will be.** Does this family rely heavily on your judgment? Do you just need to listen and help them sort out their thoughts? Who else will be involved in helping make decisions (e.g., chaplain or case manager)?

4. **Determine some possible courses of action (go "out of the box"—think about as many alternatives as you can).** Would it be possible to have the daughter come in to discuss caring for her mother? Could social services help? Should you request an ethics consult?

5. **Determine the outcomes (consequences) of each of the courses of actions you thought about.** For example, what would happen if the daughter is incapable of caring for her mother—what role could the daughter have in this case?

6. **List the courses of action, and rate them according to which choice is most likely to produce an outcome that gives greatest balance of benefits over possible harm.** To do so, don't consider "good" versus "bad." Instead, ask where each choice fits on the following scale.

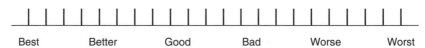

| Best | Better | Good | Bad | Worse | Worst |

7. **Together with the main stakeholders,** develop a plan of action aimed at achieving the best outcomes based on the circumstances.

8. **Put the plan into action, and monitor patient and family responses closely.** Modify the plan if needed. The following are great Internet resources to learn more about moral and ethical reasoning.

ONLINE ETHICS RESOURCES

- American Nurses Association, Center for Ethics and Human Rights: www.nursingworld.org/ethics/
- National Reference Center for Bioethics Literature: http://bioethics.georgetown.edu/
- American Society of Law and Ethics: www.aslme.org
- American Society of Bioethics and Humanities: www.asbh.org
- Nursing Ethics of Canada: www.nursingethics.ca
- Markkula Center for Applied Ethics, Santa Clara University: www.scu.edu/SCU/Centers/Ethics/

OTHER PERSPECTIVES

TWO WOLVES IN EACH OF US

An old Indian told his grandson about a battle that goes on inside people. He said, "My son, there is a battle between two 'wolves' inside all of us. One is *Evil*. It is anger, envy, jealousy, sorrow, regret, greed, arrogance, self-pity, guilt, resentment, inferiority, lies, false pride, superiority, and ego. The other is *Good*. It is joy, peace, love, hope, serenity, humility, kindness, benevolence, empathy, generosity, truth, compassion, and faith." The boy thought about it and then asked his grandfather: "Which wolf wins?" The old Indian replied simply, "The one you feed."

DYING IS HARD WORK

"There's a lot of push and pull on the part of family members, especially the members who haven't been on the spot. They parachute in at the last minute and want everything done…. The revelation to me was that dying is hard work. It can take a long time."

—*Gail Sheehy*

UNHEARD SCREAMS

I was working in a clinic and had to persuade an HIV-positive, pregnant teenager to agree to highly active antiviral therapy (HAART). After taking a deep breath to calm my emotions, I said, "I can't tell you what to do. I can only support your decision. But I can tell you that infants have a much worse time dealing with HIV than adults. Whatever difficulties you have with the virus or the medication, multiply them and think about your baby having them. You must be prepared to deal with the consequences of whatever choice you make." The doctor and I waited for a response. There was none. The young patient snatched the prescriptions and left the room. In that quiet room, I felt that there were silent screams. The patient was screaming her fear. I was screaming my anger. The physician was screaming his frustration. As loud as our screams were, in that little room you couldn't hear a sound.[5]

—*Jacqui Scipio-Bannerman, RNC*

EVIDENCE-BASED PRACTICE

Thanks to informatics and the hard work on the part of committed experts and researchers, care has shifted from approaches based in tradition ("we do it this way because that's the way it's always been done") to evidence-based approaches ("we do it this way because the most current research and evidence shows we get the best outcomes when we do it this way").

This section addresses the interrelated topics of evidence-based practice (EBP), research, and QI. Before we go on with this topic, let's talk about a key skill you'll need to be able to apply EBP: knowing how to access, analyze, and apply information.

Accessing, Analyzing, and Applying Information

Whether you access information from a computer, iPhone, BlackBerry, or a Personal Assistive Device (PDA), knowing how to find and use reliable, relevant information makes the difference between drowning in TMI (too much information) and quickly finding what you need to know. It makes the difference between whether you give care that's unsafe or care that's safe, efficient, and based on the best available knowledge.

How to Access and Use Information Effectively. The following gives key points on learning how to access and use information effectively.

☐ Learn how to use Internet and library resources: indexes, interlibrary loan services, circulation and reference departments, audiovisual services, and electronic databases (recommended search engines and websites are listed in Box 4-2).

☐ Get to know your human resources—introduce yourself to the librarian and informatics nurses. Ask for help if you get stuck. Remember that Internet search engines have "help buttons" to assist you with questions.

☐ Whether you're using printed references or Web-based information, learn how to evaluate the reliability of your resources. The shaded section below summarizes the ABCD approach to evaluating Internet resources. You can also find detailed information on evaluating information resources at the following URLs:

- Evaluating Internet Information: http://guides.library.jhu.edu/evaluatinginformation
- Evaluating Web Sites: Criteria and Tools: http://www.library.cornell.edu/olinuris/ref/research/webeval.html

---

ABCDs of Evaluating Websites and Other Works*

Authority: How well known is the author?

- Is the author a well-regarded name you recognize? What are the author's qualifications?
- Does the document contain an e-mail address?

---

*Adapted from Schrock, K. ABC's of website evaluation. Retrieved January 2, 2011, from http://school.discovery.com/schrockguide/eval.html)

BOX 4-2 RECOMMENDED SEARCH ENGINES AND HEALTH-RELATED WEBSITES*

Agency for Healthcare Research and Quality (AHRQ): www.ahrq.gov
AHRQ Guideline Clearinghouse: http://guidelines.gov/
Cumulative Index to Nursing and Allied Health Literature: www.cinahl.com
Directory of Healthcare Sites: http://www.lib.uiowa.edu/hardin/md
Google Scholar: http://scholar.google.com
Google Health: http://health.google.com
Health on the Net: www.hon.ch
Healthfinder: http://www.healthfinder.gov/
Mayo Clinic: http://www.mayoclinic.com/
Microsoft Health Vault: http://www.healthvault.com
NurseLinx.com: www.NurseLinx.com
MedlinePlus: http://www.medlineplus.gov
Medical videos, images and sounds: http://www.medicalvideos.us/
PubMed: www.ncbi.nlm.nih.gov/entrez/query.fcgi
Canadian Health Network: http://www.canadian-health-network.ca
Health Insite: http://www.healthinsite.gov.au
NHS Direct Online: http://www.nhsdirect.nhs.uk/
See also *Evidence-Based Resources* on pages 149 to 150.

*These are just a few of the many excellent online references.

- Did you link to this site or document from a site you trust?
- Are you led to additional information about the author?
- Are there statements about the review process? (e.g., is there a peer review process?)

Bias: Does the site or document try to *persuade,* rather than *inform?*

- What organization sponsors the site or document? Is the organization reliable?
- Is the page actually an ad disguised as information?

Citations:

- Are full citations given to support the work?
- If so, did you compare the author's content with the content in the citation?

Dates:

- How recent are the dates that are listed?
- Does the information you need demand more current data than is given in the documents you have?
- Is there a seal of approval posted? For example, the Health on the Net Foundation (www.hon.ch/) gives a seal of approval to websites that meet high standards. TRUSTe (http://www.truste.com/) gives a seal that guarantees privacy.
- Whether you use a website or a print reference, use the following strategies:
  1. Always try to verify information with the primary (original) sources. For example, cite this book directly if there's no credit to another reference. But, if I give a citation for a specific sentence or idea, check that citation, since it is the primary (original) source.

2. If you're unsure about the information you have, compare it with at least two other reputable sources on the same topic. Remember, "more than one source, more likely of course."

3. When overwhelmed, ask for help. Nurse educators, pharmacists, librarians, and other professionals can point you in the right direction.

4. Develop information processing skills so that you can focus on what's important and keep data available in a way that helps you access the most important information quickly.

Strategies to Process, Manage, and Remember Information

■ Never read without taking notes—your notes help you process the information so you understand and remember it better. Don't highlight your way through articles—it doesn't help you process, unless you pick out only a few main ideas.

■ Make the information your own by asking yourself questions like, "How well do I understand what's known and what's unknown about this topic?" "What are the relationships between key concepts?" and "What questions does this information raise for me?" Think about what you're reading!

■ Draw maps to identify relationships between key concepts.

■ Revise your notes and maps at least once to force yourself to do more in-depth thinking about what's most important. Organizing and reorganizing information to find new relationships gives you more in-depth understanding and will help you *remember* the content better.

■ Get rid of irrelevant or unimportant information. It clears your mind of clutter.

Relationship of Research to Evidence-Based Practice

To understand the relationship between research and EBP, study the following definitions:*

■ **Research:** A systematic, objective approach to creating new knowledge—or refining current knowledge—by using rigorous data-collection and testing conditions.

■ **EBP:** Care practices that are based on the most current research and clinical expertise. EBP bridges the gap between *scientific evidence* and its *practical use* in the clinical setting. EBP integrates (1) the best research evidence, (2) knowledge from clinical experts, and (3) patient preferences into clinical practice. It aims to give the most consistent and best possible care by creating clinical guidelines that are based on current evidence.

Transforming Knowledge to Evidence-Based Practice

EBP requires that knowledge be transformed by the systematic study of how evidence from research can best be *applied in practice*. Transforming knowledge from research to practice is something you don't do alone. The volume of scientific information is such

---

*Definitions compiled from several resources.

that no one can do it all. You need the collaborative knowledge of a team of experts to interpret the data and decide how it can best be applied to practice.

Clinical Summaries and Practice Alerts

Because reading and critiquing research studies is time-consuming and requires significant expertise, clinical summaries are now a common way to make research more useable.[6] Practice Alerts—important evidence-based information that affects patient care—give cutting-edge, evidence-based information to busy staff nurses. Many nurses receive practice alerts via e-mail, in the form of newsletters. The American Association of Critical Care Nurses articulates the importance of practice alerts in the following way: "Practice alerts are succinct, dynamic directives that are supported by authoritative evidence to ensure excellence in practice and a safe and humane work environment. Practice alerts help nurses and other health-care practitioners carry their bold voices to the bedside to directly impact patient care."[7]

The next section explains the work that goes into transforming knowledge from research into useful clinical information that's integrated into actual care practices.

ACE Star Model of Knowledge Transformation

Figure 4-1 shows the Academic Center for Evidence-Based Practice (ACE) Star Model of Knowledge Transformation. In this model, research evidence moves through the following cycles and then is combined with other knowledge and integrated into practice.[8]

1. **Discovery:** New knowledge is discovered through traditional research and scientific inquiry.

ACE STAR MODEL® OF KNOWLEDGE TRANSFORMATION

FIGURE 4-1 The star shows the process for developing Evidence-Based Practice (EBP)—how evidence from research moves through several cycles (discovery, summary, translation, integration, and evaluation). Reprinted with permission from Stevens, K. R. (2004). *ACE Star Model of EBP: Knowledge transformation.* Academic Center for Evidence-Based Practice. The University of Texas Health Science Center at San Antonio. Retrieved January 2, 2011, from www.acestar.uthscsa.edu.

2. **Evidence Summary:** A single, meaningful statement of the state of the science is developed (this is a complex task that takes a lot of critical thinking on the part of knowledgeable experts).
3. **Translation:** Evidence summaries are translated into practice recommendations and integrated into practice. Recommendations are made in clinical practice guidelines, care standards, clinical pathways, protocols, and algorithms.
4. **Integration:** Individual and organizational practices are changed through formal and informal channels.
5. **Evaluation:** The impact on patient health outcomes, provider and patient satisfaction, efficacy, efficiency, and economic costs is continually examined.

The ACE Star Model helps ensure that care is driven by evidence, rather than tradition: It combines the best of what we know from research with the best of what we know from clinical practice to give current information that's clinically relevant. Box 4-3 addresses how to find the most up-to-date information on clinical practice guidelines and evidenced-based practice.

BOX 4-3 CLINICAL PRACTICE GUIDELINES AND EVIDENCE-BASED PRACTICE*

What are clinical practice guidelines (CPGs)?
CPGs are recommendations for how to manage care in specific diseases, problems, or situations (e.g., how to best manage smoking cessation or neonate umbilical cord care). CPGs are developed for specific use and are designed by a collaborative panel of clinical and scientific experts. When scientific evidence is sufficient, practice guidelines are obvious and clear. When scientific evidence is insufficient, other sources of knowledge—for example, wisdom gained from clinical experts or specific cases—must be brought to bear on the recommendations to fill in the gaps in the research evidence. Evidence summaries and CPGs are the essence of evidence-based practice (EBP). EBP provides mechanisms for fulfilling our social responsibility to provide the best care in the most effective and affordable way. You will find many helpful links and resources at www.acestar.uthscsa.edu/.

What are the best EBP websites for updating practice standards?
For evidence summaries, the two best resources are the Agency for Healthcare Research and Quality (www.ahrq.gov) and the Cochrane Library (www.cochrane.org). For CPGs, the most definitive source is the National Guideline Clearinghouse (http://www.guideline.gov/index.aspx). This a publicly available electronic repository of clinical practice guidelines, easily searchable by topics.

How do you best use the information on these websites?
The AHRQ offers free access to evidence summaries and reports (on its home page, click on Evidence-Based Practice). They also archive CPGs. If you access archived CPGs, use the information only after updating them with the latest research on the topic. The Cochrane Library produces systematic reviews, which give a single statement that summarizes the state of the science and draws on all research on a given topic. A systematic review is the strongest level of evidence for clinical decisions.

---

*Answers to questions provided by Kathleen R. Stevens, RN, EdD, ANEF, FAAN, Director, Academic Center for Evidence-Based Practice (ACE), University of Texas Health Science Center at San Antonio (www.acestar.uthscsa.edu).

Research: All Nurses Play a Part

To give nursing care that's based on the best available knowledge, we must continue to question current practices and develop new knowledge through nursing research. Yet many nurses don't understand the value of research. Often, they feel this way because they had little or no research training, the courses they took were overwhelming, or they don't have enough time and resources.

One way to get excited about research is to start by looking at some of the significant research findings we have gained in recent years. For example, think about the importance of the results from the following studies:

- **Traditionally, we have taught that mouth care must be done for hygiene and to prevent problems in the mouth.** Research shows that poor mouth care can result in microbes colonizing the oropharynx. This colonization is a critical factor in the development of nosocomial (hospital-acquired) pneumonia. We now know that if we don't have evidence-based guidelines for giving oral hygiene, we put patients at risk for deadly *pneumonia*.[9]

- **Nurses are concerned about inadequate registered nurse (RN) staffing.** Research shows that having more RN staff reduces the number of infections, pressure ulcers, falls, and other adverse events such as failure to rescue (deaths after complications). It reduces the length of hospital stays and promotes early detection of complications and patient and nurse satisfaction.[10,11] This type of data is very persuasive when justifying the need to hire more nurses.

- **Restraining patients often creates the very problems we're trying to avoid.**[12] Many assume that restraining patients protects them from injury. On the contrary, we now know that applying restraints increases the incidence of costly, dehumanizing outcomes (e.g., serious injuries, pressure ulcers, depression, anger).

- **Cancer patients who receive palliative care (care that focuses on quality of life) early in their treatment course may live longer than those who receive only standard treatments.** A recent study found that patients who started on palliative care— along with usual cancer care—soon after their lung cancer diagnosis lived nearly three months longer than people given only standard cancer care, even though this second group had more chemotherapy.[13]

Nursing research is a rigorous, disciplined use of critical thinking. Researchers need highly developed critical thinking skills—from knowing how to clearly identify the issue to be studied to determining the best way to collect meaningful data, to analyzing and interpreting statistical data.[14] Although it's beyond the scope of this book to address how to actually *conduct research studies,* this section addresses novice and staff nurses' roles in research and EBP. Let's start by addressing frequently asked questions.

Frequently Asked Questions on Staff Nurses' Role

Q. If I'm a student or staff nurse, what are my responsibilities related to research and EBP?

A. **As a staff nurse, you have five main responsibilities:**

1. **Think analytically about the patients and situations you encounter**—seek out evidence of findings that might improve nursing care. For example, if you

frequently care for people with postoperative leg edema after heart bypass surgery, you should be asking, *I wonder if there are any new studies explaining why this happens and what can be done about it?*

2. **Know the rationale behind your actions and the level of evidence that supports the rationale.** For example, are the rationales behind your actions supported by national clinical practice guidelines? A textbook? Your instructor or another clinical expert?

RULE

There are different forms of evidence that may support clinical practices—from expert opinion to meta-analysis (analysis that combines data from all available studies on a certain topic). Each form is not equally persuasive in making the case that a certain clinical procedure should become a part of recommended care for a specific problem or population. Greater scientific rigor in producing clinical evidence gives stronger evidence for influencing clinical practice. The more important and unchanging the outcomes of care practices are, the greater the need for sound supporting evidence (e.g., care practices for postoperative cardiac patients need supporting evidence that is much stronger than if you were trying to decide the most efficient way to deliver meals to patients on a certain unit).

The following gives an example rating scale for EBP.

EXAMPLE RATING SCALE FOR EBP
- **Level A:** Actions are supported clinical practice guidelines (CPGs). CPGs are designed by a collaborative panel of clinical and scientific experts, and give recommendations for how to manage care in specific diseases, problems, or situations to achieve the best outcomes, from safety, efficiency, satisfaction, and cost perspectives. The most definitive source for CPGs is the National Guideline Clearinghouse (http://www.guideline.gov/index.aspx). CPGs may also come from the AHRQ Evidence-based Practice Centers (http://www.ahrq.gov/clinic/epc/) or from clinical specialty organizations—for example, the American Association of Critical Care Nurses (AACN).
- **Level B:** Actions are supported by a high-quality randomized controlled trial (RCT) that considers all important outcomes.
- **Level C:** Actions are supported by other evidence (e.g., well-designed clinical trials; lower quality RCTs; case-controlled studies with nonbiased selection of study participants and consistent findings; other evidence).
- **Level D:** Actions are supported by consensus viewpoint (agreement among *all* consulted experts) or expert opinion (agreement among *most* consulted experts).

  Find a summary of the systems used to evaluate the strength of evidence at http://www.thecre.com/pdf/ahrq-system-strength.pdf.[15]

3. **Raise questions** that might prompt a researcher to formulate a question to guide a study. For example, you could ask your manager, "Since we seem to be having

an increase in infections, should we study our procedure for hand sanitizing. Is it convenient? Are we applying EBP?"

4. **Help researchers collect data.** If you're asked to complete a questionnaire or to chart specific data for research purposes, it's your professional responsibility to do so, diligently and accurately, as long as it doesn't interfere with nursing care.

5. **Acquire and share knowledge** related to research and EBP. We must constantly ask ourselves questions like "Am I making time to become familiar with EBP related to the clinical situations in which I'm involved?" and "Do I interact with others (peers, educators) to learn more about research and EBP?" If you find reading research articles tedious, get started by talking with peers and educators or perhaps joining a journal club. This helps you to learn in a dynamic, stimulating environment. Once you learn the basics, reading research articles becomes easier, more interesting, and even an enjoyable challenge!

Q. If I have limited knowledge of research, how do I know whether there are results from research studies that I should be using in my practice?

A. As a student or staff nurse, it's important that you ask your leaders and educators for help with finding and using research articles. However, be sure that you understand the following basic facts about choosing useful research articles and information:

1. Choose refereed or peer-reviewed journals (journals that publish articles only after they've been reviewed by peer experts; whether or not a journal is peer-reviewed is usually found in the front of the journal where you find the editorial board, the publisher, and so on).

2. Remember that only a small percentage of the published literature contains evidence that is ready for clinical application. It's estimated that only 1 in 5000 ideas eventually makes it through all of the trials and the research stages to produce evidence with clinical outcomes.[16]

3. Always ask, "How valid and reliable are these results?" "How sure am I that this study was conducted in such a way that I can trust that the results are accurate?" Consider whether there's vested interest on the part of the researchers or publishers. For example, how often have you heard a commercial that proclaims, "In a recent research study, our product was proven to be more effective than the other leading products"? Do you believe every one of these commercials? Probably not. Think independently, and ask questions. To help you with these issues, you can find excellent self-paced tutorials and refreshers on research and EBP at the following URLS:

   □ Beginner's Research Guide—Searching Steps: http://library.nyu.edu/research/subjects/health/tutorial/steps.html

   □ Guide for using online resources: http://library.nyu.edu/research/health/tutorial/

   □ Research Utilization and Evidence-Based Practice; http://library.nyu.edu/research/subjects/health/tutorial/researchutilization.html

   □ Also see URLs in Boxes 4-2 and 4-3 (pages 137 and 140)

Scanning before Reading Research Articles

Knowing how to scan research articles saves you time. You can quickly eliminate irrelevant articles, giving you more time to focus on ones that *are* relevant. Here are some steps to systematically scan articles so you can choose the ones most relevant to your needs.

1. **Read the abstract first:** This summarizes the issues, the methods, and the results. If the abstract isn't applicable to your clinical problem, you might choose to read no further.

2. **If the abstract seems applicable, skip to the end of the article,** and then scan the article by reading the content under the following headings, in the order listed here:
   - Summary (may also be listed as Conclusions)
   - Discussion
   - Nursing Implications
   - Suggestions for Further Research

   You may be able to eliminate articles just by reading the content under any of the above headings.

3. **If what you scanned is relevant, go on to read the entire study.** Give yourself plenty of time, and don't be discouraged if you find sections you don't understand. Instead, take notes on what you do understand. Come back to the more difficult sections at another time, after getting help from an expert or textbook (or both).

4. **After you read the article,** ask yourself whether you understand the following:
   - What's already known about the topic?
   - What did the researchers study, and why and how did they study it?
   - What did they find out, and are the results valid?
   - What do results imply, and how do they apply to my particular clinical situation?
   - Might the study be biased (for example, when drug companies fund a study, there may be a vested interest)?
   - How do the results of the study compare with the results of other, similar studies? (If other studies produced similar findings, the probability that the results are reliable increases.)

QUESTIONING CARE PRACTICES: PROMOTING INQUIRY AND CREATIVITY

Too many nurses continue to do things based on tradition without going "out of the box" and questioning care practices. Don't settle for the status quo. Question what you do, why you do it, what your patients' experiences are, and how patient care and nurses' jobs can be improved. Use the following strategies to promote inquiry and creativity:

- ☐ On a bulletin board, post a blank paper with "What Do You Want to Know?" at the top. For example, someone might write, "Does anyone know the best programs on managing wound infections?"

☐ Make reading research articles convenient. If you find a good article, post it on the bulletin board, and ask people to initial that they've read it. Reward nurses who bring in useful literature.

☐ Encourage nurses to critique practice protocols, and make suggestions for improvement.

☐ Keep a real or virtual suggestion box. On performance evaluations, recognize nurses who raise questions or come up with creative, practical solutions.

☐ Join an Internet listserv where nurses with common interests share questions and information.

SURVEILLANCE AND QUALITY IMPROVEMENT

Most facilities have risk managers and QI nurses who are in charge of surveillance and improving care quality. Surveillance, in the context of QI, is defined as *monitoring patients and systems for the presence of factors that cause delays in treatment or increase the likelihood of illness or harm.*

Frontline nurses are in the unique position of being able to identify overall system problems that affect patient care. They bring important insights into deciding whether care practices are practical, consistent, and timely. For example, in one case, nurses noted that medications were always arriving late from the pharmacy. They did a study that showed that delays in medication administration increased the length of hospital stays. As a result, policies and procedures changed to ensure that medications came to the units in a timely way, ultimately shortening patients' length of stay.

To ensure a comprehensive way of examining how we can improve care practices, QI studies three different aspects of care: outcomes, process, and structure, described in the following shaded section.

Three Approaches to Quality Improvement Studies

1. **Outcomes** evaluation (studies *results*). *Example:* Studying the number of respiratory complications in postoperative patients
2. **Process** evaluation (studies *how* care was given). *Example:* Studying how frequently the respiratory status of patients was assessed and whether care was managed by a registered nurse
3. **Structure** evaluation (studies *the setting* in which care was given). *Example:* Studying the locations of the rooms of patients who had respiratory complications in relation to closeness to the nurses' station

Studying *all three* of these aspects gives you a comprehensive analysis that helps you improve practice. If you only examine outcomes (results), you won't be able to improve efficiency. You could be getting great outcomes, but there may be more efficient, cost-effective ways to achieve them.

The ANA National Center for Nursing Quality (NCNQ®) addresses safety, nursing care quality, and nurses' work lives. The center advocates for nursing quality through quality measurement, innovative research, and collaborative learning. The center tackles issues such as how staffing affects patient outcomes and nurses' job satisfaction.[17]

Your responsibilities related to surveillance and QI are the same as the previously listed responsibilities for research and EBP. You can find ready-to-use tools for measuring and improving the quality of health care by entering "Quality Improvement Tools" in the search box at http://www.ahrq.gov/.

CRITICAL MOMENTS

SUPPORTING A SPIRIT OF INQUIRY

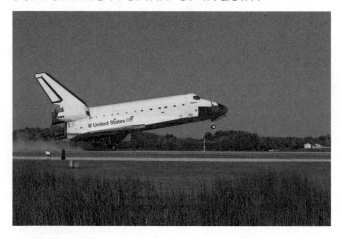

Source: NASA Images Gallery, www.nasa.gov.

Being curious and inquisitive is a hallmark of critical thinking. Inquisitive researchers have a challenging mission. Do what you can to support researchers, as you never know what knowledge their work will bring—studying one thing for a specific purpose often brings knowledge for another. For example, the following are just a few of the spin-off technologies we gained from National Aeronautics and Space Administration (NASA) research: heart monitors; laparoscopes; voice-controlled wheelchairs; portable x-rays; magnetic resonance imaging (MRI); ultrasound; automatic insulin pumps; and light-emitting diode (LED) lights (give light for laparoscopes and are being studied for use in promoting bone growth and removing tumors that are hard to reach). **Source:** Health and Medicine NASA Spinoffs (http://www.thespaceplace.com/nasa/spinoffs.html#health).

OTHER PERSPECTIVES

RESEARCH—PROMOTING A CULTURE OF INQUIRY

Research skills developed in a culture of inquiry can become part of individual professional practice. The face of nursing practice today continues to evolve as the profession moves toward seamlessly intertwining research and technology with high-quality and compassionate care. To assure this challenging objective is met, nurses have a personal responsibility to apply research and own their clinical practices.[18]

Critical Thinking Exercises

Moral and Ethical Reasoning Exercises

Example responses are on page 269.

1. What would you do if you were "Me" in the following scenario?*

My father was admitted to an intensive care unit and wasn't expected to live. I was approached by a physician, who asked, "Do you want us to resuscitate him if he arrests again?" Since my father never wanted to talk about these things, I didn't know what he'd want. I also didn't feel it was my place to answer. I called my mother and asked her the question. Here's how the conversation went:

Me: "Mom, they want to know if they should resuscitate Dad if he arrests again."

Mom: "You don't know what you're asking me."

Me: "Yes, I do. I know it's hard, but you're supposed to speak in his voice. Not what you want—what you think he wants."

Mom: "That's the problem. All my life when I've tried to guess his decisions, he's always done just the opposite. Even when I've said to myself, 'I think he'll do (whatever) only because it's the opposite of what I think he'd do,' I've still been wrong."

Scenario
CODE OR NO CODE: WHAT WOULD YOU DO?

2. Which of the seven moral and ethical principles (autonomy, beneficence, justice, fidelity, veracity, confidentiality, accountability) apply to the following statement? *By choosing to be a nurse, you must see that your patients receive competent care.* (More than one principle may apply.)
3. Fill in the blanks in the following statement. Ethical reasoning differs from moral reasoning in that it requires you to apply _____ standards rather than _____ standards.

Think, Pair, Share

With a partner, in a group, or in a journal entry:

1. Consider the ethical issues involved when parents try to sneak medication into their child's meals (See "Treating a Son's O.C.D." by Randy Cohen at http://www.nytimes.com/2010/04/18/magazine/18FOB-Ethicist-t.html)
2. Download and discuss your state-specific Advance Directives by clicking on your state at http://www.caringinfo.org/stateaddownload. How do these

directives make you feel? How do you feel about discussing them with clients, colleagues, or friends?

3. Consider the ethics and issues involved in the following.

> *"In Crises, Silence Is Golden! I see too many fundamental errors in handling crisis situations. Simple principles such as maintaining "one voice" to the client and providing enough space and time for a patient or client to de-escalate are often ignored. Two common mistakes I've noticed when observing staff responding to clients in crisis are the use of too much verbal interaction and premature use of intrusive intervention strategies. Our first instinct is to talk to a client; however silence can be an extremely effective strategy to de-escalate a crisis situation. When I am training direct care staff, I stress that they should never try to force a situation to resolution if time and space may solve the problem. Many people intervene before it is necessary instead of allowing time to solve the problem."*
>
> —**Matthew Riley, MA, BCBA, Co-Owner,** Behavior for Life

1. Discuss the Palliative and End-of-Life Assessment tool posted at http://www.aacn.org/WD/Palliative/Docs/Player/main.html

2. Grief is difficult and continues after people die. Contact your local hospice and find out what services are available for families after patients die.

3. Identify the implications of the Other Perspectives on page 135.

4. Decide where you stand in relation to achieving the following learning outcomes from page 129.
   a. Develop or adopt a personal code of conduct based on your personal values and content in this chapter.
   b. Compare and contrast the terms *moral reasoning* and *ethical reasoning*.
   c. Make prudent decisions based on ethical principles, codes, and practice standards.

Research, Evidence-Based Practice, and Quality Improvement Exercises

1. Fill in the blanks in the following sentences:
   a. Research is an objective, orderly process that uses _____ data collection and testing conditions.
   b. EBP integrates the best research, knowledge from clinical experts, and patient _____ into clinical practice.
   c. EBP requires that knowledge be _____ by the systematic study of how evidence from research can best be _____ in _____.

2. What is the purpose of clinical summaries and practice alerts?

3. Is the following statement true or false, and why? *Staff nurses must make finding and critiquing applicable research results a part of their daily work.*

4. Explain why it's important to do QI studies from the following perspectives, and then give an example for each type of study:
   a. Outcomes evaluation (focuses on results)
   b. Process evaluation (focuses on how care was given)
   c. Structure evaluation (focuses on setting)

Think, Pair, Share

With a partner, in a group, or in a journal entry:

1. Read the following article and address the ethics, research, and clinical challenges involved in restraining patients: Green, C. Moving toward a restraint-free environment. Retrieved January 11, 2011, from http://www.americannursetoday.com/Article.aspx?id=6984&fid=6848

2. Discuss how the information in the following research article may be applied: Bankhead, C. (2010). Score predicts morbidity risk in preterm infants. Retrieved January 2, 2011, from http://www.medpagetoday.com/Pediatrics/GeneralPediatrics/22116

3. Find a research article on a topic you find interesting. Then discuss the following:
   a. What did the researchers study?
   b. What were the key points listed in the discussion, nursing interventions, and summary sections?
   c. What questions does this article raise?
   d. How do you feel about applying the results to your practice?
   e. Where can you find out more about this topic?

4. Go to www.noodletools.com/ and examine some of the different ways you can narrow your Internet search to find what you really need. For example, is it timeliness or history that you need?

5. Visit some of the following websites, and discuss how you might be able to use the information found there.

Resources for Evidence-Based Practice
- Journal descriptions with links to their websites: http://www.rss4medics.com/rss_directory/nursing_feeds.html
- AHRQ Quality Indicators: http://www.qualityindicators.ahrq.gov/
- America Association of Critical Care Nurses Evidence-Based Resources: http://www.aacn.org/wd/practice/content/ebp.pcms?menu=practice&lastmenu=divheader_evidence-based_resources

- Beginner's Research Guide—Searching Steps: http://library.nyu.edu/research/subjects/health/tutorial/steps.html
- Guide for using online resources: http://library.nyu.edu/research/health/tutorial/
- National Institute of Nursing Research: www.nih.gov/about/almanac/organization/NINR.htm
- National Data Base of Nursing Quality Indicators: https://www.nursingquality.org/
- Research Utilization and Evidence-Based Practice: http://library.nyu.edu/research/subjects/health/tutorial/researchutilization.html
- Resource Guide for Evidence-Based Practice: http://www.library.ualberta.ca/subject/evidence/guide/index.cfm
- The Joint Commission (enter "evidence-based practice" into the search field): www.jointcommision.org
- University of Washington Health Links: http://healthlinks.washington.edu/ebp/ebpresources.html
- Joanna Briggs Institute: http://www.joannabriggs.edu.au

6. Learn more about transforming knowledge to evidence-based practice. Go to www.acestar.uthscsa.edu/acestar-model.asp and discuss the eight underlying principles of knowledge transformation, and the various phases of the ACE Star Model shown on page 139. Finally, draw the star model without looking at it.
7. Decide where you stand in relation to achieving the following learning outcomes from page 129.
   a. Explain (or map) the relationship between nursing research and EBP.
   b. Describe your responsibilities for nursing research, EBP, surveillance, and QI.
   c. Choose refereed (peer-reviewed) journals and reliable websites to learn more about up-to-date EBP on specific topics.

TEACHING OTHERS: PROMOTING INDEPENDENCE

Your role as a teacher—helping patients, families, and peers to acquire the knowledge and skills they need to be independent—can be one of the most rewarding, time-saving, and cost-effective things you do. Patients are discharged "quicker and sicker" than they were in the past, and many manage complex problems independently at home—they need competent, knowledgeable teachers.[19]

Whether you're dealing with patients, students, or peers, being an effective teacher requires working closely together with learners to identify (1) what must be learned, (2) how they want to learn it, and (3) what resources can best be used to facilitate learning. The following steps can help you think critically about how to teach others.

10 Steps for Teaching Others

1. Determine the desired outcome(s) together with the learner. What exactly must the person be able to do when you complete your teaching? *Example:* Sam will be able to regulate insulin dosage based on blood glucose readings.

2. Find out what the person already knows, and then decide (1) what exactly the person must learn to achieve the desired outcome and (2) how much time you have before the person must know it.
   - Determine readiness to learn (e.g., How ready are you to learn this? What are your biggest concerns?).
   - Ask about preferred learning styles (e.g., doing, observing, listening, or reading on page 32) and use this information to plan teaching. *Example:* If you're teaching injection technique to *doers,* have them start by doing something, like handling a syringe. If they'd rather read, start by giving them a pamphlet.
   - Identify barriers to learning (e.g., consider language, reading skills, developmental problems, or problems with motivation).
   - Encourage people to ask questions, get involved, and let you know how they'd like to learn. *Example:* "Let me know if you have a better way of learning this. Not everyone learns the same way."

3. Reduce anxiety by offering support. *Example:* "Everyone is nervous when first learning to change dressings, but once you've done it a couple of times, it will be much easier."

4. Minimize distractions, and teach at appropriate times. Pick a quiet room, and choose times when the learners are likely to be comfortable and rested.

5. Use pictures, diagrams, and illustrations to promote comprehension and retention. Have them draw their own pictures and maps—ask them to explain them to you.

6. Create mental images by using analogies and metaphors. *Example:* "Insulin is like a key that opens the cell's door to allow sugar to enter. If you don't have the key (insulin), sugar can't get in to feed the cell. The cell starves, and sugar accumulates in the blood, damaging kidneys and vessels."

7. Help people process and remember by using whatever words best trigger their mind. *Example:* "I need to have three things: the soaking-dressing stuff, the scrubbing stuff, and the after-dressing stuff."

8. Keep it simple. The explain-it-to-me-as-if-I-were-a-10-year-old approach works especially well for complex situations. If you can't make it simple, you're not ready to teach it.

9. Tune into your learners' responses and change the pace, techniques, or content if needed. If they don't remember important content, take time to review it; if they don't seem to understand what you're saying, write it down or draw a picture.

10. Summarize main points, and don't leave learners empty-handed. Give them the important points in print or on videotape so that they can refresh their memory later.

TEACHING OURSELVES: GRAB THE SPOON

I used to love to be spoon-fed information. I didn't know how to learn independently, and I wanted teachers to do it all. Then I learned how to teach myself. I realized that often teachers were trying to "feed me" more than I could learn at one time. Sometimes they "fed me" in a different order than I wanted, and sometimes it felt like I got "food" all over my face but not in my brain. Now I know that I can teach myself better than anyone else can—I grab the spoon and feed myself.

When you know how to teach yourself, you save time and feel more intelligent and confident. You learn in ways that help you understand deeply. You *remember* what you learn. When you encounter something new, take charge and reason your way through the learning experience. Apply the strategies in this section and be confident in your ability to learn. Don't be afraid to ask questions. Remember, you are your own best teacher.

Memorizing Effectively

Critical thinking takes more than memorizing facts—you must know how to *apply* information in context of various situations. Still, learning how to memorize effectively does enhance your ability to think critically: You must be able to *recall facts* to progress to *higher levels* of thinking, such as knowing *how to apply and analyze information*. For example, if you aren't able to recall what *normal* health assessment findings are, you won't be able to analyze your patient's data to decide whether there are any *abnormal* findings. Because nursing requires a lot of memorization, especially in the beginning, use the following strategies to memorize and learn efficiently.

Strategies to Boost Your Memory

☐ **Remember the "use it or lose it" rule.** If you haven't been using information, refresh your memory by using it again. An example of "use it or lose it" is when you forget your multiplication tables because you depend on calculators without doing the math on your own now and then.

☐ **Work to *understand* information before you try to memorize it.** Once you make sense of the information, you can identify the most important things to remember.

☐ **Don't try to memorize *everything*.** Separate the most important things from all the other information. Looking at the most important things, lifted out, removes clutter and helps you avoid the problem of TMI (too much information).

☐ **Look for *relationships* between the facts, and group related facts together.** Your brain remembers *groups of information* better than *isolated facts*. This is like putting information in folders, rather than cluttering your desktop with individual documents. Looking for relationships between and among the facts also helps you *remember* because you are *using* the information. Drawing maps is great for helping you see relationships (see Appendix A).

☐ **Create a memory hook—put the information into context.** For example, suppose you're studying *pneumonia* in class, and you cared for "Fred" who had pneumonia when you were doing your clinical experience. Visualize "Fred" and how he compared with the textbook picture ("Fred" becomes your memory hook). If you don't have a real situation to connect with, play around with the information until something comes to mind that helps you remember (e.g., a rhyme, a picture, a story). For example:

1. **Use a mnemonic** (a memory jog that makes an association between something that's easy to remember and something that's hard to remember). *Example:* **TACIT** helps you remember what to assess for medications (Therapeutic effect, Allergic or Adverse reactions, Contraindications, Interactions, Toxicity/overdose).

2. **Create an acrostic** (a catchy phrase that helps you remember the first letters of the information you're trying to remember). *Example:* M*aggie* c*hewed* n*uts* e*very* p*lace* s*he* w*ent* gives the first letters of things you must assess in neurovascular assessment: movement, color, numbness, edema, pulses, sensation, and warmth.

☐ **Use your preferred learning style and as many senses as possible.** Examples: Say words as you write and read them. Sing what you're trying to remember to the tune of a favorite song. Light a scented candle. Play your favorite music.

☐ **Organize and reorganize information.** This helps you see different patterns, and you remember because you're *using* the information.

☐ **Review the information briefly before going to sleep.** Studies show that even if you're a "morning person," information moves into long-term memory better if reviewed late in the day, immediately before going to bed.[21]

☐ **Quiz yourself without your notes.** Just because you can *recognize* information in your notes, it doesn't mean you'll be able to *recall* it without your notes.

☐ **Know yourself and use self-discipline.** Identify the circumstances that help you retain information, and plan your schedule to include those circumstances. If you study better in the morning, go to bed early enough that you can get up early and feel rested. If you're easily distracted or sidetracked, turn off your cell phone and e-mail. Go to the library or put a *Don't Disturb* sign on your door.[20]

☐ **Seek out mentors and role models**—teachers, other nurses, friends, and peers. They help you clarify your thoughts and set goals better than any textbook.

> As long as there are tests, there will be prayer in schools.
>

TEST-TAKING: IMPROVING GRADES AND PASSING THE FIRST TIME

Test-taking can be frustrating and anxiety-producing.[22] We all have been in the position of knowing something well, yet feeling lost on the test. Many complex, creative critical thinkers struggle with trying to "match" right answers on a test. Lots of us can reason well in real situations but struggle with test-taking. As a friend once said to me, "I need to be in real situations to think well." This section helps you use critical thinking to identify the best way to prepare for—and take—tests. Using the strategies in this section helps you reduce test anxiety, improve your confidence and grades, and pass tests on the first try.

Strategies for Successful Test-Taking

Staying up on course work and studying each week—rather than cramming at the end of courses—is the key for doing well on exams. But it isn't the *only* key. Good test-taking skills are equally as important. This section gives general strategies to use when taking any test, followed by specific strategies for taking the NCLEX® and other standard tests.

Preparing for Tests

■ **Know yourself.** Identify your usual test-taking behaviors (e.g., do you get overly anxious? Do you tend to run out of time? Are you better at one type of test than another?). Seek help for areas you'd like to change.

■ **Know the test plan.** Find out what types of questions are going to be asked and what information is the most important to study. If the teacher doesn't share this information, review course objectives, text objectives, and summaries—often these will help you decide what's most important.

■ **Find out how long you have to take the test,** what resources you're allowed to bring, and whether you get penalized for guessing.

■ **Prepare with an attitude of, "I can do this—I just have to figure out how."** You *are* capable. Sometimes you need to remind yourself of this to gain the positive attitude that's so important. Anxiety and lack of confidence are self-defeating brain-drains— take a deep breath and focus on doing the best you can.

■ **Get organized and budget your time.** Decide what you need to study, what your resources are (for example, notes, books, tutors, peers), and when and how you'll prepare for the test.

■ **Join a study group**—be sure the group stays on task and on time.

■ **Know the parts of a question, how to read questions, and how to make educated guesses** (Boxes 4-4 and 4-5).

■ **Practice taking the test under the same conditions you will experience when you actually take it.** For example, if it's a computerized test, practice on the computer.

Taking Tests

■ **Arrive early for warm-up.** Give yourself time to calm down, get focused, and scan your review materials. Reviewing practice questions is also a good way to get your brain in test-taking gear.

■ **Pay attention to verbal and written instructions.** Jot down notes to be sure you remember the instructions.

■ **If allowed, skim the whole test and plan your approach.** For example, begin by answering the types of questions you *like* before tackling types you *don't like* (you may like matching questions better than essay). *Completing what you like and know first*

BOX 4-4   PARTS OF A TEST QUESTION

1. **The background statement(s):** The statements or phrases that tell you the *context* in which you're expected to answer the question (e.g., the words in italics in the following example):
   Example test question: You're caring for *someone who has severe asthma, is wheezing loudly, is confused, and can't sleep.* You check the orders and note that a sedative can be given for sleeplessness. Knowing the possible effects of giving a sedative to an asthmatic, <u>what would you do?</u>
   a. Give the sedative to help the patient relax.
   b. Withhold the sedative, because it aggravates asthma.
   c. Withhold the sedative, and monitor the patient closely.
   d. Give the sedative, but monitor the patient carefully.
2. **The stem:** A phrase that asks or states the intent of the question (e.g., the underlined words above)
3. **Key concepts:** The most important concepts addressed in the background statement(s). In the example above, the key concepts are "severe asthma," "wheezing loudly," and "effects of giving a sedative to an asthmatic."
4. **Key word(s):** The words that specify what's being asked and what's happening. In the example above, the key words are "severe," "loudly," and "confused." These words specify that the asthma problem is severe. "Would you do" specifies that you're being asked for an appropriate action to take.
5. **The options (choices):** These include one correct answer (called the *keyed response*) and three to five distracters (incorrect answers). In the example above, (c) is the keyed response, and the rest are distracters.

See also: Parts of a Question and How to Read Test Questions at http://passnclex.drexel.edu/study_resources.aspx.

reduces anxiety and gets your brain in the test-taking mode before you tackle more difficult questions.

- **Watch your time, and note how the questions are weighted.** If a question is worth 50% of your grade, you might want to save 50% of your time to work on that question.
- **Focus on what you know.**
  1. If allowed, skip difficult questions and come back to them later. Mark the easy questions and do them first.
  2. For short-answer and essay tests: (1) Jot down main points you need to address before writing your essay. When you finish, check your essay to be sure you hit all the major points. (2) If you have time at the end, come back to these questions and ask yourself, "What else can I say?" or "What did I miss?"
- **If you don't understand a question, ask for clarification.** If you're not allowed to ask questions during the test, write something like, "I wasn't sure what you meant, so I'm answering the question assuming you meant...." If allowed, write this on your answer sheet.
- **When in doubt, don't change answers.** Your first response is more likely to be correct.
- **For case history questions, read the questions about the case history *first*.** Then read the histories, looking for the answers.

BOX 4-5   GUIDELINES FOR MAKING EDUCATED GUESSES*

Definition of an educated guess: *Applying test-taking strategies to choose a right answer when you're unsure from content alone (when none of the options seem to jump out at you)*

1. Be sure you understand the test directions.
2. Find out whether you're penalized for guessing.
3. Read the question *twice,* asking yourself the following:
   - **What** does the stem ask (see Box 4-4, Parts of a Test Question, on previous page)
   - **Who** is the client? (e.g., age, sex, role)
   - **What** is the problem? (e.g., diagnosis, signs, symptoms, behavior)
   - **What rationale** is offered in the question? (e.g., to prevent respiratory complications... Because the cast is damp...)
   - **What time frame** is being addressed? (e.g., immediately before surgery, on the day of admission, or when?)
4. Study all the answers.
   - Eliminate answers you know are outright wrong.
   - Look for answers that are wrong based on the directions.
   - Look for clues in the questions or answers that might help you narrow it down further to the most likely best answer (see strategies 5 and 6 below).
5. Use the following rules together with your knowledge to make educated guesses:
   - **Initial = Assessment.** The word *initial* used in a question usually requires an assessment answer. (What would you assess?)
   - **Essential = Safety.** The word *essential* used in a question usually requires a safety answer. (What's required for safety?) Remember: "Keep them breathing, keep them safe."
   - **Opposites Attract Right Answers.** If you have two answers that are opposite to one another, the *right* answer is usually *one* of the two opposites.
     Example: The correct answer below is likely to be (a) or (b) because they're opposites.
     a. Turn the client on to the right side.
     b. Turn the client on to the left side.
     c. Encourage fluids.
     d. Ambulate the client.
   - **Odd Man Wins.** The option that's most different in length, style, or content is usually the right answer. The *right* answer is often the longest one or the shortest one. *Example:* The correct answer below is likely to be (b) because it's the "odd man."
     a. Decreased temperature
     b. Rapid pulse
     c. Decreased respirations
     d. Decreased blood pressure
   - **Same Answer = Neither One.** If two responses say the same thing in different words, they can't both be right, so neither one is right. *Example:* Tachycardia and rapid heartbeat as two answer options.
   - **Repeated Words Means Right.** If the answer contains the same word (or a synonym) that appears in the question, it's more likely to be a correct response. *Example:* The word *hypotension* in question, the word *hypotension* or *shock* in answer.
   - **Absolutely Not.** Answers that use "absolutes" aren't usually the right response. *Example:* always, never, all, none.
   - **Generally So.** Answers that use qualifiers that make the response more "generally so" tend to signify right answers. *Examples:* usually, frequently, often.
6. When answering questions about setting priorities, remember Maslow's Hierarchy of Needs (see Box 5-2, page 199).

*Strategies developed with the help of Judith Miller (http://judymillernclexreview.com) and Deanne Blach (www.DeanneBlach.com).

■ **If you're stuck on a question**, try sketching a picture, map, or diagram to help you conceptualize the answer.

After the Test

■ **If you do poorly, don't think it's the end of the world.** Even the best minds have failed tests (Einstein flunked algebra; Edison was considered unteachable). Instead, *do* something. Explain your difficulty to your instructor; ask for suggestions on how to prepare better or whether you can do extra credit work.

■ **If there's a test review, be sure to go—you'll** *learn.* Too many students think that this is an opportunity to skip class, since "nothing much will be happening."

Strategies for the NCLEX® and Other Standard Tests*
The following summarizes important points on the NCLEX® and gives strategies for taking standard tests such as certification exams.

Fast Facts on the NCLEX®

■ Based on surveys of skills that new graduates must have (surveys are done every 3 years)
■ Taken on a computer; takes up to 6 hours. As soon as you answer enough questions to predict that you will pass or fail, the computer shuts down. You answer a minimum of 75 questions, 15 of these are being tested for reliability and are not a part of your score. The maximum number of questions is 265.
■ The following are the main activities tested on the NCLEX®.

Main Activities Tested on NCLEX® RN Exam[22]
NCLEX® tests ability to:
● Apply principles of infection control (e.g., hand hygiene, aseptic/sterile technique)
● Provide care within the legal scope of practice
● Maintain patient confidentiality
● Ensure proper patient identification
● Practice in a manner consistent with a code of ethics for a registered nurse
● Protect a patient from injury (falls, malfunctioning equipment, electrical hazards)
● Review pertinent data prior to medication administration
● Prepare and give medications applying the rights of medication administration
● Prioritize workload to manage time effectively
● Use approved abbreviations and standard terminology when documenting care
● Perform and manage care of a patient receiving peritoneal dialysis
● Provide intrapartum care and education
● Facilitate group sessions
● Identify and report occupational/environmental exposures
● Provide care and/or support for a patient with non–substance-related dependencies

*Strategies developed with the help of Judith Miller (http://judymillernclexreview.com) and Deanne Blach (www.DeanneBlach.com).

- Questions require analysis and application. If you answer easy questions correctly, you move on to higher-level questions. You can't go back and change answers. Don't skip questions—try your best on each one.

> **RULE**
>
> **The NCLEX® is a power test, not a speed test.** Work slowly and accurately, rather than rapidly and carelessly. Careless wrong answers can "dig a hole that is hard to climb out of."[23]

- Types of questions you will encounter:
  1. The majority are multiple-choice questions that require selection of one answer.
  2. There are a few "alternate item questions": these require selecting one or more responses, filling in the blank (including calculation and prioritizing questions), or clicking and dragging the mouse to select a "hot spot."
  3. All items may include charts, tables, or graphs.
- The test integrates four processes throughout:
  1. Nursing process
  2. Teaching and learning
  3. Caring
  4. Communication and documentation

> **NCLEX® TEST CATEGORIES**
>
> The test plan is based on the results of the RN Practice Analysis that was conducted in 2008, evaluated in 2009, and implemented in April 2010, and tests the following categories.
> 1. Safe, effective care environment—management of care (16% to 22% of the test)
> 2. Safe, effective care environment—safety and infection control (8% to 14% of the test)
> 3. Health promotion and maintenance (6% to 12% of the test)
> 4. Psychosocial integrity (6% to 12% of the test)
> 5. Physiologic integrity (around 50% of the test)
>   - Basic care and comfort and assistance in performance of ADLs (6% to 12% of the test)
>   - Pharmacology and intravenous (IV) therapy (13% to 19% of the test)
>   - Risk reduction (10% to 16% of the test)
>   - Physiologic adaptation (11% to 17% of the test)

- Stresses assessment and monitoring (safe, effective care)
  1. Before procedure, during procedure, and after procedure assessment
  2. Before drug administration, during drug administration, and after drug administration assessment
  3. Delegation (what should you delegate, to whom, and when?)
  4. Prioritization (what should you do first?)

- Includes questions on all major specialties, as well as advance directives, injury prevention, family systems, cultural diversity, legal rights and responsibilities, error prevention, bioterrorism, disaster response, human sexuality, and mental health.

Preparing for the NCLEX®

- Get review books early, and use them as you progress through your program. This helps you be familiar with the types of questions you will have to answer and also helps you learn.
- Complete at least 2000 computerized practice questions, since this will significantly increase your chances of passing the first time. Appendix F (pages 290 to 297) gives example practice questions you can try.
- To increase learning and retention, when you get a question wrong, look up the information immediately so that you understand *why* you chose the incorrect response.
- Be sure you reviewed the general strategies for test-taking listed earlier in this section.
- Complete a tutorial before the exam (http://www.vue.com/nclex/). This helps you deal with various question types and helps keep you grounded.
- For Internet resources for studying, test-taking, and the NCLEX®, see http://evolve.elsevier.com/Alfaro-LeFevre/CT or http://www.alfaroteachsmart.com/handouts.html

CRITICAL MOMENTS

TEACHING OTHERS HELPS YOU LEARN
When you want to learn something, offer to teach it to someone else. You learn and recall best what you teach someone *else.*

TEACHING "WHY" PROMOTES INDEPENDENCE
Knowing why something must be done empowers people to problem solve independently. Always explain the principles and rationales for treatments. If they know the reasons behind the treatments, they'll be able to make decisions about what to do when things go wrong.

OTHER PERSPECTIVES

HOW LITERATE ARE YOU?
"The illiterate of the twenty-first century will not be those who cannot read and write, but those who cannot learn, unlearn, and relearn."
—*Alvin Toffler, author of* Future Shock[24]

FIGURING THINGS OUT FOR YOURSELF: THE BEST WAY TO LEARN
Figuring things out for yourself goes something like this: "Let's see, how can I understand this? Is it to be understood on the model of this experience or that? Shall I think of it in this way or that? Let me see. Ah, I think I see. It's just so ...

but, no, not exactly. Let me try again. Perhaps I can understand it from this point of view … OK, now I think I'm getting it."[25]

> —*Richard Paul, Author of* Critical Thinking:
> How to Prepare Students for a Rapidly Changing World

ATTENDING CLASS SAVES YOU TIME
Every hour you spend in class saves you 3 hours of study time. If you're going to cut corners somewhere, go to class and skimp on study time. Attend every class.[26]

> —*Melodie Chenevert, Author of* Mosby's Tour Guide to Nursing School:
> A Student's Road Survival Kit

A PATIENT COVERED IN PATCHES?
As I escorted "Bob" into one of our examining rooms, he said, "I was told to put on a new medication patch every six hours, but I'm running out of room." When he took off his shirt, he was covered in patches. Needless to say, the instructions for this drug now say "remove previous patch and apply the next one in a different spot."

> —*Posting on a Nursing Listserv*

PATIENT EDUCATION: DON'T ASSUME
The most dangerous mistakes in patient education are assumptions. You assume they can read. You assume they understand. You assume they have no more questions. You assume they can do it. You assume they will do it.[27]

> —*Fran London, MS, RN, Author of* No Time to Teach:
> The Essence of Patient and Family Education for Health Care Providers

NEW TWIST ON AN OLD PROVERB
Give a man a fish and he eats for a day. Teach a man to fish, and he leaves you alone every weekend. ☺

Critical Thinking Exercises

Example responses are on page 269.

Teaching Others, Teaching Ourselves, and Test-Taking

1. Explain why knowing how to teach others and yourself efficiently is essential to meeting nursing outcomes.
2. When studying for a test, why is it important to be sure you know the content without looking at your notes?

3. Fill in the following blanks:
   a. Two main steps to teaching others are: finding out what they _____ _____ and determining whether they are _____ to learn.
   b. You learn and recall best what you _____ someone *else*.
   c. Doing well on a test requires you to not only have the required knowledge, but to _____ taking the test under the_____ conditions you will experience when you actually take it.

Think, Pair, Share

With a partner, in a group, or in a journal entry:

1. Giving examples from your life experience, discuss what the *Critical Moments* and *Other Perspectives* on pages 159 to 160 mean to you.
2. Discuss the strategies given in: "Ticket to Home" tool helps patients and families prepare for discharge. Retrieved January 6, 2011, from http://www.strategiesfornursemanagers.com/ce_detail/254410.cfm
3. Share your thoughts on the strategies for learning and memorizing addressed in this chapter.
4. Using page 33 as a guide, discuss how you can best teach someone who has different learning preferences than your own.
5. Discuss the study skills and time management tips at http://homeworktips.about.com/
6. Discuss your experiences with using some of the strategies in Box 4-5 (Guidelines for Making Educated Guesses).
7. If you plan to take the NCLEX®:
   • Sign up to get a practice question delivered daily to your e-mail account at http://www.testprepreview.com/nclex_practice.htm.
   • Discuss the parts of a question and how to read test questions as addressed in this chapter and posted at http://passnclex.drexel.edu/study_resources.aspx.
   • Decide how you might use the Internet resources for studying, test-taking, and the NCLEX® posted at: http://www.alfaroteachsmart.com/handouts.
   • Discuss the practice questions in Appendix F.
8. Decide where you stand in relation to achieving the outcomes on page 129.

KEY POINTS/SUMMARY

• Knowing how to reason your way through moral and ethical issues is integral to everyday nursing practice.

• Practice standards, ethics codes, and bills of rights guide ethical conduct. The following are common values addressed in ethical codes and standards: maintaining client confidentiality; acting as client advocate; delivering care in a nonjudgmental and nondiscriminatory way; being sensitive to diversity and culture; promoting autonomy, dignity, and rights; and seeking resources for solving ethical dilemmas.

- Seven principles form a foundation for ethical reasoning: autonomy, beneficence, justice, fidelity, veracity, confidentiality, and accountability.
- Pages 133 to 134 gives steps for moral and ethical reasoning. Advance directives help us make decisions about cardiac resuscitation and other end-of-life treatments.
- EBP requires integrating (1) the best research evidence, (2) clinical expertise, and (3) patient preferences into clinical practice.
- ACE Star Model of Knowledge Transformation (page 139) provides a framework for transforming knowledge to EBP.
- Pages 141 to 142 addresses five main responsibilities of nurses related to nursing research, surveillance, QI, and EBP.
- ANA standards of performance stress that nurses must apply research to practice. We must continue to question current practices and develop new knowledge.

- Pages 141 to 143 answer "frequently asked questions" about staff nurses' role as it relates to research and EBP.
- QI studies examine health care from three different perspectives: (1) outcomes (evaluates results), (2) process (evaluates how care was given), and (3) structure.
- To be an effective teacher, work closely together with learners to identify (1) what must be learned, (2) how they want to learn it, and (3) what resources can best be used to facilitate learning.
- Today's workplace requires you to have excellent independent learning skills.
- Improving test performance and passing the first time requires that you know yourself, the test format, test-taking skills, and how to make educated guesses.
- Learning how to memorize effectively enhances your ability to think critically: You must be able to *recall facts* to progress to *higher levels* of thinking, such as knowing *how to apply and analyze information.*
- Pages 154 to 159 give strategies for successful test-taking.
- Scan this chapter to review all highlighted rules.

REFERENCES

1. American Association of Critical Care Nurses. Healthy work environments initiatives. Retrieved January 7, 2011, from http://www.aacn.org/WD/HWE/Content/hwehome.pcms ?menu=Practice&lastmenu
2. Riley, M. (January 2011). E-mail communication.
3. American Nurses Association. (2001). Code of ethics for nurses with interpretive statements. Retrieved January 6, 2011, from http://www.nursingworld.org/MainMenuCategories/ EthicsStandards/CodeofEthicsforNurses.aspx
4. Taylor, C., Lillis, C., Lemone, P., et al. (2011). *Fundamentals of nursing: The art and science of nursing care.* (7th ed.) Philadelphia: Lippincott Williams & Wilkins.
5. Scipio-Bannerman, J. (2007). Unheard screams. Retrieved January 11, 2011, from http:// news.nurse.com/apps/pbcs.dll/article?AID=2006610090315
6. Oermann, M., Floyd, J., Galvin, E., et al. (2006). Brief reports for disseminating systematic reviews to nurses. *Clinical Nurse Specialist,* 20(5), 233-238.

7. American Association of Critical Care Nurses. Evidence-based resources. Retrieved January 11, 2011, from http://www.aacn.org/wd/practice/content/ebp.pcms?menu=practice

8. Academic Center for Evidence-Based Practice. (Website). Retrieved January 11, 2011, from http://www.acestar.uthscsa.edu

9. American Association of Critical Care Nurses. Practice alert: Oral care in the critically ill. Retrieved January 11, 2011, from http://classic.aacn.org/AACN/aacnnews.nsf/GetArticle/ArticleThree238

10. Kalisch, B. (2006). Missed nursing care: A qualitative study. *Journal of Nursing Care Quality*, 21(4), 306-313. Retrieved January 11, 2011, from www.nursingcenter.com/prodev/ce_article.asp?tid=671279

11. Aiken, L., Clarke, S., Sloane, D., et al. (2002). Hospital nurse staffing and patient mortality, nurse burnout, and job dissatisfaction. *Journal of the American Medical Association*, 288(16), 1987-1993.

12. Green, C. Moving toward a restraint-free environment. Retrieved January 11, 2011, from http://www.americannursetoday.com/Article.aspx?id=6984&fid=6848

13. Temel, J., Greer, J., Muzikansky, A., et al. (2010). Early palliative care for patients with metastatic non–small-cell lung cancer. *New England Journal of Medicine*, 363(8), 733-742. Retrieved January 10, 2011 from http://www.nejm.org/doi/full/10.1056/NEJMoa1000678

14. Burns, N., Grove, S. (2011). *Understanding nursing research: Building an evidence-based practice* (5th ed.). Philadelphia: Saunders.

15. West, S., King, V., Carey, T., et al. (2002). Systems to rate the strength of scientific evidence. Evidence Report/Technology Assessment No. 47. AHRQ Publication No. 02-E016. Rockville, MD: Agency for Healthcare Research and Quality. Retrieved January 1, 2011, from http://www.thecre.com/pdf/ahrq-system-strength.pdf

16. Research utilization and evidence-based practice. (Website.) Retrieved January11, 2011, from http://library.nyu.edu/research/subjects/health/tutorial/researchutilization.html

17. American Nurses Association National Center for Nursing Quality. (Website). Retrieved January 6, 2011, from http://www.nursingworld.org

18. Baker, K., Martin, A., Broutron, K. (2010). Bringing research to the bedside. Retrieved January 2, 2011, from http://nursing.advanceweb.com/Continuing-Education/CE-Articles/Bringing-Research-to-the-Bedside.aspx.

19. Burkhart, J. (2008). Training nurses to be teachers. *The Journal of Continuing Education in Nursing*, 39(11), 503-510.

20. Fleming, G. Should I stay up late to study? Retrieved January 2, 2011, from http://homeworktips.about.com/od/mindandbody/qt/latestudy.htm

21. Silvestri, L. (2010). *Strategies for test success*. Philadelphia: Saunders.

22. Zerwekh, J., Claborn, J. (2010). *Illustrated study guide for the NCLEX-RN exam*. St. Louis: Mosby.

23. Miller, J. (January 11, 2011). E-mail communication. Website: http://judymillernclexreview.com

24. Toffler, A. (2000). In S. Thorpe (Ed.), *How to think like Einstein*. Naperville, IL: Sourcebooks.

25. Paul, R. (1993). *Critical thinking: How to prepare students for a rapidly changing world*. Santa Rosa, CA: Foundation for Critical Thinking.

26. Chenevert, M. (2011). *Mosby's tour guide to nursing school: A student's road survival kit* (6th ed.). St Louis: Mosby.

27. London, F. (2009). *No time to teach: The essence of patient and family education for health care providers*. Atlanta: Pritchett & Hull.

Practicing Clinical Reasoning Skills: Applying the Nursing Process

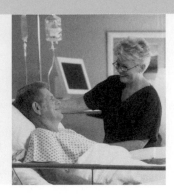

This chapter at a glance ...

---

*This skill deals with identifying risk factors in healthy people. The next skill, Diagnosing Actual and Potential Problems, deals with risk factors in people with existing health problems.

Decide where you stand in relation to the following learning outcomes.

Learning Outcomes

After completing this chapter, you should be able to:
1. Explain why each skill in this section is needed for clinical reasoning.
2. Explain how to accomplish each skill in this section.
3. Describe your reasoning in various clinical situations (e.g., how you came to a conclusion or made a decision).
4. Develop a comprehensive, patient-centered plan of care.

CHAPTER OVERVIEW

This chapter helps you practice clinical reasoning skills in patient situations that are based on real experiences (the names and some facts have been changed). Organized in logical progression according to how the skills might be used in the nursing process, each skill is presented in the following format: (1) name of the skill, (2) definition of the skill, (3) why the skill is needed for clinical reasoning, (4) how to accomplish the skill, and (5) Clinical Reasoning Exercises.

CLINICAL REASONING SKILLS: DYNAMIC AND INTERRELATED

The skills in this section are listed as *separate skills*. In real life, these skills are dynamic and interrelated. Some skills depend on—and facilitate—each other. For instance, you may *recognize inconsistencies* (Skill 8) in how someone responds to your care. This should trigger you to wonder, "Did I identify assumptions (Skill 1)?"

WHY PRACTICE THESE SKILLS SEPARATELY?

Think about this analogy: Tennis players practice interrelated *tennis skills* (e.g., foot placement, serve, forehand, backhand) separately to analyze and improve their *overall* game. This section gives practice for interrelated *intellectual skills* to help you analyze and improve your *overall clinical reasoning skills*. To keep the length of this chapter manageable, the chapter focuses mainly on reasoning in the context of *problems*. However, remember that critical thinking and clinical reasoning also focus on improving the status quo. For example, your asthmatic patient may be doing well with the current treatment plan, but you may consider whether a better exercise program would improve his lung function even more.

HOW TO GET THE MOST OUT OF THIS CHAPTER

1. To get the most out of these exercises, don't try to do too much at once. Some of these exercises, as in real life, are time-consuming. Rather, take your time and get in touch with your thinking. If possible, get at least one other person to complete the exercises with you. You learn more by discussing the skills with others.
2. Your brain is a tricky thing—describing what goes on in someone's head to complete each skill is difficult. If you have trouble with an exercise, read on and come back to it later. Explanations and exercises in later sections are likely to help you.
3. If you encounter diseases or drugs you don't know, look them up right away. This helps you build your own mental storehouse of problem-specific facts, because you

apply the information to the exercise. You remember best the information that you use.

4.   Before starting this chapter, be sure you have a good understanding of the terms in the following shaded section. These terms are listed in order of how you can best learn them (you need to know the first term to understand the second term, and so on).

REQUIRED VOCABULARY

Diagnosis: (1) The process of working to identify what disease or health problem is indicated by the patient's signs, symptoms, and health data. (2) The opinion reached by this process (usually refers to naming the disease or health problem). In this section, the terms *diagnosis* and *problem identification* may be used interchangeably.

Definitive diagnosis: The most specific, most correct diagnosis. For example, someone is admitted with an initial diagnosis of respiratory distress. Then, after studies are completed, the definitive diagnosis is congestive heart failure. To identify the best treatment, you must determine the most specific diagnosis.

Causative factor: Something known to create or contribute to a problem. For example, dizziness is known to cause falls.

Risk factor: Something known to cause, or be associated with, a specific problem. For example, smoking is a risk factor for cancer; having a family history of breast cancer is a risk factor for breast cancer.

Related factor: Used interchangeably with *risk factor*.

Potential problem or diagnosis: A problem or diagnosis that may occur because certain risk factors are present. For example, someone who's on prolonged bed rest has a potential (or risk for) *pressure ulcer*.

Data: Pieces of information about health status. Example: vital signs.

Objective data: Information that you can clearly observe or measure. Example: a pulse of 140 beats per minute. To remember this term, remember this:

O-O: Objective data = Observable data

Subjective data: Information the patient states or communicates. These are the patient's perceptions. Example: "My heart feels like it's racing." To remember this term, remember this:

S-S: Subjective data = Stated data (or written or communicated in sign language).

Signs and symptoms: Abnormal data that prompt you to suspect a health problem. Signs are objective data. Symptoms are subjective data. For example, fever is a sign of infection; chest pain is a symptom of heart disease.

Cues: Data that trigger you to think about a certain aspect of someone's health. Often used interchangeably with signs and symptoms.

Defining characteristics: Signs and symptoms usually present with a diagnosis or problem.

Baseline data: Information collected before treatment begins.

Database assessment: Comprehensive data collection performed to gain complete information about all aspects of health status (e.g., respiratory status, neurologic status, circulatory status).

Focus assessment: Data collection that aims to gain specific (focused) information about only one aspect of health status (e.g., neurologic status).

Infer: To draw a conclusion, or to attach meaning to a cue. For example, if an infant doesn't stop crying, no matter what's done for him, you might infer that *he's in pain*.

Inference: Something we suspect to be true, based on a logical conclusion. For example, the italicized words in the preceding definition.

1. IDENTIFYING ASSUMPTIONS

Definition

Recognizing when something is taken for granted or presented as fact without supporting evidence (e.g., you might assume a woman on a maternity unit has just had a baby)

Why This Skill Is Needed for Clinical Reasoning

As humans, we all have a tendency to make assumptions, especially when we're in new or unfamiliar situations. Sound clinical reasoning requires that you make judgments based on the best available evidence. This means double-checking your thinking to overcome your brain's natural tendency to grasp things at an intuitive (gut) level. By identifying assumptions, you begin to apply logic to the situation and avoid jumping to conclusions and making errors in judgment. This skill is placed at the top of the list in this section because it's one of the most commonly addressed skills in the critical thinking literature (both nursing and non-nursing).

Guidelines: How to Identify Assumptions

The best way to identify assumptions is to *look for them* by asking questions like "What's being taken for granted here?" and "How do I know that I've got the facts right?" To identify assumptions, make sure that you have *a complete picture* of what's going on with the patient (addressed in the next skill, *Assessing Systematically and Comprehensively*). Other skills that help you identify assumptions are *Checking Accuracy and Reliability* (Skill 3), *Recognizing Inconsistencies,* (Skill 8), *Identifying Patterns* (Skill 9), and *Identifying Missing Information* (Skill 10).

OTHER PERSPECTIVES

AVOID ASSUMPTIONS BASED ON CULTURE

"Giving culturally competent care means being careful to avoid making assumptions about patients' beliefs based on cultural, ethnic, or religious background, alone. For example, nurses ask me if all Hispanic patients believe in the evil eye ('el mal de ojo'). The answer is, 'No.' Each patient—regardless of culture—is an individual, with varying levels of education, experience, and assimilation into mainstream America. Learning the common beliefs, traditions, and health practices of other cultures is important. But, to truly give culturally competent care—to help patients feel respected and supported within their own beliefs—we must assess with an open mind and a true desire to understand each individual's perspective about what's influencing that individual's health."[1]

—Darlene N. Silver, MSN, RN, IBCLC

Clinical Reasoning Exercises: Identifying Assumptions

Example responses are on page 270.

1. Explain why the following statement is an assumption: *We need to teach this patient how to stick to a low-salt diet because he eats whatever he wants.*
2. What could happen if you planned nursing care based on the preceding assumption?
3. Read the following scenarios, and then answer the questions that follow them.

Scenario One

Anita plans to teach Jeff about diabetes today. She's well prepared and decides she'll create a positive attitude for Jeff by telling him about all the advances in diabetic care. She doesn't have much time, so she introduces herself and starts telling him how much easier it is to manage diabetes than it used to be. She goes on to explain how easy it is to learn the required diet, monitor blood sugar, and take insulin. Jeff listens to all Anita has to say, asks a few questions, and then leaves with his wife. As they drive off, he says to his wife in a discouraged tone, "She sure is a know-it-all, isn't she?"

a. In the preceding scenario, what assumption does it seem Anita made about creating a positive attitude?
b. What key thing did Anita forget to do that might have helped her avoid making this assumption?
c. Why do you think Jeff said Anita is a know-it-all?

Scenario Two

Four-year-old Bobby is in the emergency department with his mother. He fell off his bike and had an initial period of unconsciousness lasting about a minute. He's been examined, has no skull fracture, and is now awake and alert and ready to go home with his mother. The nurse gives his mother a computer printout of instructions for checking Bobby's neurologic status and says, "Let me know if you have questions."

a.   In the preceding scenario, what assumption does it seem the nurse has made?

b.   What might happen if the nurse's assumption is incorrect?

Scenario Three

A friend told me the following story:

I was working evenings in the emergency department of a seaside hospital. We admitted a 54-year-old man, whom I'll call Mr. Schmidt. He told me, "I just got here for vacation, and I'm not feeling so great. I had pneumonia at home, got treated, and thought I was better. Now my breathing feels lousy again." A check of his vital signs while he was sitting quietly revealed the following: T 99°, P 138, R 36, BP 168/80. As I helped him to the stretcher, he became significantly more short of breath. I checked his lung sounds and heard a lot of congestion. I notified the physician and voiced my concern that Mr. Schmidt seemed quite ill. The doctor examined him and ordered an ECG and chest x-ray study. During this time we got very busy. I was helping another patient when the physician came to me and said, "I want you to give Mr. Schmidt 80 mg of furosemide (a diuretic) IV now and discharge him. "I looked at him skeptically and said, "Discharge him?" He said, "Yes. I'm sure the diuretic will help him get rid of this fluid." Tactfully, I asked, "Can we give him some time to see how he responds?"

The physician responded: "No. This place is wild. I'm sending him home. He's going to a private physician in the morning. He'll be fine once he gets rid of some fluid. Discharge him with instructions to call if he doesn't feel better." Reluctantly, I went to give Mr. Schmidt the furosemide. I still had trouble with the idea of sending this man home before knowing his response to the IV diuretic. Then I decided to use my own clout as a nurse: I had established a rapport with the Schmidts, and they trusted me. Before I gave the drug, I said, "I realize the doctor has discharged you, but I'd be interested to see if there's any change in blood pressure after you get rid of some fluid. How would you feel about sitting in the waiting room, and I'll check your blood pressure in an hour?" The Schmidts thought this was a good idea and went off to the waiting room. Only 45 minutes had passed when there was a shout for help. I ran to the waiting room and found Mr. Schmidt on the floor having a grand mal seizure. He then stopped breathing.

We were able to resuscitate Mr. Schmidt. He was admitted to the hospital, diagnosed with electrolyte imbalance and heart failure, and discharged a week later.

a.   In the preceding scenario, what assumption does it seem the physician made about Mr. Schmidt's response to the furosemide?

b.   Why do you think the nurse was so concerned about the assumption the physician made?

c. What assumption does it seem the nurse made about how the physician would respond to her if she cautioned him about discharging Mr. Schmidt?

2. ASSESSING SYSTEMATICALLY AND COMPREHENSIVELY

Definition
Using an organized, systematic approach that enhances your ability to discover all the information needed to fully understand a person's health status (e.g., What are the actual and potential problems? What needs aren't being met? What are the person's strengths and resources?)

Why This Skill Is Needed for Clinical Reasoning
Making judgments or decisions based on incomplete information is a leading cause of clinical judgment errors. Having an organized approach to assessment prevents you from forgetting something. For example, you might be interrupted while doing a physical assessment. If you use a printed or electronic assessment tool to record your assessment, you know exactly where you left off and where to continue. If you consistently use the same organized approach, you also form habits that help you be systematic and complete.

Guidelines: How to Assess Systematically and Comprehensively
Being *purposeful and focused* is the key to knowing how to assess systemically and comprehensively: You must decide the purpose of your assessment and use an approach that gets the information needed to *achieve your purpose*. For example, medical assessments focus on identifying diseases or organ or system problems, rather than problems with human responses or activities of daily living (key nursing concerns). If you use only a medical approach to assessment, you may miss key information needed to determine *nursing* needs (e.g., whether the person has a risk for falls). If you use only a nursing approach, you may miss signs and symptoms that indicate the presence of medical problems that need to be reported to the physician immediately (e.g., acute chest pain).

RULE

Always consider *your direct assessment of the patient* to be the *primary source* of information. Also collect information from *secondary resources* (patient records, caregivers, significant others, and print and electronic references (e.g., using drug references to determine side effects of patients' medications).

In compliance with health care regulations and standards, in most settings, you'll use standard print or electronic assessment tools to promote systematic and complete assessment. Some tools are designed for *database assessment* (see Appendix E, page 286). Others are designed for *focus* assessment (see the *Neurologic Focus Assessment Guide* below).

NEUROLOGIC FOCUS ASSESSMENT GUIDE

VITAL SIGNS Temp.____ Pulse____ Resp.____ BP ____
(Check the boxes that apply below)

EYE OPENING
☐ Spontaneous ☐ To command ☐ To pain ☐ No response

MOTOR RESPONSE
☐ Obeys commands ☐ Localizes pain ☐ Flexion withdrawal
☐ Abnormal flexion ☐ Abnormal extension ☐ No response

BEST VERBAL RESPONSE
☐ Oriented ☐ Confused ☐ Inappropriate words
☐ Incomprehensible words ☐ No response

PUPIL REACTION
☐ Right eye:____ Size of pupil____ Reaction to light (brisk, sluggish)
☐ Left eye:____ Size of pupil____ Reaction to light (brisk, sluggish)

GAG REFLEX
☐ Present ☐ Absent ☐ Weak

PURPOSEFUL LIMB MOVEMENT

Right arm
☐ Spontaneous ☐ To command ☐ Paralysis
☐ Visible muscle contraction but no movement
☐ Weak contraction; not enough to overcome gravity
☐ Moves against gravity, not to external resistance
☐ Normal range of motion; can be overcome by increased gravity
☐ Normal muscle strength

Right leg
☐ Spontaneous ☐ To command ☐ Paralysis
☐ Visible muscle contraction but no movement
☐ Weak contraction; not enough to overcome gravity
☐ Moves against gravity, not to external resistance
☐ Normal range of motion; can be overcome by increased gravity
☐ Normal muscle strength

Left arm
☐ Spontaneous ☐ To command ☐ Paralysis
☐ Visible muscle contraction but no movement
☐ Weak contraction; not enough to overcome gravity
☐ Moves against gravity, not to external resistance
☐ Normal range of motion; can be overcome by increased gravity
☐ Normal muscle strength

Left leg
☐ Spontaneous ☐ To command ☐ Paralysis
☐ Visible muscle contraction but no movement
☐ Weak contraction; not enough to overcome gravity
☐ Moves against gravity, not to external resistance
☐ Normal range of motion; can be overcome by increased gravity
☐ Normal muscle strength

Limb Sensation (prick limb with sterile needle)

Right arm:	☐ Normal	☐ Decreased	☐ Absent
Right leg:	☐ Normal	☐ Decreased	☐ Absent
Left arm:	☐ Normal	☐ Decreased	☐ Absent
Left leg:	☐ Normal	☐ Decreased	☐ Absent

Seizure Activity: Describe in nurse's notes.

Electronic and print tools help you develop habits that promote an organized and comprehensive approach to assessment. But, keep in mind that these tools can't *think* for you. Just as you need basic mathematics "in your head" to use a calculator safely, you need to have some approaches "in your head" to give safe and effective care (and to pass the NCLEX®). The following are some points that can help you develop independent critical thinking and clinical reasoning skills related to assessment.

- Before using a tool, make the connection between what information is requested on the tool and *why* it's relevant. For example, suppose you use a neurologic focus assessment tool, and it says to collect data about how the pupils react to light. Ask *why* do I need to check the pupils, and what is the significance of how pupils react to light in context of determining neurologic status?
- Consider both *subjective data* (patient's perceptions) and *objective data* (your observations).
- Remember that assessment tools don't prompt you to use all your resources. After you interview and examine your patient, ask, "What other resources might provide additional information about this person's health status (e.g., medical and nursing records, significant others, other health care professionals)?"
- No *single* tool fits all situations. Think independently. Change your approach to assessment, depending on the person's health status:
  1. If the person is acutely ill, assess urgent problems first (see Skill 13, *Setting Priorities*, page 198).
  2. If the person has a specific complaint, assess that problem first, and then go on to complete the assessment in the same way you would if the person were healthy (next number).
  3. If the person is generally healthy, choose the method that meets your purpose and is most convenient. For example, use the head-to-toe approach, the body systems approach (page 115), or the functional health patterns approach (page 115), or follow a preprinted or electronic assessment tool (page 172).
  4. Practice using various assessment tools, and be sure you understand *why* you collect each piece of data. This will help you learn *what's relevant* to various situations.
- Keep in mind that a body systems approach to assessment helps you collect data about medical problems. Nursing frameworks, such as functional health patterns, help you collect data about human function, activities of daily living, and human responses (nursing problems).
- Always assess the four major vital signs: temperature, pulse, respirations, and blood pressure. Also assess the "fifth and sixth" vital signs: pain and cough, respectively.*Ask about the presence of pain or discomfort, and assess closely as indicated. Ask the

---

*Some consider *pulse oximetry* to be the sixth vital sign. *Pulse oximetry*—using a probe attached to the patient's finger or ear and linked to a computerized unit—monitors the percentage of hemoglobin saturated with oxygen.

person to cough. Although asking the person to cough doesn't replace a thorough lung assessment, you can learn a lot from brief encounters. Say something like, "Can you cough for me, so I can hear how it sounds?" The person's ability (or inability) to comply with this request gives you a lot of information (for example, whether the person has pain with coughing, whether there's congestion, or whether the person coughs well enough to clear the airway). These brief encounters can flag patients that need more in-depth monitoring and assessment.

Clinical Reasoning Exercises: Assessing Systematically and Comprehensively

Example responses are on page 270.

1. Imagine that you're a school nurse and have been asked to do physical exams to screen students for possible medical problems. Identify an organized, comprehensive approach to assessing for signs and symptoms of medical problems.

2. Suppose you make a home visit to a woman who has a newborn child and seven other children younger than 12 years old. Both the baby and the mother are healthy. Identify an organized and comprehensive approach to assessing for nursing and medical problems.

3. Memory-jogs—also called *mnemonics*—can help you remember important information. In the clinical setting, your thinking will be guided by standard evidence-based tools. But, if you ever need to have things "in your head" (e.g., for a test), memory-jogs really help. In the following scenarios, you can practice using both memory-jogs and standard tools. As you read the following scenarios and complete the questions that follow them, think about the difference between using a mnemonic and a standard tool.

Scenario One

Pearl, an 89-year-old grandmother, is admitted with a fractured ankle. She has surgery, and a cast is applied. The cast goes from her toes to the knee. Her toes are visible, and she can wiggle them freely. A small window was cut in the cast over the dorsalis pedis pulse. Routine hospital protocols state that anyone with a cast must have neurovascular checks every 2 hours. You have a standard tool to follow for neurovascular checks, but you also want to remember assessment parameters for a test you're going to take.

Use the following memory-jog to memorize the things you need to check when performing a neurovascular assessment:

Maggie **C**hewed **N**uts **E**very **P**lace **S**he **W**ent, which stands for this:
Movement, **C**olor, **N**umbness, **E**dema, **P**ulses, **S**ensation, **W**armth

a. Based on the preceding memory-jog, how would you assess the neurovascular status of Pearl's injured leg?
b. Why is it necessary to monitor each of the assessment parameters listed in the memory-jog to determine neurovascular status?
c. What would you do if Pearl told you her toes felt numb and cold?

Scenario Two

You have to give Mr. Wu digoxin by mouth. You know that using the memory-jog **TACIT** explained below helps you remember what you need to monitor in patients taking medications.

MONITORING MEDICATION REGIMENS

T—Therapeutic effect (Is there a therapeutic effect?)
A—Allergic or adverse reactions (Are there signs of allergic or adverse reactions?)
C—Contraindications (Are there contraindications to giving this drug?)
I—Interactions? (Are there possible drug interactions?)
T—Toxicity or overdose (Are there signs of toxicity or overdose?)

Assuming that you followed medication reconciliation standards (i.e., you made sure that Mr. Wu's drug regimen is correct and up-to-date), use **TACIT** to systematically gather information about how Mr. Wu is responding to the digoxin, and answer the following questions:
a. What, specifically, would you assess to decide whether to give the digoxin?
b. Why is it important to determine all of the things listed in the mnemonic **TACIT**?

Scenario Three

You just admitted Gerome, who fell off his bike, hit his head, and had a short period of unconsciousness. He is now awake and alert but is admitted for 24 hours of neurologic monitoring. The physician orders neurologic assessments every hour.

Using the *Neurologic Focus Assessment Guide* on page 172, respond to the following questions:
a. How would you assess Gerome to determine the status of each of the neurologic assessment parameters addressed in the guide?
b. Why is each piece of data on the focus assessment guide relevant to determining neurologic status?
c. What would you do if, on admission, Gerome demonstrates normal neurologic assessment findings but 2 hours later demonstrates extreme drowsiness (that is, he awakens only if you shake him and call his name)?
d. What would you do if one pupil started to become more sluggish in its response to light than the other?
e. What would you do if you noted a general pattern of the pulse getting slower than the baseline pulse?

Think, Pair, Share

With a partner, in a group, or in a journal entry, share your thoughts on the following article: Garcia, T. A. (2006). Life of a nurse: An oh-so-simple-tool for nurse educators, preceptors, and mentors. Retrieved January 9, 2011, from http://community.nursingspectrum.com/MagazineArticles/article.cfm?AID= 20107.

3. CHECKING ACCURACY AND RELIABILITY (VALIDATING DATA)

Definition
Collecting more data to verify whether information you gathered is correct and complete.

Why This Skill Is Needed for Clinical Reasoning
Clinical reasoning and judgments must be based on evidence. Verifying that your information is accurate, factual, and complete helps you avoid making assumptions and making decisions based on incorrect or incomplete data. Checking accuracy and reliability also promotes *comprehensive data collection* because you gather more data to double-check your information.

Guidelines: How to Check Accuracy and Reliability
1. Review the data you gathered, and ask questions like these:
   - Do the **objective data** (what you observed) support the **subjective data** (what the patient stated)? For example, if the patient complains of rib pain, how are the breath sounds, and are recent X-rays posted on the record?
   - How do I know this information is reliable?
   - How does this information compare with similar data collected in a different way or at another time (e.g., how does an oral temperature compare with a rectal temperature)?
   - Does this information make sense in the context of this particular patient's health status and situation?
2. Focus your assessment to gain more information about whether your information is correct. For example, an elderly person may have told you that she took her medicine. To verify this, interview significant others or caregivers, check pill containers to see if pills are gone, and ask whether there is any record kept when pills are taken. Remember the following rule.

> **RULE**
>
> **More than one source, more likely of course.** The more information you have coming from different sources, indicating the same thing, the more likely it is that your information is valid and reliable. For example, verify *what your patient says by checking with family members and patient records.*

Clinical Reasoning Exercises: Checking Accuracy and Reliability (Validating Data)

Example responses are on page 272.

For each of the following, determine how to validate whether the information is accurate and reliable:

1. The off-going nurse tells you that Mrs. Molina is depressed and angry about being in the hospital.
2. Mr. Nola tells you his blood sugar was 240 when he tested it an hour ago.
3. You take a blood pressure from the left arm and find it to be abnormally high.
4. A team member tells you that Mr. McGwire needs teaching about diabetic foot care because this is his third admission for foot ulcers.

4. DISTINGUISHING NORMAL FROM ABNORMAL AND IDENTIFYING SIGNS AND SYMPTOMS

Definition
Analyzing patient data and deciding what's within normal range and what's outside the usual range for normalcy; then deciding whether abnormal data may be signs or symptoms of a specific problem.

Example: If a 62-year-old man who takes no medications has a pulse of 42 beats per minute, this is *abnormal* because a normal pulse rate rarely drops below 55 to 60 beats per minute (in someone this age who takes no medications—some cardiac medications lower heart rate). Consider that this may be a *sign* of a heart problem.

Why This Skill Is Needed for Clinical Reasoning
Recognizing abnormal data (signs and symptoms) is the first step to problem identification: Signs and symptoms are like red flags that prompt you to suspect a problem. If you miss these red flags, you allow problems to go untreated.

> **RULE**
>
> If you identify signs and symptoms, but are unsure about what they indicate, activate the chain of command (report them to your instructor, supervisor, or appropriate care provider).

Guidelines: How to Distinguish Normal from Abnormal and Identify Signs and Symptoms

Identifying signs and symptoms requires you to apply knowledge of what are considered to be normal findings. If your patient's findings are *outside the normal range*, then you have identified an abnormality—a *possible sign or symptom*. Use all your senses (sight, hearing, touch, and smell) to gain all the relevant information you need (e.g., if you see cloudy urine, smell it to check its odor).

Ask the following questions:

1. **How does my patient's information compare with accepted standards for normal for someone of this age, culture, disease process, and lifestyle?** If the patient's information isn't within normal accepted standards, this is a possible sign or symptom of a problem.

2. **Does my patient take any medications or have any chronic conditions that change normal function?** For example, if someone is taking a medication that lowers heart rate, this abnormally low heart rate may be normal for him or her. Check action and side effects of all medications.

3. **How does my patient's current information compare with the previously collected data?** This question is especially helpful in situations where the patient has chronic signs and symptoms and you need to decide whether the signs and symptoms are getting *worse*. For example, an asthmatic may always be slightly wheezy. However, if this same person is now wheezier than before, this increased wheezing is a sign of *increasing problems*.

Clinical Reasoning Exercises: Distinguishing Normal from Abnormal and Identifying Signs and Symptoms

Example responses are on page 273.

1. Place an *S* next to the data below that are signs or symptoms of a possible problem or signs or symptoms of a problem that's getting worse. Place an *O* if it's neither a sign nor a symptom. Place a question mark if you need more information to decide.
   a. _____ Temperature of 99.68° F
   b. _____ Bilateral pulmonary rales

   c. _____ Someone tells you she rarely sleeps more than 3 hours at a time
   d. _____ Someone's nasogastric drainage has turned from brown to red
   e. _____ Someone's abdominal incision is slightly red around the sutures
   f. _____ A 2-year-old is inconsolable when his mother leaves the room
   g. _____ Someone with no health problems has developed ankle edema
   h. _____ Someone tells you he bathes every other week
   i. _____ Someone on kidney dialysis never urinates
   j. _____ Pulse of 54 per minute

2. For each question mark you placed above, explain what else you want to know before you decide whether the information is abnormal (and therefore a sign or a symptom).

5. MAKING INFERENCES (DRAWING VALID CONCLUSIONS)

Definition

Making deductions or forming opinions that follow logically, based on patient cues (subjective and objective data)

EXAMPLES OF CUES AND INFERENCES

Cue	Corresponding Inference
Frowning	*Seems worried*
White blood cell count = 14,000	*Probable infection*
Deaf	*Probable communication problems*

Why This Skill Is Needed for Clinical Reasoning

Your ability to interpret data and draw valid conclusions (make inferences) is essential to determining health status. If you draw incorrect conclusions, your clinical judgments will be flawed, which may cause the entire treatment plan to be flawed.

    Making correct inferences helps you focus your assessment to look for additional relevant information. For example, if you infer that an elevated white blood cell count may indicate an infection, you know to look for signs and symptoms of infection (or vice versa).

Guidelines: How to Make Inferences (Draw Valid Conclusions)

Making correct inferences requires knowledge of:
- Signs and symptoms of common complications and health problems
- How humans often behave when faced with health problems (human behavior)

- The common needs of certain age groups (e.g., elderly versus young)
- Cultural and spiritual influences
- Knowledge of *the patient as a person*

For example, to make the inference of *probable infection*, you must know the signs and symptoms of infection. To draw conclusions about someone's lack of eye contact, you must know how eye contact is used in his particular culture (in some cultures, direct eye contact may be disrespectful). To draw conclusions about how to help a diabetic manage his care, you need to know what's important to him as person.

To avoid jumping to conclusions, begin your statements about inferences by saying, "I suspect this information indicates...." Using this phrase reinforces that you to need to collect more data to decide if your suspicions are correct. Once you have enough evidence to support your inference, you can know that you are probably correct. Also remember that principles of critical thinking require you to think about *alternate conclusions and ideas*. If you make an inference, try to think of some other things that you could also reasonably infer. For example, you may infer that a patient is angry with you because she is shouting and irritable. Ask yourself, "Could she really be mad about something else?" **When drawing conclusions about signs and symptoms, remember "MMA"** (medications, medical problems, allergies). Consider whether the signs and symptoms could be related to medications, medical problems, or allergic responses that you need to report.

RULE

More than one cue, more likely it's true—more than one source, more likely of course. Avoid making inferences based on only one cue or only one source (the more facts and sources you have to support your inference, the more likely it is that your inference is correct). After you make an inference, verify whether it's correct by gathering more information and looking for additional cues.

Clinical Reasoning Exercises: Making Inferences (Drawing Valid Conclusions)

Example responses are on page 273.

Make an inference about each of the following data (begin your inference by writing, *I suspect this information indicates* …).

1. Temperature of 102.8° F for 3 days
2. A mother tells you she can't afford prenatal care.
3. A diabetic is 100 pounds overweight and says his blood sugar is always out of control, even though he watches his food intake and takes his insulin regularly.

4. A 6-year-old child whose mother told you he broke his leg falling down the stairs keeps looking at his mother before answering your questions.
5. A usually active, alert grandmother has unkempt appearance and seems a bit confused.

6. CLUSTERING RELATED CUES (DATA)

Definition
Grouping data together in a way that you can see patterns and relationships among the data.

Example: Suppose you grouped the following cues together: 2 years old; temperature 100.8° F; pulse 150 per minute; rash all over trunk; recent measles exposure; never had measles; screaming that he wants his mother. If you consider the relationship among this data, you should suspect that the child's rapid pulse is related to his screaming and elevated temperature rather than a sign of cardiac problems. If you consider *all of the data*, you'll probably suspect that these symptoms indicate the child may have measles.

Why This Skill Is Needed for Clinical Reasoning
Grouping information applies the scientific principle of classifying information to enhance ability to see relationships between and among data. It helps you get a beginning picture of patterns of health or illness. A good way to remember the importance of clustering related data is what I call "the puzzle analogy." When you put together a puzzle, you begin by putting all the edges of the picture in one pile, all the pieces of a certain color in another pile, and so on. Putting the pieces in piles helps you begin to see patterns. The same principle applies to health assessment data, but in health care you cluster *signs and symptoms*.

Guidelines: How to Cluster Related Cues (Data)
1. How you cluster data depends on your purpose:
   - If you're trying to determine the status of medical problems or physiologic responses, cluster the data according to body systems (page 115).
   - If you're trying to determine the status of nursing problems, cluster the data according to a nursing framework (e.g., functional health patterns on page 115).
2. Concept mapping is especially helpful for identifying relationships. Mapping relationships between and among patient cues helps you get a picture of how factors contribute to one another.

Clinical Reasoning Exercises: Clustering Related Cues (Data)

Example responses are on page 274.

Read the following scenarios, and then answer the questions that follow them.

Scenario One

The baby-sitter next door calls and tells you that Jack, the 8-year-old she's watching, was stung by a bee on the ear an hour ago. She tells you the ear is swollen and asks you to come and check him. You go over and examine the child. He asks you if he might die "like the kid on TV did." The baby-sitter tells you she's afraid because she doesn't know where the mother is. You check the ear and find it red, swollen, and free of the stinger. When asked, Jack tells you he was stung before but that it wasn't as scary. Jack has no rash and no wheezing. He asks if he could have a Popsicle and watch TV. His pulse and respirations are normal.

Cluster the information that will help you determine the following:
a. Jack's physical health status
b. Jack's human responses
c. The baby-sitter's learning needs

Scenario Two

Imagine that you just admitted Mr. Nelson, a 41-year-old businessman who has acute abdominal pain. He's never been in the hospital and tells you he hates everything about hospitals. He's been vomiting for 2 days and is unable to keep any food down. His abdomen is distended, and he has no bowel sounds. He is scheduled to go to the operating room at 2 pm for emergency exploratory surgery. He tells you he's worried because his brother died in the hospital. Suddenly he doubles over and says, "This is really getting worse!" You take his vital signs, and they are as follows: T 101°, P 122, R 32, BP 140/80. These signs are the same as those taken an hour ago, except that before, his pulse was 104.

Cluster the information that will help you determine the following:
a. Mr. Nelson's physical status
b. Mr. Nelson's human responses

7. DISTINGUISHING RELEVANT FROM IRRELEVANT

Definition

Deciding what information is pertinent to understanding the situations at hand and what information is immaterial.

Why This Skill Is Needed for Clinical Reasoning

When faced with a lot of information, narrowing it down to only the *pertinent facts* prevents your brain from being cluttered with unnecessary facts. *Deciding what's relevant* is also an example of one of the principles of the scientific method: classifying or categorizing information into groups of related (relevant) information.

Guidelines: How to Distinguish Relevant from Irrelevant

This skill is closely related to Skill 6, *Clustering Related Cues*. Here, however, we're looking at this skill a little differently. In *clustering related cues*, you simply put related information together (for example, you put all the respiratory data in one place, all the nutritional data in another, and so on). In this skill, you *analyze* the data you put together and decide what information is related to a specific health concern. For example, if you suspect constipation, and you note that the person has a sedentary life, poor fiber intake, and takes iron supplements, it's likely that this information is relevant to the constipation.

Distinguishing *relevant from irrelevant* is especially difficult for novices because being able to do **this** depends on having *problem-specific knowledge and experience*. If you're a novice, you'll find that this skill will get easier as you gain more clinical experience.

Here are some strategies that can help you determine what's relevant, even with limited knowledge:

1. List (or map) the abnormal data you collected.
2. Then ask yourself, "Could there be any connection between this (abnormal data) and that (abnormal data)?"
3. As appropriate, ask the person or significant others, "Do you think there's any relationship between this (abnormal data) and that (abnormal data)?"

Clinical Reasoning Exercises: Distinguishing Relevant from Irrelevant

Example responses are on page 274.

Read the following scenarios, and then answer the questions that follow them.

Scenario One

Imagine you work in community health and make a visit to Mrs. Roberts, who is 80 years old and had a cerebrovascular accident (CVA) a month ago. Today you notice she seems to be increasingly confused: She knows where she is, but forgets what day it is and doesn't seem to remember her daily routine. You know that confusion in the elderly can be caused by any of the following: medications, infection, decreased oxygen to the brain, electrolyte imbalance, and brain pathology.

In relation to the preceding scenario, imagine you gathered the data listed in choices *a* through *f* below. Decide its possible relevance to the problem of confusion. Put an *R* in front of the things that are relevant.

a. _____ Recently started taking buspirone hydrochloride for anxiety
b. _____ Temperature: 100.8° F orally
c. _____ History of myocardial infarction 5 years ago
d. _____ Seems dehydrated
e. _____ Has no allergies
f. _____ Regular diet

Scenario Two

You assess Mrs. Clark, a 32-year-old diabetic who is in for a routine visit. When you ask how the new diet is going, she breaks down into tears, saying, "I'm never going to be able to do this!"

Consider the following data, and decide its possible relevance to her problem with sticking to the diabetic diet. Put an *R* in front of the things that are relevant.

a. _____ Diagnosed with diabetes 2 months ago
b. _____ Vital signs within normal limits
c. _____ Complains of constipation
d. _____ Married with three school-age children
e. _____ Loves to cook
f. _____ Has always been 50 pounds overweight
g. _____ Allergic to aspirin

8. RECOGNIZING INCONSISTENCIES

Definition

Realizing when pieces of information contradict each other.

Example: Imagine that you're caring for Fred after chest surgery and he tells you that he has no pain. However, he moves very little and barely breathes when you ask him to take a deep breath. The way he's moving is *inconsistent* with his statements of being pain-free.

Why This Skill Is Needed for Clinical Reasoning

Recognizing inconsistencies prompts you to investigate issues more closely. It sends up a red flag that tells you to probe more deeply to get to the facts. It also helps you focus your assessment to clarify the issues. For example, with Fred in the preceding section, you might say, "It seems to me that you aren't moving very well.... I suspect you have more pain than you admit. I want you to be comfortable, so that you move well and can take deep breaths to clear your lungs. Are you sure there isn't a particular spot that's bothering you?"

Guidelines: How to Recognize Inconsistencies

One way to recognize inconsistencies is to compare what the patient states (subjective data) with what you observe (objective data). If what the *person states* isn't supported by what *you observe*, you have inconsistent information and need to investigate further.

    Recognizing inconsistencies requires problem-specific knowledge. For example, suppose you have the following data:

Subjective Data: Patient states, "I must have strained my back lifting my child. My right side is killing me."

Objective Data: Fever of 102.4° F; cloudy, foul-smelling urine.

    If you know how back injuries usually present themselves, you know that the subjective and objective data are *inconsistent* with a back injury and *more consistent* with a urinary tract infection.

To Recognize Inconsistencies with Limited Knowledge

1. Determine the signs and symptoms of the problem you suspect by looking up the problem in a reference. For example, if you suspect pneumonia—something you should report immediately—look up the signs and symptoms of pneumonia.

2. Compare the information in the reference with your patient's data. If your patient's signs and symptoms are *different* from those listed in the reference, you have *inconsistencies* and must investigate further. Assess the person more closely, and consider other problems that the signs and symptoms might represent. For example, are the signs and symptoms more consistent with a cold or flu than pneumonia?

> ### Clinical Reasoning Exercises: Recognizing Inconsistencies

Example responses are on page 274.

Read the following scenarios, and then answer the questions that follow them.

Scenario One

You interview Cathy in the prenatal clinic 2 weeks before delivery. You ask her how she feels about the baby coming. She tells you she's happy that she gets to see the baby in only 2 weeks. When you ask her if she has any questions about the delivery, she tells you she's been going to birthing classes with her boyfriend and feels like she knows what to expect.

You review her records and notice that her first clinic visit was 2 weeks ago, when she came with her mother.

a. Identify inconsistencies in the preceding scenario.

b. Explain what you might do to clarify the inconsistencies you identified.

Scenario Two

You're in the grocery store and a 20-year-old woman comes up to you and says, "Please help me! I can't breathe, and my heart is racing." She is sweating profusely and says, "I feel like I'm having a heart attack and I'm going to die!" You help her sit down, then take her pulse, and find it to be 100 per minute, regular, and strong. Her respirations are 36 per minute. She tells you she has no pain, but wants you to call an ambulance. You offer emotional support and ask someone to call 911. As you wait for the ambulance, she tells you this has happened to her several times before and that she has had an electrocardiogram, which showed normal cardiac function.

How consistent are this woman's signs, symptoms, and risk factors with those of a cardiac problem?

9. IDENTIFYING PATTERNS

Definition

Deciding what patterns of health, illness, or function are indicated by patient data.

Example: Suppose you cluster together cues of chronic productive cough, wheezing, and exercise intolerance and decide that they indicate a pattern of respiratory problems. Keep in mind that *identifying patterns* means looking at signs and symptoms *over a period of time,* not just as single incidences. You may have a headache, but this isn't considered *a pattern* (unless you are having a lot of headaches).

Why This Skill Is Needed for Clinical Reasoning

Identifying patterns helps you (1) get a beginning picture of problems, and (2) recognize gaps in data collection. Once you recognize gaps in data collection, you can decide how to focus your assessment to gain that missing information. Using the puzzle analogy, when you put some pieces together, you start to see what the end picture will be.

Here's an example of how *identifying patterns* helps you discover missing pieces of information. Suppose you clustered together the following data:

- No bowel movement in 3 days
- Abdominal fullness
- States he's been "constipated off and on for the past month"

You'll probably decide that the preceding cues represent a pattern of bowel elimination problems. Having recognized this pattern, you know to focus your assessment to gain more information and decide exactly what the problem with bowel elimination is. For example, you ask, "What does *off and on* mean?" The person responds, "I get so constipated I have to take laxatives, and then I get diarrhea." This added information is likely to make you suspect that the bowel elimination problem may be caused in part by laxative abuse. You then explore his knowledge of how diet, fluids, and exercise influence bowel function. You also need to ask when the person had a physical exam by a doctor and whether this bowel problem was evaluated, as changes in bowel elimination is one of the danger signs of cancer.

Guidelines: How to Identify Patterns

To identify patterns:

1. Analyze the cues you put together and decide which of the following patterns they represent:
    - **Normal Pattern** (no signs and symptoms of the pattern present)
    - **Risk for Abnormal Pattern** (risk factors for the pattern present)
    - **Abnormal Pattern** (signs and symptoms of an abnormal pattern present)
2. After you get a beginning idea of the patterns, look for gaps in data collection by asking, "What other information might clarify my understanding of this pattern?"

Clinical Reasoning Exercises: Identifying Patterns

Example responses are on page 275.

Matching: Decide which numbers best match the phrases in the letters that follow on the next page.

1. Potential (risk) for impaired bowel elimination pattern
2. Potential (risk) for ineffective sexual-reproductive pattern
3. Probably normal sleep-rest pattern
4. Impaired respiratory function pattern
5. Probably normal coping pattern

a. Bilateral rales; respirations increased to 34 per minute; coughing up thick, white mucus

b. States, "I can cope with my illness, so long as I have help from my husband." Manages daily self-care; has husband cook all meals; passes the time by knitting blankets for the homeless

c. Eats little fiber; just started taking codeine every 4 hours; drinks about three glasses of water daily; spends most of her time in bed; normal bowel function

d. Works nights; sleeps 4 hours in the morning and 3 hours just before going to work at night

e. Has just been diagnosed with genital herpes; single; worried about transmitting herpes to future sex partners and future children (during delivery)

10. IDENTIFYING MISSING INFORMATION

Definition
Recognizing gaps in data collection and searching for information to fill in the gaps

Why This Skill Is Needed for Clinical Reasoning
Recognizing gaps in information and filling in those gaps prevents you from making one of the most common clinical reasoning errors: making judgments based on incomplete information. It also helps you gain a deep understanding of the situations at hand.

Guidelines: How to Identify Missing Information
1. Don't try to do it all in your head—reflect *on recorded data* and ask, "What's missing here?" You may have to print out electronic information so that you can see more of it at once.
2. If you're not sure if you really need more information, ask questions like, "What difference will it make?" or "How will knowing this information change the approach to treatment?" If the information won't change your approach, then you may not need to take the time to gather it.
3. Other strategies for recognizing missing information include accomplishing all of the following clinical reasoning skills: *identifying assumptions; checking accuracy and reliability; clustering related cues; recognizing inconsistencies; identifying patterns;* and *evaluating and correcting thinking.*

Clinical Reasoning Exercises: Identifying Missing Information

Example responses are on page 275.

Go back to the Clinical Reasoning Exercises for the previous skill, *identifying patterns*. For each pattern represented by the information listed in *a* through *e* on page 188, decide what information might be missing that could add to your understanding of the pattern.

11. PROMOTING HEALTH BY IDENTIFYING AND MANAGING RISK FACTORS

Note: This skill deals with *identifying risk factors* in healthy people. The next skill, *diagnosing actual and potential problems* deals with identifying risk factors in the context of people with existing health problems.

Definition
Maximizing well-being by detecting and managing factors that evidence shows contribute to health problems (e.g., sedentary lifestyles contribute to many health problems)

Why This Skill Is Needed for Clinical Reasoning
You don't wait for problems to appear to put a plan into action. By identifying risk factors, you apply the proactive *predict, prevent, manage, promote (PPMP)* approach, rather than the reactive *diagnose and treat (DT)* approach (see Chapter 3, pages 84 to 85).

Guidelines: How to Identify and Manage Risk Factors
1. Assess people's awareness of—and motivation for—identifying and managing risk factors. For example, do they know what's required for adequate nutrition, rest, exercise, and spiritual and psychological well-being? Are they able and willing to do what's needed to reduce risks? *Not knowing about risk factors* and *not wanting do something about them* are risk factors in themselves.

2. Keep growth and development in mind. **Examples:**
   - A woman who is pregnant or planning on becoming pregnant must consider risk factors for both herself and the fetus when taking medications. She should know that inadequate intake of folic acid increases risk of spontaneous abortion and other problems such as spina bifida in the infant.
   - After menopause, women should be aware that they should be screened for osteoporosis (decreased bone density).

3. Look for risk factors that are known to put people at risk for a variety of common problems. **Examples:** Obesity, poor diet, high cholesterol, tobacco use, immobility, sedentary life, stressful life, poor sleeping habits, allergies, chronic illness, extremes of age (very young or old), low socioeconomic status, illiteracy, sun exposure, and excessive use of medications, alcohol, or illicit drugs.

4. Also assess for the following:
   - Genetic, cultural, or biologic factors (e.g., race, family history, and personal history predisposing one to health problems)
   - Behavioral factors (e.g., problems with anger management, attention-deficit disorders)
   - Psychosocial and/or economic factors (e.g., lack of significant others, poverty)
   - Environmental factors (e.g., air quality)
   - Age-related factors (e.g., women after menopause are at risk for osteoporosis; infants are at risk for ear infection)
   - Sexual-pattern factors (e.g., whether one is sexually active and with whom)
   - Safety-related factors (e.g., whether seat belts are worn, whether the home environment is safe for children)
   - Disease-related factors (e.g., someone with chronic lung disease is at risk for pneumonia; someone with diabetes is at risk for skin problems)
   - Treatment-related factors (e.g., complicated medication or treatment regimen)

5. Teach the importance of managing risk factors to prevent costly, debilitating illnesses.

6. **For more strategies on risk management,** go to the following Web pages:
   - Harvard Center for Risk Analysis (www.hcra.harvard.edu), which is dedicated to promoting reasoned public responses to health, safety, and environmental hazards. It also gives statistics and approaches for problems like stroke, heart disease, suicide, cancer, and drowning and other accidents.
   - The Centers for Disease Control and Prevention (www.cdc.gov), which has a wealth of information on disease and disability prevention.
   - Healthy People (http://www.healthypeople.gov/), which challenges individuals, communities, and professionals to take specific steps to ensure that good health and long life are enjoyed by all.

You can also look up "risk factors" in the index of up-to-date textbooks or on Google. Usually you can find excellent tables on common diseases and risk factors that present information in an easy-to-grasp format.

Clinical Reasoning Exercises: Promoting Health by Identifying and Managing Risk Factors

Example responses are on page 275.

1. You assess a 25-year-old man and determine that he is healthy. What questions might you ask to identify risk factors for possible problems?
2. You assess a 72-year-old woman and find that she is healthy, but she says "I tend to be a little clumsy—I lose my balance." Why should you be concerned about this?
3. A 50-year-old man says, "I'm getting to the age where I should be doing more to look after myself, and I want to know more about my risk factors." How do you respond?

12. DIAGNOSING ACTUAL AND POTENTIAL PROBLEMS

This skill deals with *identifying risk factors* in the context of people with existing health problems. The preceding skill deals with risk factors in the context of healthy people.

Definition
Ensuring that the actual and potential problems your patient has are correctly named, based on evidence from the health assessment and patient records.

This skill includes: (1) ensuring that signs and symptoms of health problems that are beyond your practice scope are referred to the appropriate health care professional, (2) choosing the name that best describes the problem (the definitive diagnosis), (3) determining the cause(s) and contributing factors of the problem, and (4) providing the evidence that leads you to believe the diagnosis, problem, or issue is present.

Why This Skill Is Needed for Clinical Reasoning
This skill is important for the following reasons:
1. Making *definitive diagnoses* (the most specific, correct diagnoses) is key to being able to determine the *specific actions* designed to prevent, manage, or resolve them. If you miss problems, are too vague about the problems, or name them incorrectly, you have made a diagnostic error that may cause you to:
    - Initiate actions that *aggravate* the problems or *waste time.*
    - Omit essential actions required to prevent and manage the problems.
    - Allow problems to go untreated.
    - Influence others to make the same mistake you did.

> **RULE**
>
> **Ensuring accurate problem identification is the key to specific treatment.** If you suspect a problem, but are unsure, don't jump to conclusions. Instead report the problem by saying something like this: "I am not sure, but there seems to be some sort of issue with [fill in the blank] or....there seems to be a pattern of [fill in the blank]."

2. You don't fully understand the problem(s)—or know what to do about them—until you clearly identify what's *causing or contributing* to them.
3. Predicting potential problems and complications helps you:
   - Know what signs and symptoms to look for when monitoring the patient.
   - Anticipate what could happen if things get worse (therefore allowing you to plan ahead to be prepared)
4. *Providing the supporting evidence* that led you to the diagnosis helps others understand the problem better. For example, compare the two following problem statements, and decide which one gives a better picture of the problem.
   - Potential for violence
   - Potential for violence related to anger management problems as evidenced by history of previous violence and refusal to attend anger management programs.

The above gives a summary statement for a diagnosis. Alternatively, use a diagram or map as shown in Figure 5-1.

Guidelines: How to Diagnose Actual and Potential Problems

As with Skill 5 *(Making Inferences)*, your ability to identify and predict problems depends on your knowledge of common health problems, human behavior, needs of certain age groups (e.g., elderly versus young), and cultural and spiritual influences. It also requires knowledge of *the patient as a person*. Experts can usually identify problems more quickly than novices because they've "seen it all before." They have better hunches about what the problems might be, and they move through problem identification in rapid, dynamic ways.

If your knowledge and expertise are limited, you are at risk of making any one of the following diagnostic (problem identification) errors:

- Making a diagnosis or naming the problem without considering whether the data may represent a *different problem altogether* (e.g., assuming indigestion signifies gastric reflux or upset stomach instead of possible coronary problems)
- Not considering all the relevant data because of a narrow focus (e.g., not looking for other coronary symptoms because you decide that the person simply has indigestion)

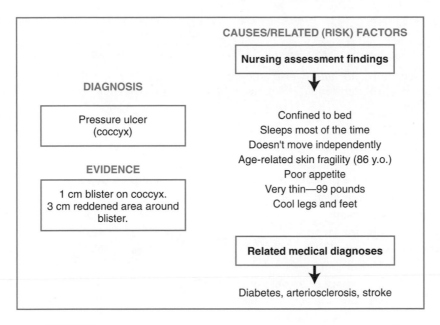

FIGURE 5-1 Using diagrams and maps to illustrate diagnosis.

■ Failing to recognize personal biases or assumptions. For example, thinking that someone is faking pain because he doesn't *look* like he's in pain. (Knowledgeable nurses know that people handle pain differently and that often outward signs of pain are not present, even though the person is experiencing significant discomfort. This is especially true for people with chronic pain.)

■ Overanalyzing ("analysis paralysis") and delaying taking action

Identifying Actual Problems

1. Verify that your information is correct and complete. If you're not sure what to do next, *make patient safety number one*: Report signs and symptoms to a more qualified nurse before going on to complete problem identification.

2. Avoid drawing conclusions or identifying problems based on only *one cue* or one source ("More than one cue, more likely it's true. More than one source, more likely of course").

3. Cluster abnormal data (signs and symptoms): Cluster according to body systems to identify medical problems and according to a nursing framework to identify nursing problems. Looking at data from *both* medical and nursing perspectives helps you see *different* problems.

4. Consider the signs and symptoms, and ask yourself what information you could have missed.

5. Create a list of problems that may be suggested by the signs and symptoms. Box 5-1 (next page) gives an example checklist to consider possible problems.

BOX 5-1 CHECKLIST FOR IDENTIFYING ACTUAL AND POTENTIAL PROBLEMS

1. List current medications (include over-the-counter and herbal drugs). Ask yourself whether any of the patient's problems could be related to any of the medications (remember **SODA**).
   S—Side effect?
   O—Overdose?
   D—Drug interaction?
   A—Allergy or **A**dverse reaction?
2. List current and past allergies, diseases, surgeries, or trauma.
3. Consider whether any of the patient's current problems are related to Questions 1 or 2 above.
4. Complete the following checklist: (Circle those that apply)

Is there a problem with breathing?	Yes	No	AR[1]	Pos[2]
Is there a problem with circulation?	Yes	No	AR	Pos
Is there a problem with comfort?	Yes	No	AR	Pos
Is there a problem with nutrition?	Yes	No	AR	Pos
Is there a problem with urinary or bowel elimination?	Yes	No	AR	Pos
Is there a problem with fluid or electrolyte balance?	Yes	No	AR	Pos
Is there a problem with ability to think or perceive environment?	Yes	No	AR	Pos
Is there a problem with communication?	Yes	No	AR	Pos
Is there a problem with safety (risk for injury or falls)?	Yes	No	AR	Pos
Is there a problem with sleeping or exercising?	Yes	No	AR	Pos
Is there a risk for infection (self or transmission to others)?	Yes	No	AR	Pos
Is there a risk for impaired skin integrity?	Yes	No	AR	Pos
Is there a problem with coping or stress?	Yes	No	AR	Pos
Is there a psychological, developmental, self-esteem problem?	Yes	No	AR	Pos
Is there a socio-cultural problem?	Yes	No	AR	Pos
Is there a problem with roles, relationships, or sexuality?	Yes	No	AR	Pos
Does the person have a problem with taking medications?	Yes	No	AR	Pos
Does the patient require teaching?	Yes	No	AR	Pos
Is there a problem with health maintenance at home?	Yes	No	AR	Pos
Is this admission going to cause difficulties at home?	Yes	No	AR	Pos
Is there a problem with personal or religious beliefs?	Yes	No	AR	Pos
Is there a problem with coping or managing stress?	Yes	No	AR	Pos
Could this person be pregnant?	Yes	No	AR	Pos

[1]AR = At risk for problem (no signs and symptoms present, but risk factors are evident).
[2]Pos = Possible problem (insufficient data, but you suspect a problem).
Copyright 2011 by R. Alfaro-LeFevre. www.AlfaroTeachSmart.com

6. After you complete your list of suspected problems, compare your patient's signs and symptoms with the signs and symptoms of the problems you suspect. Some call this phase "testing hunches (hypotheses)."
7. Name the problems by using the term that most closely matches your patient's signs and symptoms. **Example:** If your patient's signs and symptoms match the signs and symptoms of *anxiety,* better than *fear,* label the problem *anxiety.*
8. Determine what's causing or contributing to the problems.

> **RULE**
>
> **Diagnosis is <u>incomplete</u> until you identify not only the problems, but also the <u>underlying causes and contributing factors</u> of the problems.** You can't adequately prevent or treat the problems unless you understand both the problems and what's causing or contributing to them.

   ■ Always ask yourself whether it's possible that medications, medical problems, or allergies are causing the problems. If so, activate the chain of command to notify the professional most qualified to manage the problem.
   ■ Ask the patient and significant others if they can identify factors that are contributing to the problems.
   ■ Consider whether there are factors related to age, disease process, treatments, medications, or life changes that could be contributing to the problems.
9. As appropriate, use the following strategies:
   ■ Draw a map to clarify relationships between problems and signs, symptoms, or risk factors.
   ■ Use the Systematic Problem Analysis Worksheet (next page) to systematically consider possible causative factors.
10. If a summary diagnostic statement is required:
   ■ Use the memory-jog **PRE** (**p**roblem, **r**elated or **r**isk factors, **e**vidence) to describe the following:
   P—Problem
   R—Related factors (risk and contributing factors)
   E—Evidence (patient data) that led you to conclude the problem exists
   ■ Use "related to" to link the problem and its cause. **Example:** *Acute pain related to left rib fracture as evidenced by statements of extreme tenderness in the left rib cage area.*

Predicting Potential Problems/Complications
1. Find out the patient's allergies, current and past medical and nursing problems, medications, treatments, or experiences of invasive monitoring.
2. Look up problems and complications often associated with the above. Chapter 3 (pages 103 to 105) helps you predict potential complications.

SYSTEMATIC PROBLEM ANALYSIS WORKSHEET

Instructions:

1. List the focus problem, diagnosis, issue, or in box below.
2. Put a check mark in all boxes on the right that correspond to factors that contribute to the problem, diagnosis, or issue you identified.
3. Decide what factors must be managed and who will manage them.
4. Use back of page or figure of man as needed.

CONTRIBUTING OR RELATED (RISK) FACTORS

Actual / potential diagnosis, problem, or issue

1. Main reason for admission or contact?

2. Vulnerability—constitutional or age-related factors?
☐ Age ____ Weight ____ Height ____ Mental Status? ____
☐ Communication ability? ☐ Smoker? ☐ Drinker (alcohol)?
☐ Skin status? ☐ Nutrition-hydration status?
☐ Mobility or self-care problems?
☐ Bowel elimination or urine elimination problems?
☐ Immune system status? ☐ Overall health status/resilience?
☐ Other?

3. Allergy, medication, or treatment-related factors?
☐ Allergies? ☐ Considered all meds (Rx, OTC, herbal)?
☐ Treatments?

4. Co-existing medical problems, injuries, or pathophysiology?
☐ Neuro? ☐ Resp? ☐ Cardiac-circulatory? ☐ GI? ☐ GU?
☐ Diabetes? ☐ Hypertension? ☐ Depression? ☐ Other?

5. Environmental factors? Patient identified factors?
☐ Current environment (include work)? ☐ Role-related?
☐ Other factors?

6. Comfort factors? Mobility problems? Self-care problems?
☐ Pain level? ☐ Pain management? ☐ Self-mobile? ☐ Other?

7. Socioeconomic, spiritual, cultural factors?
☐ Family issues? ☐ Coping problems? ☐ Support systems limited?
☐ Other?

Examples: If the person has diabetes, there is a risk for foot ulcers and poor healing. If your patient just had a myocardial infarction (MI) and has an arterial line in place, determine common potential complications of MI (e.g., congestive heart failure, arrhythmias, pericarditis, MI extension, and cardiac arrest) and of the arterial line (e.g., thrombus or emboli).

3. Look for common risk factors as addressed in Skill 11, *Promoting Health by Identifying and Managing Risk Factors* (page 189). If the person has common risk factors for a problem but does not actually have signs and symptoms, name the potential complication. For example, if someone is taking an anticoagulant, they have a *potential for bleeding*.

CRITICAL MOMENTS

TOLERATING AMBIGUITY: A GOOD THING—OR NOT

Acceptance of ambiguity is often listed in the literature as a critical thinking characteristic. Certainly there are times, as the saying goes, that there is "no black or white—only gray." But you must ask, "How much ambiguity is acceptable in this particular situation?" For example, if you were sick, would you be happy with an ambiguous diagnosis, or would you want it to be specific? Remember that clearly and specifically defining *the problem and its cause* helps you identify *specific* treatment and interventions to resolve it.

Clinical Reasoning Exercises: Diagnosing Actual and Potential Problems

Example responses are on page 276.

1. Write a summary statement that best describes the potential problem in the following scenario (state the problem and the related factors). Alternatively, draw a map or diagram.

Scenario

You just admitted Nigel to the psychiatric unit. He is agitated but won't talk to anyone. You check previous records and note that he has a history of striking caregivers.

2. Based on the information given in the following scenario, predict the potential complications Elaine might experience.

Scenario

Elaine is in the recovery room after having an emergency appendectomy under general anesthesia. She's very groggy and extremely nauseated.

3. Based on the information in the following scenario, write a summary statement that best describes the problem, using the PRE format (see Point 10 on page 195).

Scenario

Susan is a single working mother of three children. She tells you that she has never been a very organized person and is having trouble coping with the many demands on her time. Her children look healthy and happy, but her house is cluttered and she appears disheveled.

4. Imagine that you're caring for a 41-year-old man with four fractured ribs. What other information might you need to determine if he is at high risk for respiratory problems?

 Think, Pair, Share

Learn how to assess and diagnose various problems by using the "working backwards strategy" as explained here: A major clinical reasoning principle is "assess before you diagnose." In a postclinical conference or study group, get a list of 10 commonly encountered problems or diagnoses (e.g., risk for infection, postoperative complications) and "work backwards"—assess whether your patients are at risk for any of the diagnoses problems, or actually have those problems. To choose your 10 common problems, ask your instructor, mentor, or manager. Or, use the boxes that address common problems and complications on pages 103 to 105 in Chapter 3. When you assess for specific problems over and over again, these problems become priority problems "in your head." You get good at assessing those particular problems and will not forget.

13. SETTING PRIORITIES

Definition

In this section, *setting priorities is defined in two ways:* (1) *differentiating between problems needing immediate attention and those requiring subsequent action,* and (2) *deciding what problems must be addressed in the patient record.*

Why This Skill Is Needed for Clinical Reasoning

This skill is important for the following reasons:

1. If you don't know how to set priorities, you may cause life-threatening treatment delays. For example, if you don't assign high priority to dealing with symptoms of congestive heart failure (CHF), it can progress to *pulmonary edema and death.*

2. If you give equal attention to *major* and *minor* problems, you won't be able to devote the time you need to manage the *most important* problems. Not only will your patients suffer, but you will constantly feel disorganized and overwhelmed.

3. To communicate care priorities to the health care team, all problems that *must* be managed to achieve the *overall outcomes* must be recorded in the patient record.

Guidelines: How to Set Priorities

Note: *Managing Your Time* (in Chapter 6, pages 240 to 245) gives additional strategies setting priorities inside and outside of the clinical setting. *Delegating Safely and Effectively* (pages 111 to 112) addresses how to make decisions about what care must be done *only by you* and what care you should delegate.

Strategies for Setting Priorities

1. Ask patients to name the three main problems they are experiencing right *now*.

RULE

Patients rarely present with an isolated problem. Rather, they have several *interrelated* problems that contribute to one another (e.g., *dehydration* contributes to *weakness,* which contributes to *increased risk of falls*). Developing a problem list and determining *relationships* among the problems is key to setting priorities.

---

2. Apply the principles and strategies listed in Boxes 5-2 and 5-3 (page 201). Note that there's more than one way to set priorities. Choose the one that makes the most sense to you in context of each situation.

RULE

Always give safety issues (e.g., medication safety, fall and injury prevention, infection prevention, safety with activities of daily living, prevention of skin problems, hazards related to immobility, and patient education needs) high priority.

BOX 5-2	SETTING PRIORITIES USING MASLOW'S HIERARCHY OF NEEDS
PRIORITIES	**PROBLEMS**
No. 1	**Survival needs** (e.g., food, fluids, oxygen, elimination, warmth, physical comfort)
No. 2	Safety and security needs (e.g., risks of injury or infection, threats to feeling secure, emotional discomfort)
No. 3	**Love and belonging needs** (e.g., family problems, separation from loved ones)
No. 4	Self-esteem needs (e.g., need for privacy, respect, independence, and positive self-image)
No. 5	**Self-actualization needs** (e.g., need to grow and achieve personal goals; self-efficacy)

Summarized from Maslow, A. (1970). *Motivation in personality.* New York: Harper & Row.

3. To determine what problems *must* be recorded in the patient record:
    - Clarify the *overall* expected outcome(s). **Example:** Mrs. Garcia will return home and be able to manage diabetic regimen independently. (How to determine expected outcomes is addressed in the next skill. To help you complete this section, outcomes are provided for you.)
    - Decide *what problems must be addressed* in order to achieve the *overall outcomes.* For example, for Mrs. Garcia above, she may have the following two problems, but only the first one relates to the *overall outcome* (and therefore must be addressed in the plan of care).
        1. Patient Education: Diabetes management, blood glucose, and insulin administration
        2. Ineffective coping related to marital problems

RULE

Set priorities by applying the "80/20 Rule." Think of all the things you have to do for your patients as 100%. Then figure out the 20% that *must get done* to stay on track and keep patients safe. This is where you need to spend 80% of your time.

Clinical Reasoning Exercises: Setting Priorities

Example responses are on page 276.

1. If the expected outcome is *will be discharged home in 5 days and able to manage colostomy care,* which of the following problems *must* be addressed in the patient record?
    a. Anxiety related to inability to return to work for 6 weeks
    b. Patient Education: colostomy care
    c. Risk for impaired skin integrity related to colostomy drainage
2. Applying the information on setting priorities in Box 5-3, what is the *most immediate* priority in the scenario below.

Scenario   Mr. Potter, a 64-year-old construction worker, is admitted with a right calf thrombophlebitis. He is a smoker and has a cold, which is causing frequent sneezing and a productive cough. The doctor has ordered bed rest, warm soaks, and anticoagulants, and bathroom privileges for bowel movements only. Mr. Potter tells you he needs to use the bathroom. Then he mentions that he has been having chest discomfort.

BOX 5-3 PRINCIPLES AND STEPS OF SETTING PRIORITIES

Principles of Setting Priorities
1. **Make sure you have "the big picture" of all the patient's problems.** Make a list of current medications, medical problems, allergies, and chief complaints. Refer to them frequently because they may affect how you set priorities.
2. **Determine the *relationships* among the problems**: If problem Y causes problem Z, problem Y takes priority over problem Z. **Example:** If pain is causing immobility, *pain management* is a high priority.
3. **Setting priorities is a dynamic, changing process**; at times, the order of priority changes, depending on the seriousness and relationship of the problems. **Example:** If abnormal lab values are at life-threatening levels, they are likely to be highest priority; if your patient is having trouble breathing because of acute rib pain, managing the pain may be a higher priority than dealing with a rapid pulse, because the pain is causing the rapid pulse.
4. Develop a multidisciplinary problem list, and refer to it frequently. These types of lists promote team communication by giving the big picture of all patient problems that *must* be addressed.

Steps for Setting Priorities
1. Ensure patient and caregiver safety and infection prevention.
2. Assign high priority to *first-level* priority problems (immediate priorities): Remember "ABCs plus V":
   A—**A**irway problems
   B—**B**reathing problems
   C—**C**ardiac and **c**irculation problems
   V—**V**ital signs concerns (e.g., high fever; hypertension, hypotension)
   EXCEPTION: With CPR for cardiac arrest, begin chest compressions immediately (see www.americanheart.org, for the most current CPR guidelines).
3. Attend to *second-level* priority problems:
   • Mental status change (e.g., confusion, decreased alertness)
   • Untreated medical problems requiring immediate attention (e.g., a diabetic who hasn't had insulin)
   • Acute pain
   • Acute urinary elimination problems
   • Abnormal lab values
   • Risks of infection, safety, or security (for patient or for others)
4. Address *third-level* priority problems (later priorities):
   • Health problems that don't fit into the above categories (e.g., problems with lack of knowledge, activity, rest, family coping)

14. DETERMINING PATIENT-CENTERED (CLIENT-CENTERED) OUTCOMES

Definition

Describing exactly what results will be observed in the patient to show the expected benefits of care at a certain point in time.

Example: Twenty-four hours after endotracheal intubation for open-heart surgery, the patient will be able to breathe independently without the tube. Before going on to complete this section, be sure you have studied pages 89 to 90 in Chapter 3, which describe various types of outcomes (clinical, functional, and other types) and address the role of outcomes in the context of evidence-based practice.

Why This Skill Is Needed for Clinical Reasoning

On a daily basis, outcomes (results) are often *implied*—if you're doing something to fix a problem, you obviously expect to see an improvement in the problem. However, in complex situations and when developing formal or standard plans, outcomes are stated according to *very specific rules* as noted in this section. Following the rules forces you to think things through and helps you to record very specific outcome that can be used to guide and evaluate care.

Identifying individualized patient-centered outcomes promotes efficiency because they help you:

■ Explain why the treatment plan is worthwhile (they delineate the expected benefits of care).

■ Keep the focus on *how the person is responding* to care, the most important measure of how well the plan is working.

■ Motivate key players—knowing the benefits and time frame for outcome achievement prompts patients and caregivers to initiate actions in a timely fashion.

■ Determine priorities. You need to know *exactly what you aim to do* before you can decide what's most important and what must be done first.

■ Determine specific interventions designed to achieve the outcomes. As the saying goes, "If you don't know where you're going, it's hard to figure out how to get there."

Guidelines: How to Determine Patient-Centered (Client-Centered) Outcomes

Study the following principles, and then go on to the following section, which addresses how to individualize outcomes when using standard plans and critical pathways.

Principles of Patient-Centered (Client-Centered) Outcomes

1. To describe expected outcomes, use terms that explain the *benefits* expected to be *observed in the patient* after care is given.

2. If you don't understand the difference between clinical, functional, quality of life, and other types of outcomes, or the interplay between outcomes and problems, study pages 89 to 90 in Chapter 3.

3. Partner with key stakeholders to develop outcomes *together*. Be realistic, considering:
   - Physical health state; overall prognosis
   - Growth and development; psychological/mental status
   - Spiritual, cultural, and economic needs
   - Expected length of stay
   - Available human, material, and financial resources
   - Other planned therapies for the client

4. Expected outcomes may be identified from a *problem* or *intervention* perspective.
   - **Outcomes identified for problems** describe exactly what will be observed in the patient to show that the problems are resolved (or managed). For example, what will be observed when a patient no longer has trouble feeding himself?
   - **Outcomes identified for interventions** describe the *desired response* to the intervention. For example, what will be observed in the patient after you irrigate his nasogastric tube?

RULE

There's a dynamic relationship between problems, interventions, and outcomes: (1) If you aren't achieving desired outcomes, ask, "Are we sure that we identified the problems correctly?" "Are we sure that we're using the right interventions?" and "Have we included the patient and key stakeholders in decision-making?" (2) To prioritize care, be sure that you have clearly determined the problems, issues, and risks that must be managed to achieve the *overall* outcomes of the plan of care. Problem and risk identification is at least 50% of the work of planning care.

5. **To determine expected outcomes for problems:** Reverse the problem—describe what will be observed *in the patient* when the problem no longer exists or is managed at an acceptable level (see the following diagram).

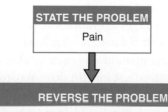

STATE THE PROBLEM

Pain

REVERSE THE PROBLEM

Expected outcome: Using a numerical or picture pain scale, **the patient will describe absence of pain** or ability to manage pain at a level that allows her to complete daily activities and get enough sleep at night.

6. **To determine expected outcomes for interventions:** Describe what will be observed *in the patient* to demonstrate that the *desired response* to the intervention has been achieved (see the following diagram).

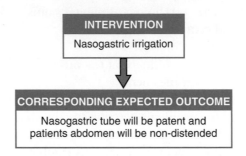

7. To ensure that outcomes are specific, they should have the following components:
   - **Subject:** Who is expected to achieve the outcome? Or, what part of the patient will be observed to demonstrate the expected benefit?
   - **Verb:** What will the person do (or what will be observed) to demonstrate outcome achievement?
   - **Condition:** Under what circumstances will the person do it?
   - **Performance Criteria:** How well will the person do it?
   - **Target Time:** By when will the person be able to do it?

   Examples: "By Friday, Jim will walk with a walker to the end of the hall." Or, "By Friday, the skin on the bottom of the heel will be intact and free from signs of irritation."

8. Use verbs for actions that are observable and measurable (actions you can clearly *see, hear, feel, or smell*).
   - **Use verbs like these:** *explain, describe, state, list, demonstrate, show, communicate, express, walk, gain,* and *lose.*
   - **Don't use verbs like these:** *know, understand, appreciate, feel* (these aren't measurable because no one can read someone else's mind to find out if they know, understand, appreciate, and so on).

9. To give a summary statement to guide evaluation, use *as evidenced by* to describe *exactly what behaviors will indicate that the outcome has been met.* **Example:** "The patient will demonstrate diabetes management *as evidenced by* ability to state how insulin works, perform glucose monitoring, adjust insulin dose according to blood sugar level, and use sterile injection technique."

10. In complex cases, develop both *short-* and *long-term* outcomes. Use short-term outcomes as stepping stones to long-term outcomes. **Example:** (Short-term) "After 1 week, Fred will be able to bathe and dress himself with assistance." (Long-term) "After 4 weeks, Fred will be totally independent in performing his morning care."

USE SMART AS A MEMORY-JOG TO REMEMBER KEY FEATURES OF EXPECTED OUTCOMES.[2]
- **S—S**pecific
- **M—M**easurable
- **A—A**greed upon by all parties
- **R—R**ealistic
- **T—T**ime-bound

Clinical Reasoning Exercises: Determining Patient-Centered (Client-Centered) Outcomes

Example responses are on page 276.

Based on the information provided, determine a specific, client-centered outcome for each of the following:
1. Risk for pressure ulcer related to age, obesity, and prolonged bed rest
2. Suction patient prn (as needed)
3. Irrigate Foley catheter every 4 hours
4. Endotracheal intubation
5. Activity intolerance related to muscle weakness secondary to prolonged bed rest as evidenced by inability to walk the length of the hall without assistance

---

15. DETERMINING INDIVIDUALIZED INTERVENTIONS

Definition
Identifying specific nursing actions that are tailored to the patient's needs and desires and designed to (1) prevent, manage, and eliminate problems and risk factors; (2) reduce the likelihood of undesired outcomes and increase the likelihood of desired outcomes; and (3) promote health and independence.

Why This Skill Is Needed for Clinical Reasoning
To prevent and resolve health problems, you must know how to develop safe, *individualized* interventions that are *specific to each patient's particular situation*. Keeping a focus on *individual patient needs and desires* gives the patient a sense of autonomy and helps you design a plan that's more likely to be followed. Knowing how to tailor the interventions

to increase the likelihood of success and decrease the likelihood of harm is the key to improving efficiency and patient satisfaction.

Guidelines: How to Determine Individualized Interventions

1. Get patients and primary caregivers (e.g., families) involved in decision-making *early*. They are the ones who can help you tailor interventions in ways that are likely to succeed. Tell patients that your role is not only to take care of them, but to help them know how to take care of themselves *when you're not there*.

2. Identify interventions that aim to monitor and manage both problems and the underlying cause(s) or contributing factors, as illustrated in the box below.

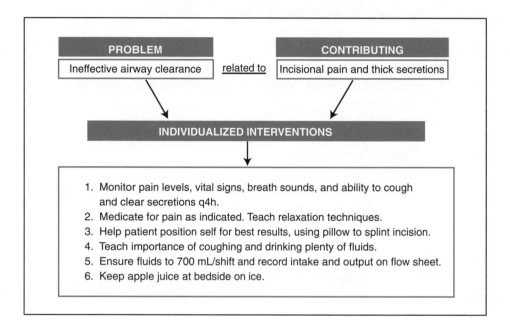

PROBLEM		CONTRIBUTING
Ineffective airway clearance	related to	Incisional pain and thick secretions

INDIVIDUALIZED INTERVENTIONS

1. Monitor pain levels, vital signs, breath sounds, and ability to cough and clear secretions q4h.
2. Medicate for pain as indicated. Teach relaxation techniques.
3. Help patient position self for best results, using pillow to splint incision.
4. Teach importance of coughing and drinking plenty of fluids.
5. Ensure fluids to 700 mL/shift and record intake and output on flow sheet.
6. Keep apple juice at bedside on ice.

3. Give high priority to designing interventions aimed at managing the factors *contributing* to the problems. For example, if your patient does not move or cough well after surgery because of incisional pain, a high-priority intervention will be to manage the pain.

4. Use the worksheet on page 196 to systematically consider all the things that may contribute to a given problem. After you identify all the things contributing to the problems, decide what can be done to manage the contributing factors and who is responsible for managing them. For example, if your patient has a pressure ulcer and is diabetic, realize that the diabetes is a contributing factor and specify who is responsible for managing the diabetes. Sometimes there are contributing factors that you can't do anything about, but you still need to consider them. For example, you can't

do anything about a risk factor of a woman being 86 years old. However, keep in mind that this woman is at risk for many potential problems and is less resilient because of her age; therefore, you should monitor her more closely.

> **RULE**
>
> **Be sure that your independent interventions are not attempting to treat a problem that needs medical management by a more qualified professional.** *Example: Unrelieved pain* may indicate that there's a life-threatening problem that needs immediate medical attention; continuing to treat the pain may mask critical symptoms and put the patient at significant risk.

5. Always ask, "Are there risk factors we need to manage?" If so, identify interventions to monitor and manage the risk factors. **Example:** If the person is bedridden, this is a risk factor for pressure ulcers. Monitor skin status carefully, and make a plan for repositioning the person.
6. Identify the problems and risk factors that must be *monitored and managed* to achieve the *overall outcomes*, and then ask the following:
   - "How will we monitor the status of the problems and risk factors?" ("What will we assess?" "Who will assess it?" "How often will we assess it?" "How will assessments be recorded?")
   - "What must be done to (1) manage or eliminate the risk (contributing) factors?" (2) "Manage or eliminate the problems?" (3) "Promote safety and reduce risk of harm?" (4) "Teach the person what he needs to know to be independent?"
7. Consider the interventions you identified, and ask the following:
   - "Have I predicted how I expect this patient *in this situation* to respond to the interventions I identified?"
   - "Have I predicted *undesired responses* and identified ways to minimize the risk of getting them?"

> **RULE**
>
> **When predicting patient responses, consider each patient's unique situation.** Identify the *desired* outcomes (the benefits of the intervention) and the *undesired* outcomes (the risks that the interventions may cause harm).

   - "Do I know the level of evidence that supports that I will get the desired results to my interventions in this situation?" For example, "Are your interventions recommended by textbooks? By policies, procedures, standard plans? By national clinical practice guidelines?"
   - "What can we do to increase the likelihood of getting desired results and reduce the risk of doing harm (getting undesired results) *in this specific patient's situation?*"

8. Remember the PPMP (predict, prevent, manage, promote) approach:
   - Predict potential complications, and be ready to manage them (pages 103 to 105) list common potential complications). Sometimes you can't do much about the *cause* of the problems, but you can prevent and manage the *symptoms and potential complications* of the problems. For instance, if someone has just had his jaws wired shut, you can't do much about it, but you must be prepared to handle the potential complication of aspiration by having suction equipment and wire cutters nearby.
   - Identify interventions that not only treat problems and risk factors, but also *promote optimum function, independence, and well-being.* **Example:** Stress the benefits of walking at least 20 minutes a day. Be sure that patients have a paper and pen to write down things they need to remember. Ask patients for things you can do to make things more convenient for them.

9. When determining nursing interventions, use the following memory-jog: *See, do, teach,* and *record.* Consider what you need to *see* (assess), what you or the patient needs to *do*, what you need to *teach*, and what you must *record*. **Example:**
   - **See:** Assess ability to walk with walker in the room before allowing the patient to go out in the hall alone.
   - **Do:** Have him walk the length of the hall three times a day.
   - **Teach:** Reinforce that research shows that walking will increase muscle strength and reduce fatigue.
   - **Record:** Record pulse and blood pressure before and after walking at least once a day.

10. Keep in mind both direct-care interventions (things you do directly for or with the patient, such as helping him get out of bed) and indirect-care interventions (things you do away from the patient, such as monitoring lab results).

Clinical Reasoning Exercises: Determining Individualized Interventions

Example responses are on page 277.

1. Determine specific interventions for each of the following problems and corresponding outcomes.

Problem	Corresponding Expected Outcome
a. Risk for dehydration related to diarrhea and insufficient fluid intake	Will maintain adequate hydration as evidenced by drinking at least 4 quarts of clear liquids per 24-hour period

Problem	Corresponding Expected Outcome
b. Anxiety related to insufficient knowledge of hospital procedures	By the end of today, will relate knowledge of hospital procedures and express ways of managing anxiety
c. Chronic pain related to arthritic joints as evidenced by statements of pain with range of motion for the past 20 years	After application of heat and assistance with range of motion, will rate pain on a scale of 0 to 10 and express that joint pain doesn't prohibit movement or sleep

2. Imagine you are doing a home visit with an 86-year-old woman who is asthmatic and is on chemotherapy for ovarian cancer. She is independent, but likes to spend much of her day reading in bed. She is 5 feet tall and weighs 93 pounds. Using the worksheet on page 196, determine all the factors she has that may contribute to a *risk for pressure ulcer.* Then decide what, if anything, will be done to manage each contributing factor.

3. Read the following scenario, and then answer the questions that follow it.

Scenario

You make a home visit to a Russian family with three children, ages 5, 7, and 10. Their home is next to a forest full of deer ticks. The mother is upset because she keeps finding ticks on the children, and she knows Lyme disease comes from tick bites. She's told the children not to go into the forest, but she suspects they disregard her instructions. Now the mother is considering punishing the children when she finds a tick on them, hoping this will make them more careful.

You look up Lyme disease and learn that the best treatment is prevention of tick bites. You then identify the following problem and expected outcome:

Problem: Risk for infection related to tick bites.

Expected outcome: The children will have a decreased risk of tick bites and infection as evidenced by their wearing insect repellent when outside, avoiding tall grassy areas, and monitoring themselves and each other for ticks.

a. Consider the risks and benefits of the following actions:
   (1) What might happen if the children are punished when a tick is found on them?
   (2) What might happen if you reward the children for finding ticks?
b. What interventions might safely motivate the children to participate in spotting ticks and avoiding bites? Write specific interventions to achieve the expected outcome listed for this situation.

16. EVALUATING AND CORRECTING THINKING (SELF-REGULATING)

Definition

Reflecting on thinking for the purpose of safety and improvement—for example, looking for flaws, deciding whether your thinking is focused, clear, and in enough depth—then making adjustments as needed.

Why This Skill Is Needed for Clinical Reasoning

Developing sound clinical reasoning skills requires you to self-regulate, which means reflecting on your thinking and asking yourself questions like "Am I clear about what's going on here? What could I be missing? How can I be surer that my reasoning is correct? Am I holding myself to high standards? Do I know what I'll do if things go wrong? What creative approaches might work here? What peers or experts can I get to dialogue with me so that I better understand the thinking that should go into a situation like this?"

RULE

To avoid errors in clinical judgment, don't settle for the first conclusion or idea you have. Reflect on thinking, and consider alternative conclusions, problems, explanations, and solutions. Successful nurses aren't successful because they can come up with one right answer or explanation—they come up with many, and then choose the best one.

Guidelines: How to Evaluate and Correct Thinking (Self-Regulate)

Evaluating and correcting thinking is an ongoing process. Because the nursing process is a major tool for clinical reasoning, the following box gives example questions you should be asking at various phases of the nursing process.

REFLECTING ON PHASES OF THE NURSING PROCESS

ASSESSMENT
- To what degree were the patient and key stakeholders involved in the process?
- How well do I understand my patient's perceptions?
- What assumptions could I have made?
- How complete is data collection?
- How accurate and reliable is my information?
- How well do I understand my patient's perceptions?
- Have I considered what data I need from both nursing and medical perspectives?

DIAGNOSIS AND OUTCOME IDENTIFICATION

- How well have I included the patient and key stakeholders in determining realistic outcomes?
- Are my outcomes clearly stated in measurable terms?
- How sure am I of the conclusions I've drawn (inferences I've made)?
- Should I be reporting some signs and symptoms immediately—could this be a medical problem that requires more qualified management?
- How well does the patient's data support that the problems I identified are correct?
- Have I missed any other problems that could be indicated by the patient's data?
- Am I clear about the underlying causes, contributing factors, and risk factors?
- How clearly and specifically are the problems and outcomes described?
- Am I clear about the definitive diagnoses?
- Have I identified "muddy issues" that may need to be clarified?
- Have I identified both nursing problems and problems requiring a multidisciplinary approach?
- Were patient strengths and resources identified?
- Have I determined the priority risks and problems that must be recorded on the plan of care?
- Have I made sure that safety issues and patient education needs were identified?

PLANNING

- To what degree did I involve the patient and key stakeholders in setting priorities and developing the plan?
- What immediate priorities could have been missed?
- Have I missed any problems that must be addressed in the plan of care?
- How well do the outcomes reflect the benefits I expect to see?
- Are the expected outcomes realistic, clear, and client-centered?
- Have I considered the undesired responses and identified interventions to reduce the likelihood of getting them?
- Did I consider both the problems and the outcomes when identifying interventions?
- Did I consider client preferences when developing the plan, and did I use client strengths and resources?
- Have I predicted patient responses and individualized interventions to this specific patient and situation?
- Have I decided where the priority problems and risks and the corresponding interventions must be recorded?

IMPLEMENTATION

- How well did I involve the patient and key stakeholders in executing the plan?
- Are the problems still the same?
- Am I missing any new problems?
- Am I keeping the focus on client responses?
- Should I be doing anything differently? Are the interventions still appropriate?
- Do I need to address safety issues?
- Have I identified and recorded changes we need to make?

EVALUATION

- Where does the patient stand in relation to achieving major desired outcomes?
- How accurately and completely have I completed each of the previous phases?
- What do the patient and the key stakeholders have to say about their progress?
- What suggestions do the patient and key stakeholders have for improvement?

There are no Clinical Reasoning Exercises for this skill, since opportunities for evaluating and correcting thinking have been provided throughout the other skills sections.

17. DETERMINING A COMPREHENSIVE PLAN/EVALUATING AND UPDATING THE PLAN

Definition
Ensuring that the priority problems and corresponding outcomes and interventions are recorded on the patient record; keeping the plan up-to-date.

Why This Skill Is Needed for Clinical Reasoning
Developing a comprehensive plan and ensuring that the major care plan components are recorded (1) forces you to think about the most important aspects of giving care, (2) promotes communication between caregivers, and (3) provides data for evaluation, research, legal, and insurance purposes.

Ongoing evaluation—continually reflecting on how the plan is working and what changes must be made—helps you make adjustments *early*, making care safer and more efficient.

The purpose of having you work through the process of determining a comprehensive plan of care is to help you gain a deep understanding of the relationship among the care plan components, and of the importance of keeping patient plans up-to-date.

Guidelines: How to Develop a Comprehensive Plan/Update the Plan
1. Being able to determine a comprehensive plan requires all of the skills listed in this section and knowing the purpose and components of the recorded plan.

PURPOSE AND COMPONENTS OF THE RECORDED PLAN OF CARE

PURPOSE
1. Promotes communication between caregivers
2. Directs care, interventions, and documentation
3. Creates a record that can later be used for evaluation, research, legal, and insurance purposes

COMPONENTS (USE THE MEMORY-JOG EASE)
Expected outcomes
Actual and potential problems that must be addressed to reach the overall outcomes
Specific interventions designed to achieve the outcomes
Evaluation statements (progress notes)

2. Identify the major problems and interventions yourself. Then:
    - Check the patient record to see whether the problems and interventions are addressed by pre-established plans, policies, or doctor's orders.
    - Compare your patient's situation with the interventions on pre-established plans. Modify or add interventions if needed.
3. To evaluate and update the plan, compare what's recorded in the plan with what you *actually find* when you assess the patient.
    - Determine progress toward expected outcomes. For example, if the expected outcome states *will be free of signs of infection around incision,* assess the incision for signs of infection (e.g., redness, drainage, heat, and tenderness).
    - Monitor problems closely; watch closely for new risk factors or problems. If risk factors or problems change, update the patient record as indicated.
    - Monitor patient responses to interventions. If you aren't seeing the expected results, together with the patient, decide what needs to change to improve results.
    - Modify interventions as needed, changing the record as needed.
4. Remember the following rule.

RULE

> **You are responsible for monitoring for care variances** (a care variance is when a patient hasn't achieved outcomes by the time frame noted on a plan of care). If you identify a care variance, ask, (1) "What additional assessment do I need to do to determine whether this delay is justified?" (2) "What can be done to improve the likelihood that the person will achieve the outcomes of the plan?" and (3) "What resources and multidisciplinary approaches might help?" Then take appropriate action.

Clinical Reasoning Exercises: Determining a Comprehensive Plan/Evaluating and Updating the Plan

Example responses are on page 277.

1. Consider each of the following expected outcomes and corresponding patient data, and decide whether the outcome has been achieved, partially achieved, or not achieved.
    a. **Expected outcome:** Will manage own wound care by day three after surgery as evidenced by ability to demonstrate how to manage wound packing. **Data:** Patient says that managing wound packing shouldn't be his concern and feels he's incapable of doing so.
    b. **Expected outcome:** Will drink at least 4 quarts of fluid as evidenced by keeping a written record of fluid intake. **Data:** Patient's record indicates 5 quarts of fluid intake daily.

c. **Expected outcome:** The baby will be discharged home with parents able to perform CPR. **Data:** Father demonstrates CPR well. Mother has trouble establishing airway.

2. Develop a comprehensive plan, identifying two priority problems for the following scenario. Include an overall expected discharge outcome, outcomes for each problem, and specific interventions.

Scenario

It's Monday, June 29. You admit Mrs. Ankiel, who has just suffered anaphylactic shock after a bee sting. She is expected to be discharged by Tuesday, June 30. The doctor gives Mrs. Ankiel an emergency epinephrine injection kit and tells her, "The nurse will teach you how to use it." Mrs. Ankiel still has hives all over her body and says her itching feet are driving her crazy. You find that placing her feet in cool water every so often helps her discomfort. She is still slightly wheezy from the bee sting reaction.

When you ask her about using the injection kit, she replies, "No way!" Her husband, who is retired, says, "I'll be glad to learn." It's decided that it's satisfactory to discharge Mrs. Ankiel on June 30, with her husband able to demonstrate how to give epinephrine in an emergency.

3. Imagine that you're using a critical pathway to guide your patient's care. It states that on the first day after surgery, the patient should have the Foley catheter out and be voiding normally. It's now the second day after surgery, and when you check the intake and output record, you see that she is voiding 30 cc every hour. What should you do, and why?

4. Suppose you're reviewing someone's chart to determine if a comprehensive plan of care is present. What four care plan components will you look for?

 Think, Pair, Share

Together with a partner:

1. Map the relationships among the key care plan components, as addressed in the memory-jog, EASE (page 212).

2. The next time you go to the clinical setting, access a patient record and find where the four main components of the plan of care are documented.

REFERENCES

1. Silver, D. (January, 2011). E-mail communication.
2. Bartle, P. SMART: Characteristics of good objectives. Retrieved January 6, 2011, from http://www.scn.org/cmp/modules/pd-smar.htm.

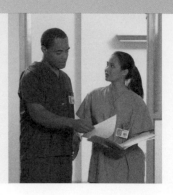

CHAPTER

6

Developing Interpersonal, Teamwork, and Self-Management Skills

This chapter at a glance ...

PRECHAPTER SELF TEST

Decide where you stand in relation to the learning outcomes at the beginning of each skill in this section.

HOW TO USE THIS CHAPTER

This chapter helps you develop interpersonal, teamwork, and self-management skills—for example, managing your time and learning how to get past "the sting" of criticism so that it helps you grow. When you know how to communicate effectively and build positive relationships with patients and team members, you spend less time getting sidetracked by interpersonal and "human nature" problems—and more time fully engaged in progress.

In the section on *Preventing and Dealing with Mistakes Constructively*, you learn how to keep patients, caregivers, and yourself safe.

Many nurses consider the skills addressed in this section to be leadership skills. Today, every nurse must be a leader. Advocating for your patients, yourself, your peers, and your community requires highly developed interpersonal and communication abilities.[1,2] Patient-centered care in the context of interdisciplinary teams is the standard for excellence. No matter what type of nursing you choose to do, you can't function effectively without developing the skills in this section as much as clinical skills.

HOW THE SKILLS ARE ORGANIZED

Listed in alphabetical order, each skill is presented in the following format: (1) name of the skill, (2) definition of the skill, (3) learning outcomes, (4) thinking critically about the skill, (5) how to accomplish the skill, and (6) critical thinking exercises.

To complete exercises, partner with at least one other person. Content is presented in a way that can help you plan a seminar for each skill to promote in-depth discussion and learning. As part of the seminar requirements, each participant should read at least two up-to-date articles on the topic. Because the all the exercises are **Think Pair Share** exercises, there are no example responses in the back of the book.

1. COMMUNICATING BAD NEWS

Definition
Knowing how to convey honesty, empathy, and responsibility when giving information that may be perceived as having a negative impact.

Learning Outcomes
After completing this section, you should be able to:
- Explain what happens when you avoid giving bad news.
- Identify strategies to minimize the impact of bad news.
- Determine how you can reduce your stress when faced with giving bad news.

- Improve your ability to give bad news related to health status and customer service issues.
- Help patients deal with bad news they receive from other health team members.

Thinking Critically About Giving Bad News

Whether bad news is related to health status or customer service issues, no one likes to give it. Many people tend to avoid this unpleasant chore altogether, making things worse. In many instances, you may not be the one to actually give the bad news yourself (for example, cancer diagnoses are given by physicians only; organ donation is requested by a skilled organ transplant team member). Still, you'll often be there when bad news has to be given, and you're responsible for deciding who is the best person to give the news and for helping people to process the information.

As you read on through this section, remember that getting bad news may be better than getting no news. Researchers report that uncertainty about a diagnosis causes more anxiety and can be more stressful than actually knowing that you have a serious illness. Once people have a diagnosis, they usually gain some understanding and control. Without the diagnosis, all they have is anxiety, and they don't know how to handle it.[3]

How you handle giving bad news—or support people when they receive bad news from others—can make the difference between making a difficult situation worse and building the supportive relationship that's so important to patients and families.

How to Give Bad News

The following shaded section gives guidelines for giving bad news in two different situations: (1) giving bad news related to health status, and (2) giving bad news related to customer service issues.

GIVING BAD NEWS RELATED TO HEALTH STATUS

STEPS	RATIONALE
1. **Determine who has the authority and qualifications to give the bad news.** Usually this is the primary care provider, such as the doctor or nurse practitioner.	Most organizations have policies related to who can give patients certain information. Depending on the impact of the news (e.g., if the news is about biopsy results, severe illness, or death), the patient and family are likely to have questions that must be answered by the most qualified professional. Always check your facility's policies regarding patient confidentiality and HIPAA privacy laws.

GIVING BAD NEWS RELATED TO HEALTH STATUS—cont'd

STEPS	RATIONALE
2. **Have the professional who is best qualified (or who has developed the best relationship with the person) give the news.**	The messenger matters. Bad news is often met with powerful emotions of disappointment and anger. Receiving bad news in a caring, straightforward way from trusted professionals softens the blow. It's easy to feel that a provider who is too busy to give the bad news has betrayed you. It takes a strong, logical mind not to want to "shoot the messenger." Making sure that those who know the patient best—for example, a trusted nurse or a chaplain—are present helps reduce feelings of being abandoned or helpless.
3. **Choose the setting—ensure privacy, and avoid using the phone.**	How and where the person gets bad news is key. Using the phone doesn't allow for appropriate assessment and support.
4. **Find out what the person already knows or suspects.**	This simplifies the process and helps clarify what you need to say.
5. **Give a warning shot.**	Saying things like, "This isn't what we wanted to hear," "I have bad news," or "I'm sorry to have to tell you this" prepares people for the emotional blow they are about to receive.
6. **Be direct, tell the news, and give time for it to sink in. (Silence is golden.)**	Being direct helps people to get the main information first, in a logical way. Bad news takes time to digest—patients often need to get through shock and anger, before they can move on to dealing with the impact of the news. Sometimes, all that is needed is someone to remain present, listening quietly as feelings are sorted out. You have to name the feelings before you can tame them.
7. **Respond to emotions with empathy.** Continue to use silence as a strategy. Use nonverbal gestures, as appropriate (e.g., put a hand on the person's shoulder). Help the person deal with feelings of blame.	Each person is unique, with a range of emotional responses that depend on circumstances. Letting people know that their emotions are *understood* helps them deal with strong feelings. Think about this analogy: Aspirin reduces fever and physical discomfort. Being allowed to express thoughts and feelings reduces anxiety and psychological discomfort. Bad news often brings feelings of blame. **Examples of statements that help:** "I'm sorry this is happening"; "There's nothing that could have been done"; "This is no one's fault"; "It's not worth blaming ... it will only make things worse ... we need to deal with the problem"; or "We'll help you through this." **Examples of statements that don't help:** "I know how you feel"; "It's God's will"; or "God only gives you what you can bear."
8. **Ask whether there are any questions or special requests, especially related to spiritual and cultural needs.**	Hearing their questions and special requests gets them involved and helps you begin to identify their most important needs. Nurses are accountable for paying attention to spiritual and cultural needs. **Examples:** "Tell me what we can do right now for you." "Is there someone we can call?" "Do you have a specific religion?" "Can I get the hospital chaplain?" or "What can I do?"

GIVING BAD NEWS RELATED TO HEALTH STATUS—cont'd

STEPS	RATIONALE
9. **Keep a positive tone, be realistic, and give hope.** End with a plan, and be sure the person has a printed list of resources.	Having hope and hearing a realistic positive attitude sets the tone for dealing with the bad news. Hope is the "tonic" that sustains people through difficult times. **Examples of what to say:** "This is tough news ... but having a positive attitude is important"; "Don't jump to conclusions or let yourself be driven by 'worst-case scenarios'"; "Don't give up hope ... we'll use all our resources." Having a plan mobilizes the patient and team toward dealing with the problem. A printed list of resources is essential for later, when the patient goes home, the information sinks in, and the patient starts thinking independently about how to handle the problem.
10. **Follow up to see how things are going.**	Some people may be mobilized in positive ways, and others may need more direction and support. Don't assume. Find out how they're doing.

Source: Alfaro-LeFevre handouts. Copyright 2010. www.AlfaroTeachSmart.com.

GIVING BAD NEWS RELATED TO CUSTOMER SERVICE ISSUES

STEPS	EXAMPLE
1. **Give bad news in a timely way.** Offer an apology, and don't try to obscure the situation.	"I'm sorry to tell you we won't be able to do your x-ray today."
2. **Showing accountability, explain what happened and why.**	"Your appointment card says today, but somehow we have you scheduled in our book for next week. I'm not sure how this happened, but you can be sure that I'll find out."
3. **Pause to give the person a chance to express thoughts and feelings.** Listen attentively.	3-5 seconds of silence encourages the person to gather his thoughts and speak his mind and tell you what's most important.
4. **Present alternative solutions, and give pros and cons of each.** Get the patient's point of view.	"I could schedule the x-ray for later today, but we get better pictures if you fast for 12 hours before the x-ray. I realize you'd have to go home and come back, and that you'd like to get it over with. I think it's worth waiting to be sure we get a good quality x-ray. Would that be okay for you?"
5. **Recommend a course of action.** Include (a) how the plan addresses the problem, and (b) how the plan addresses hardships resulting from what happened.	"I think the best solution is to schedule the x-ray as soon as possible. Since you've already had enough problems, I'll do my best to schedule you whenever it's convenient for you. I'll also find out who made this mistake and see what we can do to prevent this from happening again."

GIVING BAD NEWS RELATED TO CUSTOMER SERVICE ISSUES—cont'd

STEPS	EXAMPLE
6. **Reaffirm your goals and vision for the future.** Include (a) key points that give confidence to those involved, and (b) time frame for expected results.	"We're here to serve you the best way we can. Soon we'll have a system that allows you to confirm appointments over the phone. We hope to have the system in place by May. Everyone will be encouraged to call and confirm their appointments when they get home."
7. **Follow up to see if results were satisfactory.**	"I'll send your name to our community relations department. They will call you to see if everything was resolved to your satisfaction. Please feel free to call and discuss anything you'd like with them as well. We want you to feel satisfied with your experience with us. Please let me know if you still have problems."

Source: Alfaro-LeFevre handouts. Copyright 2010. www.AlfaroTeachSmart.com.

OTHER PERSPECTIVES

DIFFICULT COMMUNICATION: LEARN ONE SKILL AT A TIME

Researchers who examined the effects of a short course on handling difficult communications found that the course helped nurses achieve significant improvements in self-efficacy (feeling confident about ability to develop the skills needed to handle difficult communications) but not in performance. The researchers suggest that it's a good idea to focus on specific communication skills rather than a full suite of skills.[4]

Critical Thinking Exercises

Think, Pair, Share

With a partner, in a group, or in a journal entry:

1. Describe the following:
   - Your best and worst experiences with how someone gave you bad news.
   - The emotions you feel when giving bad news.
   - How you or someone you know responded to getting bad news situations and why you think they responded that way.
   - The differences between giving bad news related to customer service situations and giving bad news related to health status.

2. Imagine that you have to tell someone that their mother has been admitted to the intensive care unit after a car accident. Using the steps for giving bad news related to health status on pages 218 to 221, develop a plan for how you will do this.

3. Imagine you have to tell someone that they have to wait 2 hours to see the doctor because the doctor has other urgent problems. Using the steps for giving bad news related to customer service issues on pages 220 to 221, develop a plan for how you will do this.

4. Discuss the implications of some of the *Other Perspectives,* and RECOMMENDED listed in this skill.

5. Decide where you stand in relation to achieving the learning outcomes listed at the beginning of this skill.

Recommended

Breaking bad news. (2011). Retrieved January 20, 2011, from http://www.medceu.com/index/index.php?page=get_course&courseID=2028&nocheck

Habel, M. (2011). Emotional intelligence helps RNs work smart. Retrieved January 11, 2011, from: http://ce.nurse.com/CE373-60/Emotional-Intelligence-Helps-RNs-Work-Smart/

Lachman, V. (2011). Delivering bad news. Retrieved January 27, 2011, from http://nursing.advanceweb.com/Article/Delivering-Bad-News-3.aspx

Orlovsky, C. (2011). Workshops train providers to deliver bad news, difficult discussions. Retrieved January 20, 2011, from http://www.nursezone.com/nursing-news-events/more-news/Workshops-Train-Providers-to-Deliver-Bad-News-Difficult-Discussions_29144.aspx

See also RECOMMENDED in the sections *Dealing with Complaints Constructively* and *Preventing and Dealing with Mistakes Constructively.*

2. DEALING WITH COMPLAINTS CONSTRUCTIVELY

Definition
Using complaints as an opportunity to improve consumer satisfaction and problems with how you or your organizational systems work.

Learning Outcomes
After completing this section, you should be able to:
- Explain the value of complaints.
- Identify strategies for dealing with difficult patients and consumers.

- Express more confidence about dealing with complaints in positive ways.
- Observe an improvement in how your patients respond when they come to you with a complaint.

Thinking Critically About Complaints

Dealing with complaints makes most of us uncomfortable—often defensive. But, complaints are actually an opportunity to improve both patient satisfaction and system problems. Knowing how to deal with complaints helps you sooth angry patients and keep them from becoming angry in the first place. Think about the last time you complained about service. Was it because you wanted your situation corrected? Did you complain only for yourself, or did you think it might help them improve their service for *others*?

Complaints help you:

- Correct problems before they become worse or happen to someone else.
- Help patients and families feel like what they are experiencing matters to you and your organization.
- Identify trends in unmet needs of patients and consumers.
- Find out about complaints before people start complaining to others.

Whether you're dealing with mildly frustrated patients—or aggressive people who seem to be looking for a reason to be mad—keeping your emotions in check, using specific strategies, and staying focused on common goals can help you achieve the following key results.

1. The patient or health care consumer feels relieved that someone is willing to listen, care about their issues, and do whatever can be done to help.
2. You can resolve issues more quickly, allowing you to get on with the rest of your work.
3. You can look back and feel like you made a difference by handling the situation professionally and in the best way you could.

When someone complains, listen carefully and do something about it: Restate the person's issue, acknowledge your understanding of the issue, and offer to do your best to correct the problem.

How to Deal with Complaints Constructively

1. Pay attention to what is being said. You don't have to agree—just try to understand the person's view of what is happening.

RULE

You can often sooth angry people with just a little affirmation of their problem.[6] Angry, frustrated people need to know that there's a sensible person who really wants to help them resolve their issues. For example, you can say "Mr. Garcia, I understand how upsetting this is. I will do my best to fix it for you."

2. Don't take things personally. Rein in the natural tendency to be defensive, and assume there's a very good reason for the complaints (these reasons may be unclear at first).

3. Find out what the person really needs and wants.
   - Ask the person to clarify his issues.
   - To clarify your own understanding, repeat back what you hear.
   - Aim to give the person what he wants (this requires that you get a clear understanding from your boss about what rules you can bend or break to immediately resolve issues).
   - If you come in late to the situation, remain quiet, listen, and ask to verify your understanding of the problem.
   - Remember, you are the professional at work. Patients are there on their own time—often with few choices—and need your help.

4. Focus on *the patient's issues*, and try to learn from them.

5. If anger explodes, take a deep breath and keep your own anger in check (remember that people requiring health care often have extenuating circumstances that cause them to have "short fuses"). Some examples follow:
   - Previous bad experience with health care providers or treatment plans
   - Effects of illness or disability on self, family, and work
   - Problems of being "in limbo" (the patient may not be responding as quickly or favorably as expected)
   - Family reaction to illness or disability

6. Don't defend yourself—swallow your pride and bite your tongue. Apologize, and avoid weak excuses (e.g., we're shorthanded, nobody's perfect). Successful apologies require you to be humble, specific on the issues, and sincere.
   - Keep in mind that some people cope in ways you consider negative (abrasive or manipulative).
   - Think about whether having your manager come and talk with the person would help.

RULE

You do get a "second chance to make a first impression." When things go wrong, don't hide. Rather, say something like, "I'm sorry this happened. ...let me see what I can do to fix this. What's most important to you?"

7. Involve the person in problem-solving (ask for solutions). Report and record special needs.

8. Take immediate steps to resolve the problem. Explain what you're going to do, and let people feel like they're winning in some way.

9. When explaining your solutions or procedures, point out how it benefits the patient.

10. Keep the person informed (e.g., "I promise to let you know the minute I know more about this"). Follow up to see if solutions are working.

OTHER PERSPECTIVES

GIVE FIVE-STAR SERVICE
"Treat patients or clients as though they were your favorite celebrity, hero, friend, or neighbor, or your grandma."

—*Author unknown*

Critical Thinking Exercises

Think, Pair, Share

With a partner, in a group, or in a journal entry:

1. Imagine this: Someone tells you one of your patients has numerous complaints. You go straight to the room, introduce yourself, and inquire about the problem. The patient's wife immediately becomes hostile and tells you to "just get out." What do you do and why?
2. Share your feelings about making complaints (e.g., anger, guilt, frustration).
3. Give an example of a time when you thought about complaining but decided it just wasn't worth it. How did this make you feel? Who lost the most in this situation?
4. Describe your best and worst experiences with making a complaint.
5. Explain how you usually deal with other people's complaints, and then determine some ways to improve your response.
6. Discuss the implications of some of the *Other Perspectives* and RECOMMENDED listed in this skill.
7. Decide where you stand in relation to achieving the learning outcomes listed at the beginning of this skill.

Recommended

Goleman, D. (2006). *Emotional intelligence: 10th anniversary edition; why it can matter more than IQ*. New York: Bantam Books.

Hunt, A. (2010). Dealing with difficult customers-angry customers. Retrieved January 1, 2011, from http://www.suite101.com/content/dealing-with-difficult-customers-angry-customers-a268127

Sherman, M. Dealing with a difficult customer. Retrieved January 1, 2011, from http://www.healthsystem.virginia.edu/internet/feap/newsletters/dealing-with-a-difficult-customer.pdf

Texas Medical Association. How to handle patient complaints. Retrieved January 11, 2011, from http://www.texmed.org/Template.aspx?id=4110

University of Huddersfield: Customer care handbook: Dealing with complaints. Retrieved June 22, 2011, from http://www.hud.ac.uk/uni/customer/index_htm

See also RECOMMENDED in the sections *Communicating Bad News, Developing Empowered Partnerships,* and *Managing Conflict Constructively.*

3. DEVELOPING EMPOWERED PARTNERSHIPS

Definition
Building mutually beneficial relationships based on the belief that people have the right and the responsibility to make their own choices and to grow in their own way.[6]

Learning Outcomes
After completing this section, you should be able to:
- Compare and contrast a parental model and an empowered partnership model.
- Explain the benefits of empowered partnerships.
- Identify ways to deal with barriers to developing empowered partnerships.
- Improve your ability to build empowered partnerships with patients, families, colleagues, and peers.

Thinking Critically About Building Empowered Partnerships
Developing empowered partnerships with peers, colleagues, and patients requires a shift in thinking from a parental model ("I'll take care of you") to an empowered partnership model ("It's your life—you have rights and responsibilities as well as I do, and we both should grow and learn from our experience together"). Table 6-1 (next page) lists phrases that demonstrate these two models.

Remember that *partnering with patients and families* is central to critical thinking and getting the results you need. From getting mutual agreement on desired outcomes to identifying care approaches, apply the saying, "nothing about me without me." Keep patients involved in all decision-making.

How to Develop Empowered Partnerships
1. Be sure you can explain the concept of an empowered partnership. Although you can't completely balance power in all relationships—for example, in adult-teenager partnerships the adult usually has more power—the aim of an empowered

partnership is to balance the power *as much as possible*. The following are examples of empowered partnerships:

- Nurse-patient (or client)
- Nurse manager–staff nurse
- Educator-learner
- Nurse-pharmacist
- Expert nurse-novice nurse
- Nurse–unlicensed worker
- Nurse-nurse
- Nurse-physician

2. Partners must agree to the following statements:
   - "We're both clear about our joint purpose, and we're both responsible."*
   - "I can be trusted; I promise to be honest."
   - "We should make decisions together as much as possible."
   - "We'll both agree to rules for resolving conflict between us."
   - "We both should expect to grow and learn from our experience together."
   - "We're each responsible for our own emotional well-being (if I feel bad about something, it's my responsibility to do something about it)."*
   - "We both have the right to say no, so long as no harm is done."*
   - "I choose to be here, so nobody's to blame."*
   - "If one of us sees the other engage in unsafe or unethical conduct, we have the responsibility to address it appropriately."
   - "We're both responsible for the outcomes (consequences) of our actions."*

TABLE 6-1   PARENTAL VERSUS EMPOWERED PARTNERSHIP MODEL

Parental Model	Empowered Partnership
I want to look after you.	How can I empower you to be able to be independent?
I know what's best for you.	You know yourself best. Tell me what you'd like to see happen, what's most important to you.
You should do as I say.	I want you to be able to make informed choices.
I'm responsible for you.	We share a common purpose, and we're both responsible for what happens.

*In the context of the nurse-patient relationship, these statements aren't always so because nurses are often held more accountable than patients. Nurses don't have the right to say *no* if it jeopardizes patient care (they must find a replacement). Hospitalized patients often have few choices about where they are.

3. An empowered partnership requires choosing to do the following:
   - Rise to the challenge of taking charge over the comfort of remaining dependent.
   - Give up some of the power; take calculated, thoughtful risks; and be willing to do the work needed to be independent.
4. It also requires the following:[7]
   - Nonjudgmental acceptance
   - Space for self-expression
   - Structure for conflict resolution
   - Respect for each other's boundaries
   - Support and encouragement for growth in the areas where one is limited
   - Coaching skills that transform (coaching that truly affects the learner's attitudes and skills)
   - Growth on the part of both partners
5. Many people are uncomfortable in an empowered partnership for the following reasons:
   - They are used to being taken care of and aren't accustomed to taking responsibility.
   - They are unwilling to accept the responsibility that comes with power.
   - They are unwilling to give up some of the power they're accustomed to having.
   - They haven't made the required shift in thinking (they don't truly believe in the benefits of partnership).
6. Change takes time. Coach those who aren't accustomed to the roles and responsibilities of being in a partnership.
7. Keep the focus on mutually agreed-upon outcomes—these are what inspire you both to work together.

CRITICAL MOMENTS

REWARDING PARTNERSHIPS: TEACHER–LEARNER
Teacher-learner partnerships are rewarding personally and professionally. No one can know it all. Create a learning culture, and work to build partnerships that support learning every day

OTHER PERSPECTIVES

PATIENTS MUST BE PARTNERS
"Patients have to be partners, equally responsible for treatment."
—*Tommy Lasorda, former Los Angeles Dodgers' manager*

Critical Thinking Exercises

Think, Pair, Share

With a partner, in a group, or in a journal entry:

1. Discuss how establishing partnerships with peers is different from establishing partnerships with patients.
2. Address how establishing an empowered partnership is affected by the following:
   - How long you have contact with the patient (e.g., 1 day versus 1 week)
   - The patient's health state
   - Growth and development (e.g., How do you partner with a child or an elderly person?)
3. Explain what's meant by the following statement: Partnership is an attitude as much as a model for relationships.
4. Think of a time that you had to complete a complex task with someone. How did it go? What were the dynamics? Would you consider the experience of an empowered partnership? In relation to what you have read in this section, what went well and what would you do differently if you did it again?
5. Discuss the implications of some of the *Critical Moments, Other Perspectives,* and RECOMMENDED listed in this skill.
6. Decide where you stand in relation to achieving the learning outcomes listed at the beginning of this skill.

Recommended

Block, P. (1996). *Stewardship: Choosing service over self-interest.* San Francisco: Berrett-Koehler.

Cheeks, P., & Dunn, P. (2010). A new-graduate program: empowering the novice nurse. *Journal for Nurses in Staff Development*, 26(5), 223-227.

Mainline Health. Nursing Professional Practice Model. Retrieved March 10, 2011, from http://www.mainlinehealth.org/oth/Page.asp?PageID= OTH002321

The Empowered Patient. (Web page). Retrieved June 29, 2011, from http:// www.theempoweredpatient.com/

Yoder, L., & Restifo, V. Partnership: Making the most of mentoring. Retrieved January 28, 2011, from http://ce.nurse.com/CE190-60/Partnership-Making-the-Most-of-Mentoring/

See also RECOMMENDED in the sections *Giving and Taking Constructive Criticism, Managing Conflict Constructively,* and *Transforming a Group into a Team.*

4. GIVING AND TAKING CONSTRUCTIVE CRITICISM

Definition
Being able to give (and respond to) constructive criticism in ways that promote growth and improvement.

Learning Outcomes
After completing this section, you should be able to:
- Discuss the effect of emotional responses to criticism.
- Determine how you can turn criticisms you receive into opportunities to grow.
- Explain how being uncomfortable with giving constructive criticism can lead to mistakes, unsafe patient care, and stunted growth.
- Identify strategies for giving constructive criticism.

Thinking Critically About Giving and Taking Constructive Criticism
Giving constructive criticism is not easy. Receiving it can be devastating. Yet, if it's something you'd rather just avoid, consider the following quotes from *Silence Kills* and *The 4-1-1 on Constructive Criticism*.[8,9]
- "A group of nurses describe a peer as careless and inattentive. Instead of confronting her, they double check her work—sometimes running into patient rooms to re-take blood pressures or re-do safety checks. They've "worked around" this nurse's weakness for over a year. The nurses resent her, but never talk to her about their concerns. Nor do any of the doctors who also avoid and compensate for her."
- "A group of eight anesthesiologists agree a peer is dangerously incompetent, but they don't confront him. Instead, they go to great efforts to schedule surgeries for the sickest babies at times when he is not on duty. This problem has persisted for over five years."
- "Being critical is easy, and offering criticism seems easier still. Yet constructive criticism—the more refined and effective brand of critical feedback—is like an art when compared to nagging, nit-picking and negativity. Nothing makes most people bristle more quickly than unfair, unskillful, or unsolicited criticism. Yet there are times when offering constructively critical feedback is essential to maintaining excellence and strong relationships."[10]
- Your ability to give and take constructive criticism is crucial to:
  - Avoiding letting little issues become big ones
  - Improving performance
  - Keeping patients safe

Knowing how to give constructive criticism in a supportive way can make the difference between alienating others and motivating them to improve. Knowing how to respond to criticism—to be objective and work through the negative aspects of criticism—reduces our stress and helps us understand exactly what we need to work on.

RULE

Whether or not criticism is useful depends on the relationship you have with the person giving or taking the criticism. Without *mutual trust,* criticism is unlikely to be viewed constructively.

How to Give and Take Constructive Criticism

The following gives strategies for giving and taking constructive criticism.

Giving Constructive Criticism

- Before giving criticism, think about how you can give it in a supportive, concerned way that stays focused on the goal of improvement and success. Aim to give the criticism in the way a mentor would give it, rather than a critic.
- Be sensitive to personality differences (personalities of both the giver and the receiver of criticism greatly affect whether the criticism is viewed as constructive).
- Give feedback frequently and in a timely way (this way it's viewed as being more sincere).
- Start with what's being done right (e.g., "Here are the things I see you do right"). Next, focus on what could be improved (rather than on what's wrong).
- Stay fully engaged in the communication; listen actively to avoid misunderstandings and making false assumptions.
- Give positive feedback often to reward growth ("catch" people being effective, and surprise them with positive feedback).
- Be aware that constant negative feedback can hinder progress by making the person focus on fear of failure.

Taking Constructive Criticism

- Keep in mind that receiving constructive criticism is a complex issue that's closely linked to self-esteem. Being told we could be better thinkers, improve in some way, or approach things differently often brings up intensely uncomfortable feelings of being wrong or not good enough. These gut reactions cloud key issues and paralyze our ability to be objective.
- Realize that getting negative feedback often brings forth intense negative feelings. For example, say to yourself, "I'm getting upset. I'd better take a deep breath, calm down,

and listen. If I work to be objective and not take things personally, I might learn something when I think about this later when I'm less stressed."

- Learn to befriend criticism, evaluating it objectively. Someone wants you to succeed, or she would not have bothered to share her thoughts. Not all criticism is given constructively, but try to focus on what you can learn.
- Ask yourself, "Have I heard this same criticism from other people?"
- Keep in mind that if you agree with the criticism, you must acknowledge that the critic is right and begin to think about what you can do about it.
- Don't make excuses for yourself, don't be defensive, and sincerely try to see the benefits of the criticism.
- Practice personal feedback by monitoring your own behavior and paying attention to how others respond to you.
- Don't let false pride, rationalization, or other negative factors get in the way of your growth.
- Remember that no one's perfect, but we can all improve. Be prepared to expend some physical and emotional energy to change.
- Don't dwell on negative criticism when you're tired—wait until a day or two later when you're refreshed and more likely to be objective. Example: Suppose you give a group presentation. If you wait a day or two or revisit the evaluations a week after the presentation—when you're rested—you'll probably see what was valid criticism from the group as a whole and what was simply one or two attendees' points of view.
- If you sincerely believe the criticism is unwarranted—and more likely to be incivility—remain confident, and discuss this with your manager or human resources department.

 ## OTHER PERSPECTIVES

CRITICISM: DEAL WITH IT
Constructive criticism helps us improve. We all need to know how to give it, take it, deal with it, and accept it.[11]

—*Barbara A. Musinski, RNPC, BS*

COMPLIMENTS FEED THE SOUL
I can live for two months on a good compliment.

—*Mark Twain*

MAKE THE BEST OF PIERCING CRITICISMS
"Poor speaker ... Too nervous ... Your writing is too vague ... There was a time when barbs like these went straight to my heart, piercing it through and through. For days and sometimes weeks, I walked around mortally wounded, sure I would never dare to write or speak in public again. It was only after the sting subsided that I began to think about the criticism. And once I did, if I thought it hit the mark, I acted on it, and as a result often ended up a better editor or writer. [When you get criticism,] distance yourself and give yourself time. Thank the person if it's

valid .... Someone cared enough to take time … Let's face it. Compliments feel good, but they're often fleeting and may be about as sincere as, 'Love your dress.' It's criticism that has the potential to make you grow. I doubt that any of great ideas came as a result of the statements, 'You're doing a great job' or 'I wouldn't change a thing.' "[12]

—*Phyllis Class, RN*

Critical Thinking Exercises

Think, Pair, Share

With a partner, in a group, or in a journal entry:

1. Think about the following statement, and decide what you would do if you had to give feedback to someone you don't get along with.
   Without mutual trust, feedback is unlikely to be viewed constructively.
2. Is it criticism or advice? Words do matter! Study the following bulleted list of suggestions from my workshop participants. Then practice using their suggestions instead of saying "I want to give you some constructive criticism."
   - Ask for permission or clarification ("May I give you some constructive criticism?" or "Are you asking for ….?").
   - Change the word *constructive* to *practical, helpful,* or *useful.*
   - Replace *criticism* with *advice, recommendation, suggestion, observation,* or *opinion.*
3. Recall a time when you tried to give constructive criticism to someone to help him improve. What happened and how did you feel? Would you do it differently if you had to do it again?
4. Think about a time when someone gave you criticism. What happened, and how did you feel? What made things easier or harder? What did you learn in the long run?
5. Discuss the implications of some of the *Other Perspectives* and RECOMMENDED listed in this skill.
6. Decide where you stand in relation to achieving the learning outcomes listed at the beginning of this skill.

Recommended

Walters, J. The 4-1-1 on constructive criticism. Retrieved January 28, 2011, from www.inc.com/articles/2001/08/23257.html

McKay, D. Employee performance reviews: How to prepare for a performance review and what to do if you get a bad one. Retrieved January 11, 2011, from http://careerplanning.about.com/od/performancereview/a/reviews.htm

Receiving Criticism. (Web page). Retrieved January 11, 2011, from http://www.youmeworks.com/receivingcriticism.html

Engelbrecht, C. Dishing criticism effectively: Taking criticism with a smile. Retrieved January 11, 2011, from http://www.disclife.com/ps030301.shtml

See also RECOMMENDED in the sections *Developing Empowered Partnerships* and *Managing Conflict Constructively*.

5. MANAGING CONFLICT CONSTRUCTIVELY

Definition
Being able to make conflict work in positive ways (learning, growth, and improvement).

Learning Outcomes
After completing this section, you should be able to:
- Compare your usual approach to dealing with conflict with that of your friends, family members, and co-workers.
- Analyze what is happening to you and the other person when you're faced with conflict.
- Use conflict resolution strategies to make conflict work in positive ways.

Thinking Critically About Conflict
Conflict arises from human instinct. From the beginning of mankind, when survival of the fittest reigned, humans instinctively protected their territory and reacted with suspicion to people different from themselves. Today, many of us subconsciously protect our territory and react negatively toward others when things aren't going the way we expect.

Conflict can be mild, taking the form of subtle opposition to an idea or action, or it can be severe, taking the form of sharp disagreement and fighting. For many, the word *conflict* has negative connotations, bringing feelings of discomfort and dread. Most of us want to live in a world where everyone gets along and everything goes smoothly. Critical thinking requires being able to understand and exchange different viewpoints, wants, and needs and to come to a sincere agreement about what's most important. Knowing how

TABLE 6-2 OUTCOMES OF CONFLICT

Negative Outcomes of Conflict	Positive Outcomes of Managing Conflict Constructively
Increased stress	Reduced stress
Decreased productivity	Increased harmony and productivity
Poor relationships and feelings of isolation	Better relationships and more interaction
Wasted time and energy	Better understanding of others involved
Frustration, anger, and hopelessness	Improved ability to clarify main issues and find creative solutions
Lack of growth	Opportunity to improve bothersome things
Poor self-esteem	Improved self-esteem

to make conflict work in positive ways helps you grow. When you know how to manage conflict constructively, you are more likely to have positive outcomes and spend less time dealing with the negative outcomes of conflict (Table 6-2).

How to Manage Conflict Constructively

1. Gain insight into your natural style of dealing with conflict (Box 6-1). Make a commitment to use your strengths and work on weaknesses in an objective, purposeful way.
2. Learn to recognize patterns and appearances of conflict early. Become cognizant of verbal and nonverbal behaviors that signal that conflict may be developing (e.g., withdrawal, verbalization of problems with current state of affairs).
3. Develop skills you need to function more comfortably when faced with conflict (e.g., being assertive without being aggressive as noted in the shaded section that follows).
4. Practice using conflict management strategies (Box 6-2 on page 237).
5. Use a comprehensive approach to assessing and managing conflict:
   - Don't jump to conclusions: Hold your opinions until you're sure of all the facts. Check your strong feelings and *assume* the person has good intentions (it may not seem like it, but most people don't intend to offend or do wrong).
   - Remember that there are three ways to view the situation: (1) the way you see it, (2) the way the other person sees it, and (3) the way it *really* is.[13]

- Stay focused on the *relationship* and common values and goals. Don't nitpick on small issues—look at the big picture, and address the impact that the major behaviors have on achieving goals.

- Choose an appropriate time and place to open discussion (ensure privacy, and find a convenient time for those involved).

- Foster an atmosphere of trust and sincere desire to face issues fairly together; encourage free exchange of ideas, feelings, and attitudes.

- Be willing to persevere until you clearly understand the issues, values, and goals of the key players involved.

- Look for win-win solutions (you may have to compromise a little bit). Try to find several solutions to the problems, evaluating each solution with the key players involved.

- Make a conscious effort to stay calm, help others stay calm, and keep the focus on the positive outcomes of resolving the conflict and building the relationship.

- Take a break, or get help from outside sources as needed. Allow for time out, but keep interacting until all parties agree to the solution.

- Set up a time to revisit issues to see if the solutions are actually being carried out and helping reduce the problem.

6. Apply principles of negotiation as appropriate (Box 6-3).

BOX 6-1 MANAGING CONFLICT: WHAT'S YOUR STYLE?

AVOIDERS pull away. They ignore issues or withdraw from people they feel are causing conflict. Avoiders often get along well with others because they focus on promoting peace and harmony. However, they tend to allow problems to persist and place little importance on their own needs. As a result, they miss opportunities to make improvements and tend to "explode" when things finally get to be too much, even though the trigger issue may be minor.

ACCOMMODATORS (SMOOTHERS) give up their own needs and try to make others feel better. Members of this group often struggle with inner conflicts because they secretly wish to speak their minds. They, too, can explode, damaging relationships because of failure to honestly confront issues that are important to them.

FORCERS try to get *their* way even if it means others have to give up what they want or need. They're minimally interested in or aware of what others need and don't really care if they are liked.

COMPROMISERS give up part of their wants and needs and persuade others to give up part of their wants and needs. They think they get win-win solutions but may be settling for minimally acceptable solutions that continue the conflict (because they assume everyone has to lose something in negotiations rather than persisting to find answers that fully satisfy everyone involved).

COLLABORATIVE PROBLEM SOLVERS make it a rule to fairly face issues together. This group has equal concern for both the issues and the relationship. They see conflict as a means of improving relationships by gaining understanding and reducing tension. They look for solutions that allow everyone to win by identifying areas of agreement and differences. They evaluate alternatives, and choose solutions that have the full support of the key parties involved.

BOX 6-2 MAD ABOUT YOU: MANAGING CONFLICT CONSTRUCTIVELY

1. Listen with the intent to understand the other person's points of view before presenting your own.
2. Take a deep breath, and keep a lid on your emotions. It's hard to think clearly when your adrenaline is flowing.
3. Using "I" messages and a nonthreatening tone of voice, clearly explain how the problem is affecting you and what you'd like to happen.
   - "I feel [name the feeling]."
   - "When I see or hear [state the problem]."
   - "I would like [state the change you want to happen]."
4. Ask yourself, What can I find in this situation that *I'm* doing to contribute to the problem? You have more control over things that *you're* doing to contribute to the problem than over things that others are doing to contribute to the problem.
5. Get rid of old baggage (feelings and preconceptions you have because of things that have happened in the past); for example, thinking, *I'm just not the type of person who can handle conflict, so she knows she can get her way.*
6. Look for deep issues. For example, say, "Tell me what's really bothering you" (keep repeating this if the answer is "I don't know").
7. Be willing to hear things you don't like to hear. You need honest feedback to work through the issues.
8. Ask for help from those involved. For example, "Can we agree to not be so hard on one another?"
9. Change your approach to managing conflict depending on the situation rather than using the style you're most comfortable with. For example, many nurses use avoidance as their main approach to resolving conflicts.
   - **Use collaborative problem-solving** as the overall, optimum way to manage conflict. Because this approach takes more time than you may have at the moment, initially you may need to use one of the following approaches. You also may need to use all the methods below as stepping stones to collaborative problem-solving.
   - **Use avoidance** only when trying to delay confrontation until a more appropriate time, when a time-out is required, or when issues are of minor importance in relation to overall goal.
   - **Use accommodation or smoothing** when the goal is to preserve relationships or encourage the others to express themselves.
   - **Use compromise** when time is too limited for a full collaborative approach and there are two equally empowered sides that must reach agreement yet maintain a positive relationship. Find a common ground to achieve temporary settlement that at least satisfies each side's main objectives.
   - **Use forcing** only when there isn't time for discussion (for example, in an emergency), when you must implement unpopular changes, or when all other strategies have failed and the change is required.

BOX 6-3 HOW TO NEGOTIATE

- Clarify the results you want to achieve.
- Build and maintain a communication climate that supports problem-solving under stress.
- Let other parties know your interests, and actively work to discover theirs.
- Be willing to explore the needs of all parties and find mutually agreeable solutions.
- Determine common interests as well as conflicting needs and desires.
- Think about various proposals, and decide whether to reject, reframe, or accept them.
- Decide the worst-case scenario (what you're willing to accept even if it's not exactly what you want). Don't accept anything that's below your worst-case scenario. Consider and discuss any offer that's less than you'd like but better than your worst-case scenario.

BEING ASSERTIVE WITHOUT BEING AGGRESSIVE

- Try to understand completely before responding. To be sure you understand correctly, paraphrase what you heard.
- State your own feelings, thoughts, and needs clearly, in a nonthreatening way.
- Stand up for your own rights while showing respect for the rights of others
- Pay attention to cultural and personality differences
- Convey needs and wants by using "I" messages to address how you feel about the specific behavior that disturbs you (e.g., "I was embarrassed and hurt when I saw you walk away from our conversation" rather than, "You made me feel like such a jerk when …").
- Value yourself and act with confidence—don't feel guilty when you say "no" ("I'm sorry, but I can't do that").
- Own responsibility and speak with authority—use eye contact, a direct body posture, and a controlled voice volume and tone (may need to adapt this if cultural differences are involved).

 OTHER PERSPECTIVES

IT TAKES COURAGE TO CONFRONT

"Confrontation takes considerable courage, and many people would rather take the course of least resistance (belittling and criticizing, betraying confidences, or participating in gossip about others behind their backs). But in the long run, people will trust and respect you if you are honest and open and kind with them. You care enough to confront."[14]

—*Author Stephen Covey*

Critical Thinking Exercises

Think, Pair, Share

With a partner, in a group, or in a journal entry:

1. Gain insight into how you tend to respond to conflict and how you feel about other people's styles for resolving conflict:
   a. Describe a conflict that you can remember in some detail.
   b. In relation to Box 6-1 (page 236), identify your usual way of dealing with conflict. After considering your own style, think about what styles the other people you know use and how they affect you and the conflict resolution process.
   c. Think about how you could you have handled the situation you identified in choice *a* above differently? What style(s) may have achieved a better outcome?
2. Share your stories about conflict with others, asking for a different viewpoint on what was going on in the conflict and what styles and strategies might help.
3. Practice using "I" messages. Change the following statements to ones that send "I" messages.
   a. "You never listen to me."
   b. "I wish you wouldn't be so sloppy all the time."
   c. "You make me feel like I'm the one who causes all the problems."
   d. "You make me feel insignificant when you ignore me like that."
   e. "Why are you always attacking me?"
4. Use role-playing to practice assertive communication and conflict resolution. Get a partner. Have one of you be the manager in the following situation and the other, the staff nurse. Here's the situation:

   A staff nurse is angry because he didn't get a specific day off, even though he had put in a written request well ahead of time. He needs the weekend off for his daughter's birthday. The manager spent hours trying to find proper coverage but couldn't honor his request because two other nurses also needed to be off and were turned down for their requests the previous month.
5. Decide where you stand in relation to achieving the learning outcomes listed at the beginning of this skill.

Recommended

Mind Tools. Conflict resolution: Resolving conflict rationally and effectively. Retrieved January 11, 2010, from http://www.mindtools.com/pages/article/newLDR_81.htm

Restifo, V., & Jackson, M. Surviving and thriving with conflict on the job. Retrieved January 28, 2011, from http://ce.nurse.com/CE112-60/Surviving-and-Thriving-with-Conflict-on-the-Job/

See also RECOMMENDED in the sections *Communicating Bad News* and *Giving and Taking Constructive Criticism.*

6. MANAGING YOUR TIME

Definition
Knowing how to use time effectively by getting organized and setting priorities, and staying focused on them.

Learning Outcomes
After completing this section, you should be able to:
- Explain how an activity diary (or log) helps you manage your time.
- Describe how to set priorities based on your personal and professional goals.
- Identify ways to organize your life to make the most of your time.
- Determine ways to improve your ability to manage your time in the clinical setting.

Thinking Critically About Managing Your Time
Have you ever felt like your days are like an endless race to catch a fast-moving train? If so, you need to learn to be on that train at the controls! Taking control to manage your time helps you avoid stress and frustration. It also improves self-confidence, results, and job satisfaction because you work smarter, not harder.

How to Manage Your Time
This section is organized by the following headings: (1) Determining What Must Be Done, (2) Ranking Priorities, (3) Organizing Your Schedule and Work, and (4) Streamlining Work in the Clinical Setting.

Determining What Must Be Done
1. Develop and record your personal, professional, and work goals. Keep them in a readily accessible place. These goals serve as a guide to help you prioritize and organize.

2. Start an activity diary (or log). For several consecutive days, write down everything you do. Include what you do, the amount of time you spend doing it, and the time of day you do it. It should look something like this:

ACTIVITY LOG

Time	Activities and Tasks
8:00 to 8:30 AM	*Drive to health club*
8:30 to 9:00 AM	*Work out*
9:00 to 9:45 AM	*Drive to class*
10:00 to 11:15 AM	*Class*
11:15 AM to 1:00 PM	*Have lunch, hang out with friends*
1:00 to 2:15 PM	*Class*
2:15 to 5:00 PM	*Miscellaneous unscheduled tasks*

---

3. After a few days, analyze your log, and arrange each of the activities and tasks according to the following categories:
   - Must do (essential) activities and tasks
   - Should or could do (or could be delegated to someone else) activities and tasks
   - Nice to do (if you had more time) activities
   - Not necessary (time waster) activities and tasks
4. Be sure that things under your "must do" category reflect your personal and professional or work goals. If they don't, decide whether you truly *must* do them.
5. Decide whether there are things missing on your "must do" list. Add these to the list.
6. Find ways to spend most of your time each day on the "must do" list. Figure out how to get rid of time wasters. For example, in the activity log under point 2 of this section, you could get rid of an hour's driving by working out at home instead of at the health club.
7. Review the list of "nice to do" activities. Ask, "Are there things on this list that I could or should be delegating to someone else? If so, who is the best person(s) to do the tasks? and What would be the results in the long run?"
8. Consider whether you could combine some activities. For example, if you have specific educational goals, you might listen to educational tapes while driving.

Ranking Priorities. This section addresses ranking priorities in relation to *everyday life*. For ranking priorities in the clinical setting, see *Delegating Safely and Effectively* (Chapter 3, page 111) and *Setting Priorities* (Chapter 5, page 198).
1. Determine the following priority needs, being clear about the rationale for your choices:
   - First-order priority: Must do—important and urgent

- Second-order priority: Must do—important but not urgent
- Third-order priority: Nice to do—not as important and not urgent
2. For each priority, consider the following:
   - How much time you have
   - Whether you (and only you) can do what needs to be done, or whether you can delegate the task(s) or parts of the task(s) to others
   - Whether technology can help you be more efficient (e.g., mastering computer skills)
   - Whether paying someone to get things done better or more quickly will improve your results or give you more time to spend on tasks related to major goals
   - Whether there is a cheaper way of accomplishing the task (e.g., using a library computer is cheaper than hiring a typist)

Organizing Your Schedule and Work

- Review your personal, professional, and work goals. Organize your time to get the tasks related to your most important goals done first.
- Work on major priorities at a time when you know you perform best (e.g., some people work better in the morning; others do better at night).
- Plan break time, eat healthily, drink lots of water, and sleep regular hours. Include time for exercise and stress reduction (this helps you be more productive by avoiding low energy levels).
- Organize your environment for optimum productivity.
- Make a "to do" list for each day, and estimate the time each activity on your list will require. Be sure that your list includes only those activities that you must or should do.
- Reserve time in your daily schedule for unexpected events. Life is unpredictable.
- For long-term (or large) projects, keep a master list to refer to periodically. For each project, map out interim target dates that ensure you will complete the project in a timely way or by the designated deadline.
- Avoid the human tendency to put off large projects or find excuses to evade things you don't enjoy. Procrastination is a major time waster.
- Don't expect or demand perfection. Letting go of a task once it's done is crucial for managing time. Perfectionism can also be a time waster!
- Look for ways to streamline work, as in the following section.

Streamlining Work in the Clinical Setting

1. Reduce your stress and improve your performance: Get to work early enough to get organized and plan your day before you're "under the gun" to perform.
   - Use a daily worksheet that is legible and organized.
   - Cluster activities before entering a room—think ahead and anticipate needs (e.g., a need for pain medication).

- Avoid charting the same thing in two places. Focus most on charting what's different—for example, use charting by exception (CBE) if allowed by charting policies.
- Organize supply and medication carts so that the commonly used items are easily found.
- Label all supply shelves and cabinets clearly for easy access.

RULE

If you "hit the ground running" the minute you get to work, you are arriving too late. Give yourself at least 10 to 15 minutes to gather your thoughts, get the big picture of what's happening on the unit, and focus and plan your day (30 minutes early is even better).

2. Use tools and technology to organize your personal and professional work. For example:
   - Use a personal digital assistant (PDA) or another electronic organizer to keep your schedule and other important information handy.
   - A paper system, such as the Franklin-Covey planner, also works well. The advantage of a paper system is that it is usually less expensive and doesn't require interaction with a personal computer (PC).
   - Whatever organizing system you use, keep all scheduled activities within the *same* organizing system, rather than keeping multiple or duplicate systems. For example, don't keep your work schedule on a PDA and your social calendar elsewhere.
3. Set limits on what you agree to do.

CRITICAL MOMENTS

TAKE CARE OF YOURSELF: A TIME MANAGEMENT PRIORITY
Many nurses feel guilty about making time to care for themselves. When making your list of priorities, health promotion activities should be high on the list. As Jim Loehr—author of *The power of full engagement: Managing energy, not time is the key to high performance and personal renewal*—says, keep your "engine" in top form by making time for things like eating well, meditating, getting enough rest, and exercising regularly.[15]

OTHER PERSPECTIVES

LEARN TO SAY NO!
"Saying "no" if the request for your time is not a "must do" or "should/could do" activity is good time management. Saying something like "I wish I could help you, but I'm overloaded right now" works very well. In some cases, you may also

have to say something like, "I need a bit more time if you want me to do a good job." Does this mean shirking responsibilities or procrastinating? Not at all. It means that when you have a track record of showing responsibility, and want to do a good job, asking for more time or simply saying "No" may be good time management."[16]

—Donna D. Ignatavicius, MS, RN

Critical Thinking Exercises

Think, Pair, Share

With a partner, in a group, or in a journal entry:

1. Identify three personal or professional goals that you want to accomplish within the next year.
2. Keep an activity diary for three consecutive days during the week. Be sure to include all activities for work, school, and home. In relation to the goals you identified in number 1 above, analyze the diary and:
   - Determine the "must do" activities that will help you achieve your goals for the next year.
   - Identify time wasters, and decide how you might eliminate them.
   - Rank the "must do" activities by assigning priorities (first-order, second-order, or third-order priorities).
   - Ask yourself whether there are some things you should be doing to achieve your personal and professional goals. Add these to the list.
   - Share what you learned from doing the above.
4. Share time-management strategies that work in your personal life.
5. Describe strategies that help you manage your time in the clinical setting—include how you deal with things that are time wasters.
6. Discuss the implications of some of the *Other Perspectives, Critical Moments,* and RECOMMENDED listed in this skill.
7. Decide where you stand in relation to achieving the learning outcomes listed at the beginning of this skill.

Recommended

Loehr, J., & Schwartz, T. (2003). *The power of full engagement: Managing energy, not time is the key to high performance and personal renewal.* New York: Free Press.

McGuinness, M. Time management for creative people. Retrieved January 21, 2011, from http://media.lateralaction.com/creativetime.pdf

MindTools. Time management. (Website). Retrieved January 10, 2011, from http://www.mindtools.com/pages/main/newMN_HTE.htm

Arevalo, J. Getting a grip on time management. Retrieved January 6, 2011, from http://www.nursezone.com/student-nurses/student-nurses-featured-articles/Getting-a-Grip-on-Time-Management_18496.aspx

7. NAVIGATING AND FACILITATING CHANGE

Definition
Knowing how to chart a course to successfully adapt to change (and to help others to do the same).

Learning Outcomes
After completing this section, you should be able to:
- Recognize how you usually react when faced with change.
- Identify strategies to help you navigate change.
- Describe how to facilitate change in others.

Thinking Critically About Change
As Will Rogers said, "Even if you're on the right track, you'll get run over if you just sit there." Change is a part of life. Knowing how to plot a course through the many changes we face on a daily basis—and how to help others do the same—helps you move from feeling disrupted and frustrated to feeling a sense of progress and accomplishment.

How to Navigate and Facilitate Change
This section first gives strategies to help *you* navigate change, and then it give strategies to help you help *others* deal with change.

Strategies to Navigate Change
- Curb the tendency to keep the status quo just because it's easy and comfortable.
- When first faced with change, suspend judgment and fairly explore reasons for the required change. Navigating change doesn't mean embracing change uncritically—it means clarifying the pros and cons and making reasoned decisions about whether the change is worthwhile.

■ Make sure you understand why the change is being made and how you feel about it. If you can get something out of the change, it helps you accept it. If you have strong feelings against making the change, you need to explore and work through them.

■ Identify barriers to making the change and find ways to deal with them. For example, make yourself a "cheat sheet" when learning new technology.

■ Ask for help. If you express the problems you have, others may be able to help. You may also identify concerns that are bothering everyone.

■ Expect the following natural sequence of events often associated with adapting to change.

STAGES ASSOCIATED WITH ADAPTING TO CHANGE

1. **Losing focus.** Expect some confusion, disorientation, and forgetfulness at first. You may be unsure about boundaries and responsibilities. Ask for clarification, keep notes, and use to-do lists.

2. **Denial.** You may want to minimize or deny the effect the change has on you. However, *connecting with and dealing with feelings* helps you move forward. Acknowledge how you feel about what you lose and gain by making the change.

3. **Anger or depression.** If you feel angry, discouraged, or frustrated:
   • Vent your anger in a safe place. Be careful with whom, how, and where you ventilate. Your words can come back to haunt you. Find someone who'll listen without being affected by your feelings (e.g., someone who has gone through the change you're experiencing, not someone who also is struggling and who may be pulled down by your negativity).
   • Use stress management strategies (e.g., exercise helps diffuse anger and frustration).
   • Keep away from negative people, or soon you'll feel the same way.
   • Stay focused on what you'll gain from making the change. Be patient with yourself, let go of the past, and take it one step at a time. Make a conscious effort to think critically and not emotionally.

4. **Moving forward.** Seek opportunities to use the new skills and procedures you've learned. Celebrate small successes, recognizing how far you've come and what you learned along the way.
   • Share your experience with those who may not have come as far as you have.
   • Remember to represent your organization positively in public, even if you don't feel that way at the moment.

Strategies to Facilitate Change in Others

■ Include key stakeholders to determine how the change will affect those involved. Be clear about the positives and negatives *from their perspectives* (e.g., "This will require effort and time on your part, but when we're done we'll all have it easier."

- Clearly describe both the required changes and the expected benefits.
- Clarify changes in roles and responsibilities.
- Get support from formal and informal group leaders (they can make or break progress).
- Allow people to explore how the change will affect their daily lives (e.g., When one group moved to electronic health records, several nurses said, "You know how we love our paper!")
- Encourage involvement in finding ways to make the change easier.
- Convey an understanding of negative feelings and extra work associated with having to make changes. Provide necessary resources and support (for example, technical support) until the change has been fully implemented.
- Ask for ownership of responsibility for change (both leaders and subordinates own some of the work).
- Involving key stakeholders, identify barriers to making the change, and find ways to deal with them. For example, if workers are expected to take time to practice using a new computer system, provide extra personnel to do ordinary chores.
- Be clear about time lines: Key players must know exactly what change is expected to occur and by when.
- Be patient. Going through the stages of adapting to change takes time.

CRITICAL MOMENTS

TRANSFORM RATHER THAN CONFORM
When facilitating change, aim to transform rather than conform. Inspire, show benefits, encourage, and support. When people are transformed, they change because they *want* to.

OTHER PERSPECTIVES

BARRIERS AND BLIND SPOTS: A PART OF CHANGE
Leaders and staff experience concerns, barriers, and "blind spots" when creating and implementing change. Regardless of whether the hesitation is rooted in fear, expectations, limitations, or restricting beliefs, coaching is designed to reveal, explore and address these issues so that they won't get in the way of successful change.

—Kimberly McNally and Liz Cunningham, Authors of
Nurse Executive Coaching Manual[17]

FINDING YOUR TRUE DIRECTION
Sometimes in the winds of change we find our true direction.

—Unknown

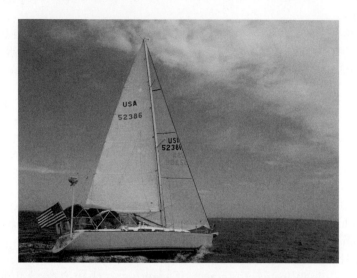

Critical Thinking Exercises

Think, Pair, Share

With a partner, in a group, or in a journal entry:

1. Share your best and worst experiences with navigating and facilitating change. Discuss the factors that made them your best and worst experiences.
2. Describe a personal or work change that you experienced that wasn't of your choice (e.g., moving to a new home, a change in job description).
   - Think about how you felt at the time and the effect it had on your ability to make the change.
   - Identify some things you could have done to make the change easier.
3. Share a time you tried to help someone else change.
   - How successful were you?
   - What, if anything, would you do differently?
4. Share your thoughts on the graphics identifying "Change Choices" found in Clemmer, J. Navigating change and adversity. Retrieved January 12, 2011, from http://www.hodu.com/change2.shtml
5. Study the following shaded section on transformational change. Discuss the difference between change that transforms versus change that conforms.

Four Ways We Change

1. Pendulum change: I was wrong before, but now I'm right.
2. Change by exception: I'm right, except for …
3. Incremental change: I was almost right before, but now I'm right.
4. Paradigm change: What I knew before was partially right. What I know now is more right, but still only part of what I'll know tomorrow.

Paradigm Change Is Transformational

Paradigm change combines what's useful about old ways with what's useful about new ways, and keeps us open to looking for even better ways. We realize:

- Our previous views were only part of the picture.
- What we now know is only part of what we'll know later.
- Change is no longer threatening: It enlarges and enriches.
- The unknown can then be friendly and interesting.
- Each insight smoothes the road, making the change process easier.

Source: Adapted from Ferguson, M. (1980). *Aquarian conspiracy: Personal and social transformation in our time.* New York: GP Putnam's Sons.

6. Discuss the implications of some of the *Critical Moments, Other Perspectives,* and RECOMMENDED listed in this skill.
7. Decide where you stand in relation to achieving the learning outcomes listed at the beginning of this skill.

Recommended

Clemmer, J. Navigating change and adversity. Retrieved January 12, 2011, from http://www.hodu.com/change2.shtml

Johnson, S., & Blanchard, K. (1998). *Who moved my cheese?* New York: Putnam Publishing Group.

McNally, K., & Cunningham, L. (2010). *Nurse executive coaching manual.* Indianapolis: Sigma Theta Tau International.

Robinson-Walker, C. Coaching: An essential skill for nurses. Retrieved January 12, 2011, from http://ce.nurse.com/60107/Coaching-An-Essential-Skill-for-Nurses/

8. PREVENTING AND DEALING WITH MISTAKES CONSTRUCTIVELY

Definition

Knowing how to prevent, detect, correct, and learn from errors.

Learning Outcomes

After completing this section, you should be able to:

- Define the terms *error, sentinel event, near miss, hazardous condition,* and *safety culture* using your own words.
- Explain how to determine the seriousness of a mistake.
- Identify circumstances that lead you and others to make mistakes.
- Identify strategies that help you be a safety net for your team members.
- Decide what to do when you make (or witness someone else make) a mistake.
- Develop a personal plan for preventing, detecting, correcting, and learning from mistakes.

Thinking Critically About Preventing and Dealing with Mistakes

Mistakes can be our worst nightmare, or they can be stepping-stones to learning and improvement. And sometimes, they can be both. Dealing with mistakes is a complex issue that includes considering legal consequences (in some states, it's the law that patients be informed of errors; mistakes sometimes end up in malpractice litigation). This section addresses how to know what constitutes a serious error, why errors happen, and how to prevent, detect, correct, and learn from errors.

There are two major types of errors:

1. **Commission**—doing the wrong thing
2. **Omission**—failing to do the right thing

There are also three common reasons for mistakes:[18]

1. **Execution errors**—doing the right thing incorrectly
2. **Rule violation**—going against current rules or policies
3. **Wrong plan**—when actions proceed as planned, but fail to achieve the intended outcome because the planned action or original intention was wrong

Too many people have a one-size-fits-all mindset when it comes to dealing with mistakes. Deep down, they believe that all errors are bad, that all errors happen because of lack of knowledge or laziness, and that the best way to deal with people who make mistakes is to punish them. However, this approach shames those involved, doesn't examine the real causes of errors, and does little to reduce the *incidence* of mistakes—it only reduces the reporting of mistakes. When errors aren't reported, opportunities to fix related problems are missed and mistakes are likely to be repeated.

Most mistakes happen for multiple reasons and in spite of good intentions. We must change the mindset from "mistakes shouldn't happen" to "when dealing with humans, mistakes *will* happen for various reasons." We must share our mistakes freely so that we can work together to find ways to prevent future mistakes. The following shaded section shows four common reasons for medication errors.

Common Reasons for Medication Errors

1. **Communication failure:** These include transcription errors, use of abbreviations, illegible handwriting, incorrect interpretation of physician's orders, use of verbal orders, failure to record medications given or omitted, and unclear medication administration records. Studies show that nearly three in four medical errors are caused by mistakes in interpersonal communication.[19] Communication issues are major causes of mistakes and adverse patient outcomes (e.g., falls, injuries, and care omissions).[20]
2. **Errors or omissions in medication reconciliation when patients are admitted or transferred from one unit to another** (medication reconciliation is a formal process for creating the most complete and accurate list possible of a patient's current medications and comparing the list to those in the patient record or medication orders).[21]
3. **Failure to ensure the "RIGHTS OF MEDICATION ADMINISTRATION":**

Right patient	Right assessment	Right to refuse
Right drug	Right route	Right evaluation (follow-up)
Right dosage	Right time	Right documentation
Right reason	Right patient education	

4. **Not complying with policies and procedures:** Lack of attention to safeguards in medication administration procedures intended to prevent errors
5. **Human and system problems:** These include things like nurses with little experience being assigned complex patients; nurse fatigue (consecutive hours worked without brakes or little time off); rotating shifts; poor staffing; distractions and interruptions; the practice of floating nurses to unfamiliar units; hospital and pharmacy design features; and drug manufacturing problems (e.g., look-alike and sound-alike drug names, look-alike packaging, confusing and unclear labeling, failure to specify drug concentrations on dose-calculation charts)

Key Terms Related to Examining Mistakes. The following terms are important to understand in the context of developing and maintaining in-depth approaches to error prevention (definitions are adapted from various documents available at www.jointcommission.org).

■ **SENTINEL EVENT:** An unexpected occurrence involving death or serious physical or psychological injury (or the risk thereof). Serious injury specifically includes loss of limb or function. The phrase "or risk thereof" means any variation from the usual process of care such that if it happens again, there is a significant chance of causing a serious adverse outcome. **Example:** a break in procedures that causes nurses to omit checking that the correct leg is marked for amputation. Whether the wrong leg is amputated or not, a sentinel event has occurred. The term *sentinel* is used because of its relationship to a sentinel guard—a soldier who stands guard to keep his people safe. Sentinel events are so serious that they signal the need for immediate investigation to ensure they don't happen again.

- **NEAR MISS:** Anything that happens during the process of care that didn't affect the outcome, but poses a significant chance of a serious adverse outcome if it happens again. **Example:** If a physician almost operates on the wrong site, but this is caught just in time, it's a near miss. Near misses are considered sentinel events, but they may not be reviewed by the Joint Commission under its sentinel event policy.

- **HAZARDOUS CONDITION:** Any set of circumstances (exclusive of the disease or condition for which the patient is being treated) that significantly increases the likelihood of a serious adverse outcome. **Example:** nurses who have too many acutely ill patients to give appropriate care.

- **ROOT CAUSE ANALYSIS (RCA):** The process for identifying deep underlying cause(s) of a mistake—the "root(s)" of errors. Requires examining in detail what happened, why it happened, who was involved, all factors that contribute to the mistake, and what can be done to prevent it. **Example:** not assuming a drug error was due to one nurse's lack of knowledge. Rather, the error is examined deeply to identify all possible contributing factors and deciding the deepest causes (e.g., the *root cause* of the nurse's lack of knowledge could be that there's no policy in place to ensure that new drugs aren't introduced unless all nurses have the required knowledge; this is considered a *system* problem).

- **FAILURE MODE EFFECT ANALYSIS (FMEA):** An approach to error prevention that aims to build systems that promote safety and prevent accidents. FMEA assumes that errors are not only possible, but also even likely, despite knowledgeable and careful health care professionals. FMEA assumes that it's too much to ask individuals alone to be responsible for errors. Instead the responsibility is placed on an interdisciplinary group that engages in a never-ending process of quality improvement to assess and correct areas where errors are likely. FMEA also aims to design a system in which critical or catastrophic errors can't happen. **Example:** wrong-site surgeries that are prevented by a strict policy that includes several "check points" to ensure that the correct surgery in the correct person in the correct body part is done.

How to Prevent and Deal with Mistakes Constructively

1. Make patient and caregiver safety a part of the health team code of conduct. The following shaded section shows an excerpt from the code of conduct on page 27:

> ## SAFETY, ERROR PREVENTION, AND CODE OF CONDUCT
>
> As a member of this group/team, I agree to work to make the following a part of my daily routine. **To keep patient and caregiver safety and welfare as the primary concern in all interactions, including:**
> * Being vigilant and monitoring for care practices that increase risks of errors
> * Remembering that no one is perfect and all humans are vulnerable to making mistakes
> * Taking responsibility for being "a safety net" when helping co-workers, anticipating what they may need and pitching in to prevent mistakes (e.g. "I think that glove is contaminated, let me get you a new one." "Here's a new needle")
> * Making it a team principle that "If we witness unethical or unsafe practices, it's our responsibility to address it (first directly with the person, then through policies and procedures if warranted)."

2. **Make it a point to look for errors and flaws in thinking.** In important or emergency situations, check, check, and check again—the more you check, the more you find.

3. **Remember that all mistakes aren't created equal**—in addition to knowing the difference between a sentinel event, near miss, or hazardous condition, you should know the following different types of mistakes, what things cause them, and how you can prevent them.

   ■ **Mental slips:** These mistakes happen when there's a lapse in your attention to what you're doing or when there's a lapse in short-term memory. **Example:** You're on the way to check an IV, but you're interrupted to help lift someone up in bed. You then forget that you were on the way to check the IV and go on to another task. **Prevention:** Keep a personal worksheet that prompts you to do important tasks (for example, check IV every hour). Get your charting done as soon as possible to help you notice when you've forgotten to do something. Checklists, protocols, and computerized decision aids all help reduce mental slips because they relieve you from relying on short-term memory, the aspect of memory that becomes most imperfect under stress or fatigue.

   ■ **Interaction (communication) errors:** These mistakes happen when people misunderstand each other. **Example:** You're working in the emergency department and just spoke to Dr. French about one of your patients, Mrs. Moran. A few minutes later, Dr. French comes to you and says, "Would you send her to x-ray?" nodding in the direction of another patient. You don't see him nod in the other direction and assume Dr. French is referring to Mrs. Moran. **Prevention:** Repeat what you hear to clarify verbal interactions ("You want me to send Mrs. Moran to x-ray?"). Check written orders to clarify verbal orders.

   ■ **Knowledge errors:** These mistakes are due to insufficient knowledge. **Example:** You cause unnecessary side effects by giving an IV drug too quickly because you didn't know it should be given slowly. **Prevention:** Be sure you find out the answers to who, what, why, when, and how in context of each individual patient situation before you give any drug or perform any intervention.

- **Learning errors:** Although these mistakes often include knowledge errors, learning errors usually are related to several different factors associated with being in a learning situation (for example, doing something for the first time or being stressed). **Example:** You change sterile dressings for the first time. You contaminate your glove by slightly touching an unsterile field. You don't notice it because you're focused on assessing the wound. **Prevention:** A surefire way to avoid learning errors is not to try anything new, which makes no sense. Many students hide from new experiences because they're afraid of making mistakes. This just postpones the inevitable. The best way to avoid learning errors is to be prepared and to practice, practice, practice in as safe an environment as possible (for example, in a skills lab). In risky situations, it's best to have a more experienced nurse guide performance, give advice, or actually handle the task at hand.

- **Relying too much on technology:** These mistakes happen when you allow technology to think for you, without wondering if there's a flaw in the system. **Example:** Someone complains that a heating pad is too hot. You check the setting and see that it's in the "low" position. Instead of carefully feeling the pad yourself, you explain that it's probably okay because it's set on low. **Prevention:** Read all instruction manuals carefully. Don't trust machines more than your own knowledge and perceptions. Don't allow technology to think *for* you: think *with* it.

- **System errors:** These mistakes are related to something wrong with the way things are accomplished within the facility as a whole. **Examples:** drugs that aren't given because the pharmacist is overloaded and unable to dispense the drug in a timely manner; errors that happen because a policy or procedure is unclear; or errors that happen because a facility uses a lot of per diem personnel who are more at risk for making mistakes. Report possible system problems to the risk management or quality assurance department. Create a multidisciplinary panel to examine possible and actual system problems.

4. **Always determine how serious the error is.** Serious errors need to be examined more closely, prevented more meticulously, and detected and corrected more quickly than less serious errors.

RULE

To determine the seriousness of a mistake, answer two questions:
1. **What harm could result if the mistake happens?** (Primarily consider harm in terms of human morbidity, mortality, and suffering. Secondarily, consider harm in terms of inconvenience, cost, and lost time. If you're unable to decide what harm could result, get help).
2. **Should this mistake be classified as a sentinel event, near miss, or hazardous condition?**

5. Follow policies and procedures, and be sure you understand the rationale behind them. These are designed by experts to prevent, detect, and correct errors early.
6. When using checklists, think about each item carefully. Checklists are supposed to jog your brain, not replace it.[22]
7. Involve patients and families in their own health care as much as possible. Educate them, and encourage them to become participants in preventing errors by verifying that they're getting the right treatments and medications and by speaking up when they have questions (see *Speak Up*, Box 3-3, page 81).
8. Never give a medication or perform an intervention without knowing why it's indicated for each *particular person*. Be careful about multitasking.
9. Involve experts. For example, if you're not sure about a medication regimen, ask a pharmacist.
10. Look after yourself. If you're rested and use stress management strategies, you're less likely to make mistakes.

What to Do When Mistakes Happen

1. Determine the seriousness of the error as soon as it's recognized, and take immediate steps to prevent or reduce harm. Get help if needed.
2. Follow policy and procedures for dealing with mistakes, including how to report and record the mistake. Standards and some state laws mandate that patients be informed when mistakes happen. Some policies also require that an apology be made (see Skill 1, Communicating Bad News).
3. Chart actions taken to address the error (for example, increasing the frequency of monitoring or a transfer to another unit).
4. Curb the tendency to focus too much on guilt and not enough on what can be learned from the mistake.
5. Explore the specifics of the incident objectively, examining the procedures and circumstances leading to the errors. Consider the value of sharing the mistake with others to alert them of the possibility of its happening again. If procedures were followed and a mistake still happened, maybe the procedures should be revised to make them more error-proof.

NOTE: For more information on error prevention, see Chapter 3, pages 78 to 84, where the following topics are addressed: Quality and safety education for nurses' competencies, safety is top priority, empowering patients: nurses as stewards for safe passage, standard tools to prevent miss-communication, use of *Read-back* and *Repeat-back* rules, and time-outs promote group thinking and prevent errors. Pages 85 to 108 address the importance of ensuring nursing surveillance through close monitoring, activating the chain of command, monitoring for (and correcting) dangerous situations, and failure to rescue. These pages also address three main strategies nurses use to identify, interrupt, and correct errors and give a map for how to monitor for technical, human, and system failures (page 108).

CRITICAL MOMENTS

EMPOWERING PATIENTS IS KEY TO SAFETY

Empower your patients by teaching them what to expect and telling them that the main thing they can do to prevent mistakes is to become actively involved in managing their own care.

APPLYING NURSING PROCESS PREVENTS MISTAKES

The nursing process steps and principles help you prevent mistakes and improve efficiency. Remember to *assess* (step 1) and *analyze* (step 2) before you *act* (step 3). To pick up problems early, pay attention to patient responses as you *implement interventions* (step 4). Use comprehensive *evaluation* (step 5) to check for mistakes and identify ways to reduce the likelihood of future errors.[23]

MAINTAIN A STERILE COCKPIT—AVOID DISTRACTIONS

Distractions are a major cause of mistakes, especially during the process of medication delivery.[24] Just as pilots maintain a sterile cockpit—no socializing on landings and takeoffs—find a quiet place to do important activities like preparing medications. Don't interrupt other caregivers when they are doing the same.

 OTHER PERSPECTIVES

MISTAKES HAPPEN SO EASILY

"Competitive cyclists have the saying, 'If you're a cyclist, you've already crashed or you're going to.' Perhaps you could substitute any other title for cyclist. If you're a nurse, you've either made a mistake or you're going to ... Crashes occur for many reasons. You can crash if you don't have the necessary knowledge, skill, or equipment. Or conditions unexpectedly become too complex, and in haste you do something you otherwise would not do. Or you or a competitor breaks the rules in an effort to gain advantage. The former would be called errors; the latter are ethical or legal violations. Sometimes that distinction is important, though not always clear ... I propose that errors and ethical misconduct are not a dichotomy of unrelated entities; they are two ends of a continuum. Some errors can be excused; misconduct is not."[25]

—*Sue Thomas Hegyvary, PhD, FAAN, Editor,* Journal of Nursing Scholarship

ERRORS: USUALLY SYSTEM FAILURES, NOT INDIVIDUAL "FAULT"

"I am a nurse scientist who studies medical errors ... I am a critical care nurse who lives in fear of making a mistake that could harm a patient ... The majority of errors are the result of system failures, not the blatant carelessness of individuals. Yet people tend to point fingers at individuals and place blame. Even when well-designed systems are in place, human errors occur. Your statement, 'I am humbled that making such an error is easy to do' will bring comfort to many clinicians and scholars who strive to do the best they can in this busy, complicated world. Acknowledging that both system failures and human fallibility contribute to errors and adverse outcomes is necessary for achieving the ultimate goal of improving the health of the world's people."[26]

—*Elizabeth Henneman, RN, PhD, CCNS*

CHANGE-OF-SHIFT AND OTHER HANDOFFS ARE RISKY POINTS IN CARE

"There's potential for miscommunication each time a patient moves from one area of care to another, for example, from the emergency department to a medical surgical inpatient unit . . . or from one set of providers to another set during a change of shift. In just one average-sized teaching hospital, for example, there are 4000 patient handoff opportunities for errors every day, "or 1.6 million a year. If you think about those staggering numbers, you think about how many opportunities there are for miscommunication."[27]

—*Cheryl Clark*

Critical Thinking Exercises

Think, Pair, Share

With a partner, in a group, or in a journal entry:

1. Address the implications of the following statements.
   a. Being ignorant doesn't merely mean not knowing; it means not knowing what you don't know. Being educated means knowing precisely what you don't know.
   b. As a nurse it's your responsibility to be alert not only to situations that might cause you to make mistakes but also to situations that may cause *others* to make mistakes.
2. Respond to the following:
   a. How do you feel when you make a mistake?
   b. What can you do to help someone else who has made a mistake?
   c. How can you help correct systems that are error-prone and increase checks to prevent medication errors?
3. Share examples of a sentinel event, near miss, hazardous condition, mental slip, knowledge error, learning error, and system error.
4. Share your personal (or a family or friend's) experiences with medical errors.
5. Visit the websites in the following box and address the roles of each of these organizations in promoting safety and preventing errors.

KEY SAFETY ORGANIZATIONS

- Agency for Healthcare Research and Quality (AHRQ): www.ahrq.gov/qual/errorsix.htm
- National Patient Safety Foundation: www.npsf.org
- The Joint Commission (TJC): www.jointcommission.org
- TJC Center for Transforming Healthcare: www.centerfortransforminghealthcare.org/
- The Institute of Medicine: www.iom.edu
- Quality & Safety for Nursing Education (QSEN): http://www.qsen.org/

6. Watch a baseball game and notice how the players back one another up and provide "safety nets" in case of overthrown balls. Notice that players who don't run to their positions to back up another player are yelled at by the crowd. Decide how this applies to what you see in the health care setting.

7. Study Figure 3-3 (page 108), and address strategies you can use to monitor to detect technical, human, and system failures. Also discuss the challenges of being a safety net and correct errors early.

8. Discuss the implications of some of the *Other Perspectives, Critical Moments,* and RECOMMENDED listed in this skill.

9. Decide where you stand in relation to achieving the learning outcomes listed at the beginning of this skill.

Recommended

Gravlin, G., & Phoenix-Bitter, N. (2010). Nurses' and nursing assistants' reports of missed care and delegation. *Journal of Nursing Administration*, 40(78), 329-335.

Good, V., & Flanders, S. (2008). Skilled communication and patient safety (webcast). Retrieved January 6, 2011, from http://www.aacn.org/DM/CETests/Overview.aspx?TestID=418&mid=2864&ItemID=411

Huges, R. (Ed.). (2008). Patient safety and quality: An evidence-based handbook for nurses. Retrieved January 12, 2011, from http://www.ahrq.gov/qual/nurseshdbk/nurseshdbk.pdf

Kosnik, L., Brown, J., Maund, T. (2007). Patient safety: Learning from the aviation industry. Retrieved January 11, 2011, from www.nursingcenter.com/prodev/ce_article.asp?tid=688333

Lambton, J., & Mahlmeister, L. (2010). Conducting root cause analysis with nursing students: Best practice in nursing education. *Journal of Nursing Education*, 49(8), 444-448.

National Patient Safety Foundation. ABCs of patient safety. Retrieved October 3, 2010, from http://www.npsf.org/download/ABCs_of_Patient_Safety.pdf

Wolf, Z. Preventing medical errors. Retrieved January 6, 2011, from http://ce.nurse.com/60150/Preventing-Medication-Errors/

9. TRANSFORMING A GROUP INTO A TEAM

Definition
Knowing how to work together to combine efforts to achieve shared goals and outcomes, within a specific time frame.

Learning Outcomes
After completing this section, you should be able to:
- Explain the common stages of team building.
- Describe strategies that transform groups into teams.
- Participate more effectively as part of a team.
- Explain why patients must be key members of the health care team.

Thinking Critically About Teamwork
How well a team works together determines whether you have frustrated, unhappy patients and staff; whether the atmosphere makes you dread going to work; or whether you have great patient outcomes, job satisfaction, and a sense of good will. Yet building a team isn't easy. Team members need to be nurtured as the team evolves from being a group of diverse, relatively insecure strangers to a group that values common goals and brings together diverse talents and strengths.

True teamwork occurs when all team members are:
1. Committed to common goals and a high level of productivity
2. Energized by their ability to work together
3. Concerned about how team members feel during the work process
4. Committed to including patients their caregivers as key team members

Consider the difference between what's going on in the two following groups:

Two Groups: Two Different Circumstances
Group 1 consists of several nurses who have worked together for the past 6 months. They don't feel like they're working as a team and want this to change. Their manager, Jane, is a busy person who has a demanding boss. Under pressure, Jane barks orders and personally takes over some tasks. The staff responds by doing what they are told or lying low until things calm down. There is minimal group participation in problem-solving and decision making. The nurses want to execute their responsibilities in a satisfactory way. But no one has given thought to the need for group goals or concerted group action. Morale is low, and everyone talks about how unhappy they are.

Group 2 consists of several nurses who also have worked together for 6 months. By contrast, these nurses are energized and proud of their successes. Like Group 1, their manager, Terri, also is a busy person with a demanding boss. However, when the pressure is on, Terri stops the action and convenes a problem-solving discussion, focusing on common goals and getting input from team members. Better solutions are found because the pressure is channeled into a spirit of "let's fix this together." These nurses enjoy a sense of growing and improving together—work is more than just a job.

How to Transform a Group into a Team

Knowing how to communicate and build trust are the cornerstones of teamwork. Early on in the team-building process, all team members must agree to a code of conduct and be aware of messages sent by their behavior. For example, if you consistently show up late for work, shirk responsibility, give excuses, or are arrogant or defensive, you need to be aware of the messages these behaviors send to the rest of the team. On the other hand, if you use behaviors like always being on time, being willing to help, accepting responsibility, and being open to suggestions, you send altogether different messages. Also remember the following rule.

RULE

Being an effective member of a patient care team requires not only building relationships with co-workers and interdisciplinary professionals, but also ensuring that patients and their caregivers are considered key members of the team.

The following gives strategies for team building first from a leadership perspective, then from the team members' perspective.

TEAM-BUILDING STRATEGIES

1. Team leaders should:
   - Create a shared vision of the team's mission or purpose: Everyone must be committed to reaching clearly defined outcomes.
   - Stress that everyone is responsible for preventing errors and improving outcomes by analyzing current practices and pointing out improvements that could be made.
   - Turn diversity to the team's advantage (e.g., assign tasks based on individual strengths and preferences as much as possible).
   - Ask for consensus in decisions (everyone agrees to agree), rather than settling for a majority vote.
   - Keep team members well-informed so that everyone understands the big picture.
   - Recognize team members for their contributions.
   - Be sure team members are familiar with the common stages of team building (Box 6-4 on next page). Although not every group goes through every stage, and the duration of each stage varies, it helps to know that there are common struggles in every team.

2. Team members should:
   - Come to agreement on roles, responsibilities, and proper lines of communication.
   - Work hard to meet responsibilities and deliver what they promise.
   - Get involved and contribute to the good of the group.
   - Stay focused on the big picture of what the team is trying to accomplish.
   - Make a conscious effort to overcome the human tendency to focus narrowly on self; too often, team members have difficulty seeing other members' struggles because they themselves are working so hard.
   - Use behaviors that promote trust and create a caring and energized environment:
     1. Follow the "Platinum Rule" (treat others as *they* want to be treated instead of assuming they want to be treated the same as *you* do).
     2. Show enthusiasm—it's contagious and it energizes others.
     3. Address and resolve conflicts early—push for high-quality communication.
     4. Pay attention to group process and where the team is in relation to the stages of team building (see Box 6-4).
     5. Recognize individual and team efforts; be a good sport and help new teammates make entry.
     6. Support creativity and new ways of doing things.
     7. Broaden your skills; offer to try new tasks or to cross-train.
     8. Promote group learning by collecting, sharing, and analyzing information.
     9. Spend fun time together (here's where relationships grow).

BOX 6-4 COMMON STAGES OF TEAM BUILDING

Forming
Group members start to get to know one another, testing each other's values, beliefs, and attitudes. Basic goals and tasks are defined, roles assigned, and ideas shared.

Storming
Conflict begins, often because of misunderstandings or disagreement about what realistically can get done and how exactly things will get done. More testing goes on in this phase, with some people asking themselves questions like "How much am I willing to do?" This is a time to maintain high standards, provide emotional support, and aim to get consensus (agreement from everyone). Beware of false consensus during this phase; some people will say they agree when they really don't (just to avoid further conflict). Because this is a stressful stage, you may need to take more breaks.

Norming
The group becomes more cohesive and really wants to work together in a positive way. Group members agree on rules—for example, when meetings will be held, who should attend, what the proper lines of communication are, and how problems and disagreements will be handled. At this point the leader needs to be sensitive to group values, asking for votes to determine common needs and desires.

Performing
Team members begin to bond to one another and function well together with a good understanding of roles, responsibilities, and relationships.

OTHER PERSPECTIVES

TEAMWORK REQUIRES EMPOWERMENT

"Teamwork requires empowerment, a willingness and commitment to 'let go' of self (one's own ideas, plans, strategies) to the benefit of the group. As I see it, there are five stages of empowerment: (1) Letting go of self-promotion; (2) Believing that others are capable and competent; (3) Trusting others; (4) Willingness to forgo one's own processes, plans, or strategies to give others a chance; (5) Sharing the outcomes and celebrating success."[28]

—*Sylvia Whiting, PhD, RN, CS*

FIRST STEP TO TEAM BUILDING

"One of the first things you need to do is realize and acknowledge that you and your co-workers are all on the same team—you are there to provide the best care to your patients and clients that you can. You don't have to become best friends with your co-workers; you don't even have to like them. What you do need to do is treat them with respect and work with them to accomplish what needs to be accomplished. Approach work with a positive attitude—negativity only adds to the stress and tension of your workday. Remember, your co-workers are in the same situation you are. If you have a problem with a co-worker, ask to speak to them privately ... One of the most difficult tasks of collaboration, the 'big picture' approach, requires repeatedly asking, 'Will this help us achieve our goal?' Continual focus on the mutually agreed upon outcome is the most likely path to success, for without it the partnership is doomed."[29]

—*Nancy Dickenson-Hazard, RN, MSN, FAAN*

FOSTERING CROSS-CULTURAL UNDERSTANDING

"Working successfully with a culturally diverse staff and patient population encompasses two sets of skills. First, nurses need the holistic skills to manage patients who are different from themselves ... However, the skill that's frequently overlooked is learning to work with diversity among staff members. Embracing cultural diversity in the workplace, as well as in the community, has to be an institutional commitment."[30]

—*Antonia Villaruel, RN, PhD, FAAN*

Critical Thinking Exercises

Think, Pair, Share

With a partner, in a group, or in a journal entry:

1. Share "your story" about a group you currently belong to, addressing what stage of team building you are in as a group in relation to the stages in Box 6-4 (page 261).
2. Share your best and worst experiences with being part of a team. Consider what went right and why you think it went right, and what went wrong and why you think it went wrong.
3. Identify what humans can learn from the geese in the 3-minute inspirational video at http://www.pullingtogethermovie.com/miami
4. Practice brainstorming as a group. Get in a group of 6 to 10 persons. Name one person the recorder and have him or her use a flip chart or blackboard. Identify a problem you'd like to resolve or a situation that could be improved (e.g., how you could get teenagers to come to a meeting on sex education). For 30 minutes, have group members each share ideas to be recorded by the recorder without interpretation. Once you're finished, spend 10 minutes discussing what happened (the group dynamics) as you brainstormed.
5. Discuss the implications of some of the *Other Perspectives* and RECOMMENDED listed in this skill.
6. Decide where you stand in relation to achieving the learning outcomes listed at the beginning of this skill.

Recommended

AHRQ. TeamSTEPPS. Retrieved January 6, 2011, from http://teamstepps.ahrq.gov/index.htm

Kalisch, B., Curley, M., & Stefanov, S. (2007). An intervention to enhance nursing staff teamwork and engagement. *Journal of Nursing Administration,* 37(2), 77-84.

Murphy, J. (2010). *Pulling together: 10 rules of high performance teamwork.* Naperville, IL: Simple Truths.

Wenckus, E., & Teinert, D. Working with an interdisciplinary team. Retrieved January 6, 2011, from http://ce.nurse.com/CE90-60/Working-with-an-Interdisciplinary-Team/

Wood, D. (2010). Changing the physician-nurse dynamic. Retrieved January 6, 2011, from http://www.nursezone.com/Nursing-News-Events/more-news/Changing-the-Physician%E2%80%93Nurse-Dynamic_34480.aspx

See also RECOMMENDED in the sections *Developing Empowered Partnerships, Giving and Taking Constructive Criticism,* and *Managing Conflict Constructively.*

REFERENCES

1. Arnold, E., Boggs, K. (2011). *Interpersonal relationships: Professional communication skills for nurses.* St Louis: Saunders.
2. Pagana, K. D. (2010). *The nurse's communication advantage: How business-savvy communication can advance your career.* Indianapolis: Sigma Theta Tau International.
3. Lowery, F. (2010). Uncertainty a huge source of anxiety in patients. Retrieved January 6, 2011, from http://www.reuters.com/article/idUSTRE6B26GJ20101203.
4. Doylea, D., Copland, H., Bush, D., et al. (2010). A course for nurses to handle difficult communication situations. A randomized controlled trial of impact on self-efficacy and performance. Patient Education and Counseling. Retrieved January 11, 2011, from http://www.pec-journal.com/article/PIIS0738399110000479/abstract?rss=yes.
5. Hunt, A. (2010). Dealing with difficult customers–Angry customers. Retrieved January 6, 2011, from http://www.suite101.com/content/dealing-with-difficult-customers-angry-customers-a268127.
6. Block, P. (1996). *Stewardship: Choosing service over self-interest.* San Francisco: Berrett-Koehler.
7. Ibid.
8. Vitalsmarts. (2010). Silence kills: The study overview. Retrieved January 20, 2011, from http://www.silencekills.com/AboutTheStudy.aspx.
9. Walters, J. (2011). The 4-1-1 on constructive criticism. Retrieved January 28, 2011, from www.inc.com/articles/2001/08/23257.html.
10. Ibid.
11. Musinski, B. (May 2010). E-mail communication.
12. Class, P. (2006). The walking wounded. *Nursing Spectrum (FL Ed),* 9(21), 3.
13. Glanz, B. (2010). *Building customer loyalty—How YOU can help keep customers returning.* Sarasota, FL: Barbara Glanz Communications, Inc. www.barbaraglanz.com.
14. Covey, S. (1989). *The seven habits of highly effective people.* New York: Simon & Schuster.
15. Loehr, J., Schwartz, T. (2003). *The power of full engagement: Managing energy, not time is the key to high performance and personal renewal.* New York: Free Press.
16. Ignatavicius, D. (April 2010). E-mail communication.
17. McNally, K., Cunningham, L. (2010). *Nurse executive coaching manual.* Indianapolis: Sigma Theta Tau International.
18. Marx, D. (2001). *Patient safety and the "just culture": A primer for health care executives.* New York: Columbia University. Retrieved January 11, 2011, from http://psnet.ahrq.gov/resource.aspx?resourceID=1582.
19. Vitalsmarts. (2011). Silence kills: The study overview. Retrieved January 12, from http://www.silencekills.com/AboutTheStudy.aspx.
20. Hohenhaus, S., Frush, S. (2005). Revolutionizing healthcare in the emergency department: Enhancing patient safety in the safety net. *Topics in Emergency Medicine,* 27(3), 206-212.

21. Barnsteiner, J. (2008). Medication reconciliation. In *Patient safety and quality: An evidence-based handbook for nurses*. Retrieved January 6, 2011, from http://www.ahrq.gov/qual/nurseshdbk/docs/barnsteinerj_mr.pdf.

22. Gawande, A. (2010). The checklist manifesto: How to get things right. *Journal of the American Medical Association*, 303(7), 671-672.

23. Alfaro-LeFevre, R. (In press). *Applying nursing process: The foundation for clinical reasoning* (8th ed.). Philadelphia: Lippincott Williams & Wilkins.

24. Hohenhaus, S., Powell, S. (2008). Distractions and interruptions: Development of a healthcare sterile cockpit. *Newborn & Infant Nursing Reviews*, 8(2), 108-110.

25. Hegyvary, S. (2006). Reflections on errors and ethics. *Journal of Nursing Scholarship*, 38(2), 107.

26. Henneman, E. (2006). Letter to the editor. *Journal of Nursing Scholarship*, 38(2), 109.

27. Clark, C. (2010). Joint Commission touts research on reducing handoff failures. HealthLeaders Media. Retrieved January 12, 2011, from http://www.centerfortransforminghealthcare.org/.

28. Whiting, S. (March, 2009). E-mail communication.

29. Dickenson-Hazard, N. (2001). Block party. *Reflections on Nursing Leadership*, 27(1), 5.

30. Campion, C. (1998). Embracing our differences. *Nursing Spectrum (FL Ed)*, 8(14), 5.

Response Key for Exercises in Chapters 1 to 5

Note: Because the exercises are open-ended questions, the following are *example* responses, not the *only* responses.

CHAPTER 1

Example Responses for Page 21

1. (a) Facts are clearly observable and easily validated as true. Opinions may vary depending on personal perspectives: They may or may not be valid. (b) The best way to determine if an opinion is valid is to ask for the *facts* (evidence) that support the opinion. Then determine the strength of the evidence.
2. You must clearly identify the problems, the issues, and the risks that must be managed to achieve the outcomes.
3. CTIs are observable behaviors that are usually seen in critical thinkers.
4. All three terms address confidence in *your own ability* to reason well. However, *confidence in reason* addresses the importance of having faith that *others* will reason best when allowed to approach things *in their own way.*
5. Your ability to demonstrate CTIs is likely to go down (because more of your brain power is going toward learning new things and gaining a comfortable state).
6. *Context* refers to the importance of paying attention to how thinking changes depending on circumstances (one size doesn't fit all). *Confident, courage, curious,* and *committed* are important characteristics needed for critical thinking.
7. Considering thinking ahead, thinking-in-action, and thinking back helps you examine thinking in a holistic way. If you look only at *one phase,* you miss important parts of thinking.

CHAPTER 2

Example Responses for Page 44

1. Communicating effectively (page 35).
2. Feelings have a great impact on what and how we think. Those of us who are driven by feelings are likely to have more problems thinking critically, especially when situations are emotionally charged. Thinking critically requires that you recognize feelings and their impact on thinking, and then use your head to apply logical and ethical

reasoning principles. All too often we aren't even aware of deep, strong feelings involved in certain situations. Those of us who are able to connect with emotions and give them the attention they deserve—to make them explicit, to accept them, and to recognize their influence over thinking—can facilitate more logical, objective thinking.

3. The *Golden Rule* and the *Platinum Rule* both aim at treating others well. The *Platinum Rule* stresses that we are all different and that others may not want to be treated the same way we do. For example, don't assume that just because you like to be "touchy-feely," others do too.

Example Responses for Page 62

1. Sometimes the terms *goals* and *outcomes* are used interchangeably. However, it's more correct to use *goals* when stating *general intent* (what you aim to do) and to use *outcomes* to clearly describe what you expect *others to observe* when the goal is observed. **Example goal:** I want to teach Juan about diabetes. **Example outcome:** After 3 weeks, Juan will be able to give his own insulin and state how he will manage his dosage based on his diet, activity level, and glucose monitor readings.

2. In the first situation, you encourage creative, off-the-top-of-your-head ideas. In the second situation, because of the risks involved, you need sound, evidence-based ideas.

3. (a) Most people say "first place," which is wrong. If you overtake the second person, you take his place and are now in the second place position! (b) Jack and Jill are goldfish, and a cat knocked the fish tank on the floor, shattering it. You could have asked, "Who are Jack and Jill?"

CHAPTER 3

Example Responses for Page 90

1. It's important to comply with *reasonable* patient requests. However, if following the patient's request is *against the plan of care* or *to the detriment of the patient's health*, explain this to the patient. Repeat the patient's request so that he knows he has been heard, and then give the reason why his request is denied. If the request is reasonable, but against the plan of care, encourage the person to speak with the primary caregivers (or appropriate team members), or speak with them yourself. In this case, after a thorough assessment of the patient's condition, you may say: "I understand that you want more medication. But I've talked with the doctor, and giving you more at this point is risky and not likely to work, as you have built up drug tolerance. I'll pay attention to the time and give you your medication as soon as I can."

2. "I don't know" isn't an acceptable answer. A critical thinker would respond, "I'll find out." Finding out will help her broaden her knowledge and help Mr. Duncan.

3. In the presence of known problems, you predict the most likely and most dangerous complications and take immediate action to (1) prevent them and (2) be prepared

to manage them in case they can't be prevented. **Example:** If you're going to care for someone with a wired jaw and you aren't familiar with the care of someone with a wired jaw, you'd look it up so that you'd know the common and dangerous complications and how to deal with them (e.g., in this case, one dangerous complication is aspiration because the person is unable to open his mouth, so you would have wire cutters nearby). You also look for evidence of risk and causative factors (things we know cause problems or put people at risk for problems). You then aim to manage these factors to prevent the actual problems. Example: In the case of the wired jaw, you assess for nausea (a risk factor for aspiration). If nausea is present, ask for an antinausea drug, hold food, and keep suction equipment and wire cutters nearby. Finally, you promote health and function by asking the person how he's handling dietary and fluid intake needs, and make suggestions as needed.

4. best results [or outcomes]; patient satisfaction.

Example Responses for Pages 121 to 122

1. (a) When you know the people you're visiting and are familiar with the surroundings, your brain isn't "bombarded" by having to get to know someone or become familiar with the environment. In familiar situations, you also spend less energy on confidence and knowledge concerns. Novices spend a lot of energy dealing with unfamiliarity and confidence concerns. (b) Each time you see the movie, you see more things and get better insights into the characters. This analogy relates to the clinical setting. Each time you go to the same clinical setting with the same co-workers and patients, making care decisions is likely to be easier and more "on target." Going to the clinical setting for a novice is like going to a movie for the first time—a lot of information may be missed. (c) Visit the setting as an observer before you have to actually function in the setting. Seek out simulated experiences so that you learn from mistakes in a safe environment. Find references on the setting that help you determine what to expect. Answer the questions in *Questions to Answer Before Going to the Clinical Area* (page 113).

2. You could irrigate a nasogastric tube if: the facility permitted it; you've received permission from your instructor; you have the required knowledge and level of competence; the procedure is reasonable, prudent, and safe; and you're willing to assume accountability for how you perform the procedure and the patient response to the procedure.

3. It's unlikely that the off-going nurse has really assessed the family's needs. It's highly unlikely that the family is doing "fine," as this is a hard time for any family. It appears as though the family has had limited involvement in the child's care. You should assess the family's needs and begin to include interventions that meet these needs in the nursing plan (e.g., allow the family to spend more time with the child).

4. MMA should trigger you to consider whether a patient's signs and symptoms may be related to <u>M</u>edication problems, <u>M</u>edical problems, or <u>A</u>llergies. EASE helps you remember the major care plan components: <u>E</u>xpected outcomes, <u>A</u>ctual and potential

problems that must be addressed to reach the overall outcomes, <u>S</u>pecific interventions designed to achieve the outcomes, and <u>E</u>valuation statements (progress notes).

5. Check with your supervisor, your instructor, and the facility's policies and procedures related to activating the chain of command.

6. Look up aspirin in a drug reference, and you will find that you don't give aspirin to a child with a fever because of the risk of developing fatal Reye's syndrome.

CHAPTER 4

Example Responses for Pages 147 to 160
Moral and Ethical Reasoning Exercises (page 147)

1. Ask for a family meeting to make the decision, and include an ethicist, trusted friends, or clergy to help.

2. Justice, beneficence, accountability.

3. professional; personal.

Research, Evidence-Based Practice, and Quality Improvement Exercises (page 148)

1. Clinical summaries and practice alerts help busy nurses use EBP to improve care practices by giving sound, simple summaries on the most up-to-date findings on a specific topic.

2. (a) rigorous (also acceptable: precise, thorough, and meticulous); (b) preferences; (c) transformed; applied (or used); practice.

3. False. Because finding and critiquing research is time-consuming, this is an unrealistic expectation. Rather, staff nurses are accountable for responsibilities listed under *Frequently Asked Questions on Staff Nurses' Role* on page 141.

4. (a) Ultimately you need to examine the *results* of nursing care (How are the patients doing in relation to desired outcomes?). But it's also important to determine whether the *process is efficient and economical,* and whether the *setting* (structure) is such that it's likely to support surveillance and care processes.

Teaching Others, Teaching Ourselves, Test-Taking Exercises (pages 160 to 161)

1. By teaching people how to manage their health, we empower them to achieve the important outcomes of being independent and achieving optimum health. In today's fast-paced clinical setting, you must be a self-starter and be able to teach yourself how to give competent care.

2. If you study only by looking at your notes, you may be misled about how much you know. Recognizing information in your notes is not the same as having the information "in your head."

3. (a) already know; ready; (b) teach; (c) practice; same.

CHAPTER 5

Example Responses for Pages 169 to 214
1. Identifying Assumptions (pages 169 to 170)

1. There's not enough evidence to indicate that the patient needs instruction. Many people are fully knowledgeable about their diet but aren't able to stick to it. It would be better to explore the main struggles with nutrition and diet.

2. You might waste your time teaching information the patient already knows. You might alienate the patient: Who likes to be taught things they already know? The patient gets the message that you don't understand the problem—that you jump to conclusions.

3. **Scenario One.** (a) She seems to have assumed that she can create a positive attitude for Jeff by talking about advances in diabetic care. (b) She needed to assess Jeff's human response to learning he's a diabetic. Jeff may be well aware of advances in diabetic care but is still having trouble coming to terms with having to regulate his diet and take insulin for the rest of his life. She didn't assess before acting. (c) Jeff probably thinks Anita is a know-it-all because she didn't take the time to find out what his point of view on the situation was. It's a real turn-off when someone starts trying to change your attitude before he or she finds out what your attitude is.

    Scenario Two. (a) She seems to have assumed the mother can read and that the mother will let her know if she has questions. (b) If the mother can't read or is embarrassed to ask questions, the child may have inadequate care from his mother. If harm results from the nurse's failure to determine the mother's understanding, the nurse may be accused of negligence.

    Scenario Three. (a) The assumption seems to be that he would have the desired response to the drug without any adverse reactions. (b) It's likely that she was concerned that Mr. Schmidt wouldn't respond to the diuretic as expected—that he might experience an adverse reaction. (c) She probably thought the physician wouldn't like it if she challenged his judgment.

2. Assessing Systematically and Comprehensively (pages 174 to 175)

1. The body systems approach to assessment (page 115) is probably the best method. Or you may choose the head-to-toe approach and cluster signs and symptoms of medical problems after you perform the assessment.

2. A nursing model approach (page 115).

3. **Scenario One.** (a) Assess the extent of Pearl's voluntary movement (Can she wiggle her toes?); color of toes and skin around cast edges; whether Pearl feels numbness or tingling in her foot or leg; whether there is any edema of the leg or toes; the quality of the dorsalis pedis pulse; whether Pearl perceives a needle prick as being sharp; and whether her toes are warm or cool. (b) Assessing each of the above helps you detect early signs of circulatory problems, nerve compression, or skin irritation: If you find one area that begins to exhibit abnormal assessment findings (e.g., edema), you

should increase the frequency and intensity of assessment of other areas (e.g., skin color). Each area of assessment has specific relevance: checking movement, numbness, and sensation monitors for nerve compression; checking for color, edema, pulse quality, and warmth monitors for circulation and skin condition. **(c)** Check circulation by assessing the dorsalis pedis pulse quality and capillary refill in toes; check for nerve compression by asking her to wiggle her toes, and ask whether there is any numbness or tingling. If these are satisfactory, you might choose to put a warm sock over the toes; encourage her to wiggle her toes frequently to increase the circulation, and continue to closely monitor her dorsalis pedis pulse, toe temperature, and toe sensation.

Scenario Two. (a) Look up digoxin in an up-to-date reference (or consult with a pharmacist). Then assess as follows. **To assess for therapeutic effect,** check to see if Mr. Wu's serum digoxin level is within therapeutic range (0.5 to 2 ng/mL). Determine status of cardiac symptoms, as compared with baseline (status of apical and/or radial pulse rate and rhythm, lung sounds, urine output, edema, activity tolerance). **To assess for allergic or adverse reactions,** check Mr. Wu for signs and symptoms of any of the allergy or adverse reactions listed in the drug reference. **To assess for contraindications,** check Mr. Wu for signs and symptoms of any of the contraindications listed in the drug reference. Most common contraindications for digoxin include serum potassium levels less than 3.5 mEq/L (increases the risk of toxicity); pulse rate less than 60 or below physician-prescribed parameters; and clinical signs of toxicity or overdose. **To assess for drug interactions,** get a complete list of medications (including herbal and holistic drugs) and check with the pharmacist to find out if there are any drug interactions. **To assess for toxicity or overdose,** check Mr. Wu for signs and symptoms of toxicity or overdose. Most common signs and symptoms of digoxin toxicity include serum digoxin level above 2 ng/mL; atrioventricular block (PR interval greater than 0.24 sec); and progressive bradycardia, nausea, vomiting, and/or visual disturbances (blurring, snowflakes, yellow-green halos around images). (b) If no therapeutic effect is achieved by giving a drug or if the person is experiencing adverse reactions, you need to question whether a change in dosage is necessary or whether the drug should be continued at all. If you identify contraindications to giving the drug, you need to withhold the drug. If you identify signs of toxicity or overdose, it's especially important to withhold the drug because you'd be adding to the toxicity or overdose problem.

Scenario Three. (a) *Vital signs:* Measure temperature, pulse, respirations, and blood pressure. *Eye opening:* Call Gerome's name. Tell him to open his eyes. If he makes no response, pinch him. *Best motor response:* Ask him to move each extremity. Use a pin prick, or pinch him and see if he can tell you where he feels it. If he makes no response, pinch him and note whether he flexes his extremity to withdraw from pain, flexes in spasm, or extends his extremity. *Best verbal response:* Ask him what his name is, where he is, and what day it is. *Pupillary reaction:* Determine the size of each pupil in millimeters before flashing a light into it. Then flash a light into each pupil and observe whether it constricts briskly. *Purposeful limb movement:* Check each extremity by asking Gerome to move it, observing for muscle contraction (attempts to move), ability to lift extremity, and ability to lift extremity even though you try to hold it down. *Limb sensation:* Prick each limb with a sterile needle, and ask Gerome what he feels (this may be unnecessary for Gerome, since he has a head injury rather than a spinal cord injury). *Seizure activity:* Observe for muscle twitching. *Gag reflex:* Place a clean tongue blade in the back of Gerome's throat, and see if it triggers gagging. (b) By monitoring all of these parameters, signs and symptoms of increased intracranial pressure can be detected early. Signs and symptoms of increased intracranial pressure are decreasing level of consciousness; increasing restlessness; irritability and confusion; stronger headache; nausea and vomiting; increasing speech problems; pupil changes (dilated and nonreactive or constricted and nonreactive pupils); cranial nerve dysfunction; increasing muscle weakness, flaccidity, or coordination problems; seizures; decerebrate posturing (muscles stiff and extended, head retracted); and decorticate posturing (muscles rigid and still, with arms flexed, fists clenched, and legs extended)—the latter two are both late signs of increased intracranial pressure. (c) Monitor other parameters of neurologic assessment closely for other signs of increased intracranial pressure. If there are no other changes and you can indeed arouse Gerome, you don't need to be immediately concerned; however, you should increase the frequency of assessment of all parameters until you're comfortable that the increased somnolence is merely a sign of the combined effects of fatigue and existing brain swelling (rather than increasing brain swelling). If you have any questions about how to proceed, report the increased somnolence to your supervisor. (d) Check other neurologic parameters closely, and report and record findings immediately; increase the frequency of assessment. (e) If the baseline pulse was rapid, this may be a normal finding. However, you should closely assess all the other assessment parameters to check for other reportable signs and symptoms. If the pulse is dropping to 60 beats/min, closely monitor all other assessment parameters and report the findings immediately (may be a sign of life-threatening increase in intracranial pressure).

3. Checking Accuracy and Reliability of Data (Validation) (page 177)

1. Talk with Mrs. Molina, and explore her feelings and concerns.
2. You may be able to turn on Mr. Nola's blood glucose monitor and check it (some monitors automatically show the previous blood glucose level). If not, ask him to take it again now (quietly observe his technique). If he is proficient at performing a check for blood glucose, it's likely his previous result was correct. If the second reading is significantly different from the previous reading, consider whether there is a relationship between the change in blood sugar reading and recent food intake or peak insulin levels. I would consider the blood sugar reading the patient took with you observing as being most valid.
3. Take it in the right arm. Take it again in 15 minutes.

4. Explore with Mr. McGwire why he thinks he got his foot ulcers. Ask him to tell you what he does to avoid getting foot ulcers. He may be very knowledgeable about diabetic care and foot ulcers and still be getting these ulcers. Review his diagnostic tests to see if the A1c (Glycohemoglobin HbA1c, A1c) is within normal range. This test indicates blood glucose levels over the long term.

4. Distinguishing Normal from Abnormal and Identifying Signs and Symptoms (pages 178 to 179)

1. (a) If you assumed this was an oral temperature, you should have placed an *S* here. You may have placed a question mark here, which is actually a more correct response. You need to ask, *"How was this temperature taken?"* (orally? rectally? tympanic?) (b) If you assumed the patient never has rales, you should have placed an *S* here. You may have placed a question mark here, which is actually a more correct response. You need to ask questions like *"What do the patient's lungs sound like when he's in his usual state of health? What is the respiratory rate? How far up the back can you hear the rales? Are there just a few rales, or are there copious rales? When the patient coughs, do the rales clear?"* (c) You may have placed an *S* here, but you really need to *ask if this is a normal pattern for the person and why the person only sleeps 3 hours at a time* (e.g., it's not unusual for mothers of newborns to sleep only 3 hours at a time because of feeding schedules). (d) *S.* (e) *O* or question mark. This is usually a normal finding, but you may have placed a question mark because you wanted to know such things as *whether there's any drainage, whether the area is hot to touch,* and *whether the patient is afebrile.* (f) *O.* This is normal for a 2-year-old. (g) *S.* (h) You may have placed an *S* here, but a question mark is a more correct response. Ask, *"What are the bathing practices of a person of this culture?"* (i) *S.* This is likely to be a normal finding, since the dialysis takes over the work of the kidney. (j) *S* or question mark. The pulse is somewhat slow but might be normal for someone who is young and athletic or older and on cardiac medication. You may have wanted to ask, *"What is this person's normal pulse?"* or *"Is the person taking any cardiac medications that slow the heart rate?"*

2. The italicized words in the preceding response are examples of what else you might want to know.

5. Making Inferences (Drawing Valid Conclusions) (pages 180 to 181)

1. I suspect this information indicates infection of some sort.
2. I suspect this information indicates financial problems.
3. I suspect this information indicates that the patient has trouble sticking to his diet.
4. I suspect this information indicates that the child wants to be sure his mother approves of his answer, or perhaps he is afraid.
5. I suspect this information indicates there is some medical reason for the grandmother's confusion.

6. Clustering Related Cues (Data) (page 182)

Scenario One. (a) Stung by a bee on the ear an hour ago; ear has no stinger, is red and swollen; no rash or wheezing; normal pulse and respirations. (b) Afraid he might die; wants to have a Popsicle and watch TV. (c) Didn't make sure she had parents' phone number down (investigate whether this was lack of knowledge or oversight); doesn't know first aid for a bee sting.

Scenario Two. (a) 41 years old; acute abdominal pain; vomiting for 2 days and unable to keep any food down; abdomen distended; no bowel sounds; scheduled to go to the operating room at 2 PM; pain suddenly getting worse; vital signs unchanged, except pulse is increased by approximately 30 beats/min. (b) 41-year-old businessman; hates everything about hospitals; scheduled to go to the operating room at 2 PM; worried because his brother died in the hospital; suddenly experiencing severe pain.

7. Distinguishing Relevant from Irrelevant (pages 183 to 184)

Scenario One. (a) May be relevant because buspirone hydrochloride can cause confusion in the elderly. (b) May be relevant because it may be a sign of infection, which can cause confusion in the elderly. (c) May be relevant because it's indicative of previous cardiovascular disease, which is a risk factor for cerebrovascular accident (stroke), which may be the cause of the confusion. (d) May be relevant because dehydration in the elderly can cause electrolyte imbalance and confusion. (e) Not relevant. (f) Not relevant.

Scenario Two. (a) Probably relevant. It takes time to adjust to a diabetic regimen. (b) Not relevant (not abnormal). (c) May be relevant (may feel constipation is caused by new diet). (d) May be relevant because she has to prepare meals for others, increasing temptation. (e) Very probably relevant. Someone who likes to cook usually takes joy in eating a variety of foods. (f) Relevant. She needs to eat even less than she will when her weight is within normal limits. (g) Not relevant (has nothing to do with sticking to a diabetic diet).

8. Recognizing Inconsistencies (pages 185 to 186)

Scenario One. (a) It doesn't make sense that Cathy has only just started coming to the prenatal clinic but has been going to birthing classes. If she hasn't had prenatal care until now, you wonder whether she's really happy about the baby coming or realizes the importance of prenatal visits. You may also wonder why her mother, rather than her boyfriend, came to the clinic visit. (b) Check her records to see if there's any mention of receiving prenatal care somewhere else for the earlier part of her pregnancy; ask her where she's been going to birthing classes; ask how her boyfriend and mother feel about the baby coming.

Scenario Two. Her age is inconsistent with usual risk factors for a myocardial infarction (MI). While sweating and feeling of impending doom may be seen with an MI, the big picture here—her age, absence of pain, normal electrocardiogram—is inconsistent with an MI. Occasionally people don't have pain when they have an MI, but usually there are other risk factors and signs and symptoms present. Her signs and symptoms are more consistent with those of a panic attack (see *Panic Attack or Heart Attack?* at http://www.womensheart.org/content/HeartDisease/panic_attack_or_heart_attack. asp). Your first responsibility here is to call 911.

9. Identifying Patterns (pages 187 to 188)

1. (c) Potential (risk) for impaired bowel elimination pattern. There are risk factors for constipation but no signs and symptoms.
2. (e) Potential (risk) for ineffective sexual-reproductive pattern. There are risk factors for ineffective sexual-reproductive pattern.
3. (d) Probably normal sleep-rest pattern. Considering that the person works nights, there are no signs and symptoms of an abnormal sleep-rest pattern.
4. (a) Impaired respiratory function pattern. Signs and symptoms of respiratory function problems are present.
5. (b) Probably normal coping pattern. There are no signs or symptoms of abnormal coping pattern.

10. Identifying Missing Information (page 189)

(a) What are the person's other vital signs (pulse, blood pressure, temperature)? Is there a history of smoking? Is the person smoking now? How long has this pattern persisted? What does the person feel is contributing to this pattern? How does the person tolerate activity? (b) How does the husband feel about helping her? (c) Who is the major caregiver? What factors are contributing to the lack of fiber in her diet and her inadequate fluid intake? What's the patient's (or caregiver's) knowledge of how to prevent altered bowel elimination? Why does the patient spend most of her time in bed? How motivated is the patient to do the things necessary to prevent altered bowel elimination? (d) Does the person feel he's getting adequate rest? Are any sleeping aids being taken? If so, what are they? (e) What are the woman's feelings about having herpes? What does the woman know about herpes transmission? How does she feel about telling prospective partners about the herpes? How does the patient plan to prevent herpes transmission?

11. Promoting Health by Identifying and Managing Risk Factors (page 191)

1. Do you have any family history of health problems? What's your ethnic background? Do you smoke or use chewing tobacco? What do your usual meals consist of? Do you exercise regularly and get enough rest? How do you manage stress? Do you drink alcohol or take drugs that aren't prescribed? Are you sexually active (if so, do you use a condom and discuss sexual history with your partner)? Do you wear your seat belt? What do you do to stay healthy?
2. Her age puts her at risk for osteoporosis. The history of falls, together with the risk of osteoporosis, put her at high risk for fractures. You need to look closely at why she

is falling (e.g., balance problems? coordination problems? weakness or fatigue? vision problems? home hazards?). You should also assess calcium intake, which has to be adequate to prevent osteoporosis.

3. Reinforce that we all live longer now and that it's good to do things to increase the likelihood of living longer and healthier. Give some examples, like the importance of staying active and eating well. Encourage him to discuss how to monitor and manage risk factors after age 50 with his primary care provider. Stress that we have many studies that support the importance of monitoring things like cholesterol, blood sugar, and prostate-specific antigen in a 50-year-old man. Suggest scheduling annual exams around specific times (e.g., birthday, Christmas) so that he remembers.

12. Diagnosing Actual and Potential Problems (pages 197 to 198)

1. Potential (risk) for violence related to agitation and previous history of striking caregivers.
2. Potential complications: hemorrhage, shock, vomiting with aspiration, pneumonia, infection, paralytic ileus.
3. Altered coping related to poor organizational skills and time management as evidence by cluttered home, disheveled appearance, and statements of having trouble coping.
4. History of smoking or lung disease, whether the fractures are stable (risk for punctured lung), whether he has pain that is preventing him from coughing and clearing his lungs (risk for pneumonia).

13. Setting Priorities (pages 200 to 201)

1. (b) and (c) should be addressed on the patient record, either through colostomy care standards, or through nurse-generated plans. The anxiety would probably be dealt with informally.
2. Assessing and reporting the chest pain should be your top priority because myocardial infarction and pulmonary embolus are potential complications of thrombophlebitis.

14. Determining Patient-Centered (Client-Centered) Outcomes (page 205)

1. The patient will maintain intact skin, free of signs of redness or irritation, and have a documented record of measures taken to prevent skin breakdown.
2. After suctioning, the mouth, the nose, and the lungs will be clear.
3. After irrigation, Foley catheter will be patent and draining clear yellow urine.
4. Endotracheal tube will be out by [date], with patient breathing independently.

5. After 3 days of practice, the patient will demonstrate increased activity tolerance as evidenced by ability to walk the length of the hall and back by [date].

15. Determining Individualized Interventions (pages 208 to 209)

1. (a) Monitor fluid intake every shift. Keep iced tea (patient's preference) at the bedside on ice. Encourage drinking at least 3 quarts during the day and 1 quart at night. Reinforce the importance of maintaining adequate hydration. Record fluid intake. (b) Monitor anxiety level. Encourage her to express feelings and concerns. Fully explain all procedures. (c) Monitor comfort level. After applying heat for 30 minutes, assist with range of motion exercises three times a day.

2. **Contributing factors:** Age, low weight, chemotherapy, spends a lot of time in bed. **Interventions:** Monitor skin for pressure points, especially coccyx, elbows, and heels. Put a foam bed pad on bed. Use a sheep skin for coccyx and heels. Teach the importance of (1) changing positions frequently, spending more time out of bed, keeping skin moisturized, maintaining hydration and a healthy diet, and having a family member monitor her back and heels for redness; and (2) reporting skin problems to the APN or physician before each chemotherapy treatment.

3. (a) (1) It's quite likely the children won't report finding ticks, increasing the likelihood that the mother won't know when the children may have been bitten. It also increases the likelihood that the ticks won't be properly disposed of. There may be no benefits from using this approach (punishment). (2) It's possible that they may go looking for ticks, increasing the likelihood of being bitten. This approach might work, but the risks outweigh the benefits. (b) Determine children's understanding of the severity of the consequences of tick bites and the importance of finding ways to avoid them. Initiate teaching as indicated. Explain to the children that they can best help by asking for insect repellent to be applied before going outside, reporting ticks found on themselves and on each other, and avoiding tall grassy areas. Start a rule that the children can't go outside without first applying insect repellent. Have the mother praise good behavior (e.g., asking for insect repellent) verbally, rather than offering rewards. Instruct the mother not to offer rewards for finding ticks.

16. Determining a Comprehensive Plan/Evaluating and Updating the Plan (pages 213 to 214)

1. (a) Not achieved; (b) Achieved; (c) Partially achieved; focus teaching toward mother's needs.

2. **Overall expected discharge outcome:** Will be discharged home with lungs clear and husband able to demonstrate administration of epinephrine by June 29. Two priority problems, expected outcomes, and interventions follow:

Priority Problems	Expected Outcomes	Interventions
1. Altered respiratory function related to allergic response as evidenced by wheezing	By June 29, lungs will be clear and free of wheezing.	Monitor lungs sounds q 4 hr. Report increased wheezing or other respiratory symptoms. Record on respiratory flow sheet.
2. Patient (husband) Education: *Epinephrine administration*	By June 29, husband will relate knowledge of action and side effects of epinephrine and when to give epinephrine, and demonstrate subcutaneous injection technique.	Assess husband's knowledge of indications, side effects, and administration of epinephrine. Initiate teaching as indicated, focusing on his preferred learning style. Record results on patient education form.

You may also have identified Altered Comfort related to itching feet. This is an important nursing concern, and could be listed as a third priority.

3. You've identified a care variance. According to the predicted care, she should be voiding normally. Assess the patient carefully, checking for bladder distention and asking the patient about urinary symptoms. Check vital signs, and bring the problem to the attention of the professional in charge of care management (e.g., APN, doctor).

4. See *Purpose and Components of the Recorded Plan of Care* (page 212).

Appendix A
Concept Mapping: Getting in the "Right" State of Mind

WHAT IS CONCEPT MAPPING?

Concept mapping is a learning strategy that uses the right brain (the creative hemisphere) to enhance your ability to deeply understand information. With concept mapping, you simply draw your personal view of key concepts and how they relate to one another. Unlike outlining, which uses the left brain (the logical hemisphere), mapping is flexible, has few rules, and is easy to learn (left brain–dominant people may struggle at first). Mapping boosts your ability to grasp and remember complex relationships because there are few words (less clutter) on the page, and you can *focus on the concepts and relationships* (without worrying about the rules of writing or outlining). The following is a simple map of key points of this paragraph. Compare how your brain handles this paragraph versus how it handles the map.

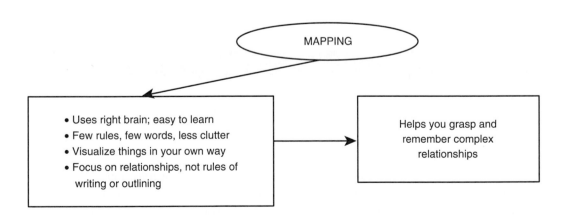

MAPPING

- Uses right brain; easy to learn
- Few rules, few words, less clutter
- Visualize things in your own way
- Focus on relationships, not rules of writing or outlining

Helps you grasp and remember complex relationships

The next page shows a map of how the brain works and gives steps for mapping.

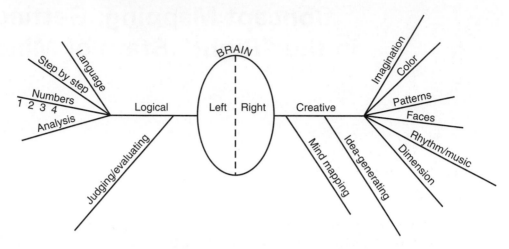

Mind map of how the brain works.

WHEN DO YOU USE MAPPING?

You can use mapping for various purposes, including the following:

- Taking notes or learning new content
- Mapping the care planning process or how symptoms relate to one another
- Writing papers or preparing presentations
- Preparing for exams
- Promoting brainstorming
- Facilitating group problem-solving

WHAT ARE THE BENEFITS?

General benefits and specific group benefits follow.

General Benefits

- Quicker than regular note-taking
- Highlights key ideas and gets rid of the irrelevant
- Helps you quickly gather, review, and recall large amounts of information
- Increases brainpower available for learning and problem-solving by reducing energy used on concerns about structure and documentation
- Encourages you to identify relationships and be creative
- Helps you retain what you learn because you "play with the information" in your own way as you make your map

Group Benefits

- Promotes communication (keeps everyone focused on the main issues)
- Facilitates problem-solving (generates more ideas, helps group suspend judgment)
- Makes ideas and relationships clear

HOW DOES IT PROMOTE CRITICAL THINKING?

Concept mapping facilitates the "productive and analytical phases" of critical thinking—the phase when you need to gather relevant information, identify relationships, and produce new ideas. After you complete this productive phase, you can get in touch with your left brain talents and move to the "judgment phase"—you can evaluate what your mind has produced, make judgments about its accuracy and usefulness, and make refinements.

STEPS FOR MAPPING TO PROMOTE CRITICAL THINKING

1. **Put central theme or concept** in the center, at the bottom, or at the top of the page, and draw a circle around it (see the example mind map above).
2. **Place the main ideas relating to the concept** on lines (or in circles) around the central theme.
3. **Add details** by putting them on lines (or in circles) connecting them to the main ideas.
4. **Use key words or simple pictures** only; keep it legible.
5. **Make sure no idea stands alone.** If you can't connect an idea with something on the page, it's irrelevant to the central theme.
6. **Don't allow yourself to slow down** over concerns about where to place words (this is your left brain habit trying to dominate). Rather let your ideas flow and use lines to show connections.
7. **Use colors** to highlight the most important ideas.
8. **Once you've completed your map,** get in touch with your left-brain talents (judging and evaluating), and evaluate what you've produced. **Revise as needed.**

Appendix B
Key Brain Parts Involved in Thinking

KEY BRAIN PARTS INVOLVED IN THINKING

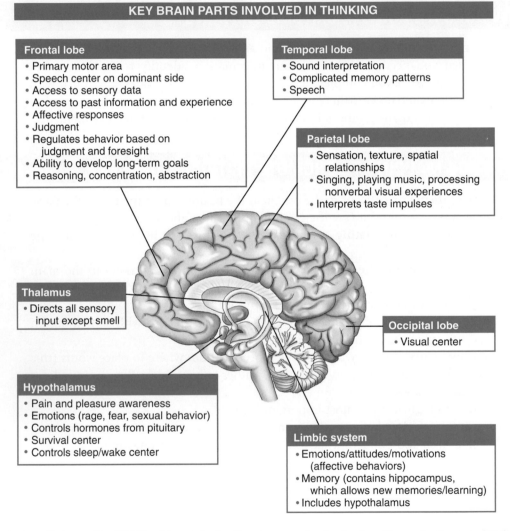

Frontal lobe
- Primary motor area
- Speech center on dominant side
- Access to sensory data
- Access to past information and experience
- Affective responses
- Judgment
- Regulates behavior based on judgment and foresight
- Ability to develop long-term goals
- Reasoning, concentration, abstraction

Temporal lobe
- Sound interpretation
- Complicated memory patterns
- Speech

Parietal lobe
- Sensation, texture, spatial relationships
- Singing, playing music, processing nonverbal visual experiences
- Interprets taste impulses

Thalamus
- Directs all sensory input except smell

Occipital lobe
- Visual center

Hypothalamus
- Pain and pleasure awareness
- Emotions (rage, fear, sexual behavior)
- Controls hormones from pituitary
- Survival center
- Controls sleep/wake center

Limbic system
- Emotions/attitudes/motivations (affective behaviors)
- Memory (contains hippocampus, which allows new memories/learning)
- Includes hypothalamus

References: Cohen, B. (2009). *Memmler's the human body in health and disease* (11th ed.) Philadelphia: Lippincott Williams & Wilkins; Ignatavicius, D., and Workman, L. (Eds.). (2010). *Medical-surgical nursing: Critical thinking for collaborative care* (6th ed.) Philadelphia: Saunders. Copyright 2010. www.AlfaroTeachSmart.com.

Appendix C
Patients' Rights*

Dear consumer:

State law requires that your health care provider or facility recognize *your rights* while receiving medical care, and that you respect *their right* to expect certain behavior on the part of patients. You may request a copy of the full text of this law from your health care provider or facility.

You have the following rights:

- To be treated with courtesy and respect with appreciation of dignity and protection of your need for privacy
- To receive prompt and reasonable response to questions and requests
- To be informed of the following:
    - Who is providing medical services and who is responsible for your care
    - What patient support services are available, including whether an interpreter is available if you have communication problems
    - Your diagnosis, planned course of treatment, alternatives, risks, and prognosis
    - Whether treatment is for purposes of experimental research (and to give or refuse your consent to participate in such research)
- To refuse treatment, except as otherwise provided by law
- To have impartial access to medical treatment or accommodations, regardless of race, national origin, religion, physical handicap, or source of payment
- To be given treatment for any emergency condition that will deteriorate upon failure to receive treatment
- To express any grievances about any violation of your rights as stated by state law, through the grievance procedure of your health care provider or facility and appropriate state licensing agency
- To file complaints against a health care professional, hospital, or ambulatory surgical center with the Agency for Health Care Administration (*Note:* Appropriate information for how to reach each state's agency must be listed here.)
- To receive the following (upon request):
    - Full information and necessary counseling on the availability of financial recourses for your care
    - A reasonable estimate of the charges for medical care before treatment
    - Information about whether your health care provider or facility accepts the Medicare assignment rate before treatment
    - To be given a copy of an itemized bill that is reasonably clear and understandable and upon request, to have charges explained

You have the following responsibilities:

- To provide your health care provider, to the best of your knowledge, with accurate and complete information about your complaints, past illnesses, hospitalizations, medications, and other matters relating to your health
- To follow the treatment plan recommended by your provider
- To report unexpected changes in your condition to the health care provider
- To keep appointments and, if you're unable to do so for any reason, to notify your provider or facility
- To ensure that the financial obligations of your health care are fulfilled as soon as possible
- To comply with health care provider and facility rules and regulations affecting patient conduct

---

*This is an example form and summary of rights. Rights may vary from state to state. Forms may vary from facility to facility.

Appendix D
ANA Standards of Practice and Professional Performance for Registered Nurses (RNs)*

Standard	What RN Must Do to Meet ANA Standard
1. **Assessment**	Collect complete data relevant to the consumer's health or situation.
2. **Diagnosis**	Analyze the assessment data to identify diagnoses or issues.
3. **Outcomes Identification**	Identify expected outcomes that are individualized to the consumer or the situation.
4. **Planning**	Develop a plan that prescribes strategies to achieve expected outcomes.
5. **Implementation**	Implement the plan, coordinating care, and using strategies to promote health and safety.
6. **Evaluation**	Determine progress toward outcome achievement.

*Summarized from American Nurses Association. (2010). *Nursing scope and standards of performance and standards of clinical practice* (2nd ed.). Silver Springs, MD: nursesbooks.org.

STANDARDS OF PROFESSIONAL PERFORMANCE

Standard	What RN Must Do to Meet ANA Standard
7. **Ethics**	Integrate ethical principles into your practice.
8. **Education**	Gain the knowledge and competencies required by current nursing practice.
9. **Evidence-Based Practice and Research**	Apply the best evidence and research finding pertinent to the consumer or situation.
10. **Quality of Practice**	Contribute to improvement of care quality.
11. **Communication**	Use the best format to communicate in all areas of practice (e.g., face-to-face, e-mail).
12. **Leadership**	Apply leadership principles in the clinical and professional setting.
13. **Collaboration**	Work together with consumers and other health team members.
14. **Professional Practice Evaluation**	Evaluate your practice in relation to professional practice standards and guidelines, relevant status, rules, and regulations.
15. **Resource Utilization**	Use appropriate resources to give care that is safe, effective, and cost-effective.
16. **Environmental Health**	Work to maintain a safe, healthy environment.

Appendix E
Comprehensive Patient Admission Tool

Main Line Hospitals

Bryn Mawr Hospital
Lankenau Hospital
Paoli Hospital

Patient I.D.

INITIAL PATIENT ASSESSMENT

Complete shaded area   **OR**   ☐ See 24 Hour Flow Sheet   ☐ See E.D. Triage Sheet

Date:	Height:	Weight:	Language spoken other than English:

Primary Care Physician/Specialist: _____

Reason for procedure/hospitalization: _____
_____

Procedure/Date: _____
_____

Upon entry to the Hospital: Correct ID band in place   ☐ Yes

Vital Signs   Temp _____   P _____   RR _____   BP _____

O2 Sat _____   O2 _____   RA _____   ☐ Not Applicable

INITIAL PAIN ASSESSMENT

Does patient have complaint of or admitting diagnosis of pain?   ☐ Patient non-verbal
    ☐ Yes (see 24 hr flowsheet)
    ☐ No

Intensity (0-10 scale) _____

Location: ☐ Head ☐ Back ☐ Upper extremity ☐ R ☐ L ☐ Lower extremity ☐ R ☐ L
    ☐ Chest ☐ Abdomen ☐ Other _____

Description: ☐ Sharp ☐ Stabbing ☐ Burning ☐ Constant Intermittent
    ☐ Other _____

Onset/Duration of Pain _____

What makes pain better/worse? _____

Impact of ADLs: ☐ Decreased Activity/Self Care _____

☐ Decreased Appetite/Nausea/Vomiting ☐ Other _____

Allergies: Drug/Food/Latex/Tape/Dyes   ☐ None Known

ALLERGIES	REACTION	ALLERGIES	REACTION

ADVANCE DIRECTIVES   ☐ NA (Patient < 18 years old)   ☐ Unable to Assess

Does the patient have an advance directive? ☐ Yes	☐ No
☐ Copy in current chart ☐ Refer to old records ☐ Patient/Family to obtain copy for record (Place reminder on Pathway until received) ☐ Patient to formulate another advance directive (sample in "It's Up To You") ☐ Substance as stated by patient: _____	☐ Information Given ☐ Information Declined ☐ Patient declines stating content ☐ Patient/family declines to bring, and/or complete advance directive information ☐ Refer to Social Work

COMPLETE THIS SECTION FOR ALL PATIENTS

Patient I.D.

PAST SURGICAL HISTORY

Past surgical History: _____

_____

Previous anesthesia: ☐ General   ☐ Spinal   ☐ Other _____
Problems with Anesthesia?   ☐ Motion Sickness
Family history/problems with anesthesia: _____

_____

HEALTH HISTORY   Check/Circle Applicable Boxes Only

NEUROLOGIC
- ☐ Stroke / TIA
  - ☐ Residual _____
  - ☐ None
- ☐ Blackouts/Fainting/Vertigo
- ☐ Seizures
- ☐ Migraine/Headaches
- ☐ Numbness/Tingling
  - Arm _____ Legs
- ☐ Speech difficulty
- ☐ Swallowing/Choking
- ☐ Head injury
- ☐ Confusion/Dementia
- ☐ Memory changes
- ☐ Other _____
- ☐ *No identified problems*

CARDIOVASCULAR
- ☐ High blood pressure/Low blood pressure
- ☐ Aneurysm
- ☐ Congenital heart defect
- ☐ Heart attack
- ☐ Heart failure
- ☐ Murmur
- ☐ Chest pain/Angina
- ☐ Irregular pulse
- ☐ Circulation problem
- ☐ Phlebitis/Clots
- ☐ Pacemaker/Defib.
- ☐ High cholesterol
- ☐ Cardiovascular intervention
- ☐ Other _____
- ☐ *No identified problems*

RESPIRATORY
- ☐ Shortness of breath
- ☐ Pneumonia
- ☐ COPD
- ☐ Asthma
- ☐ Acute Bronchitis
- ☐ Cough
- ☐ Seasonal/Environmental allergies
- ☐ Snoring/Apnea
- ☐ CPAP/BiPAP
- ☐ TB
- ☐ Post nasal drip
- ☐ Other_____
- ☐ *No identified problems*

GASTROINTESTINAL
- ☐ Constipation/Incontinence
- ☐ Irritable Bowels/Diarrhea
- ☐ Last B.M. _____
- ☐ Blood in stool
- ☐ Recent change in bowel habits
- ☐ Crohn's/Colitis
- ☐ Diverticular disease
- ☐ Ostomy _____
- ☐ Ulcers
- ☐ Hiatal hernia/Reflux
- ☐ Hepatitis
- ☐ Gall bladder disease
- ☐ Mucositis
- ☐ Other _____
- ☐ *No identified problems*

MUSCULOSKELETAL
- ☐ Arthritis/DJD
- ☐ Joint replacement _____
- ☐ Osteoporosis
- ☐ Spinal/Back problems _____
- ☐ Muscle weakness/ Spasticity
- ☐ Fibromyalgia
- ☐ Quadriplegic
- ☐ Paraplegic
- ☐ Other _____
- ☐ *No identified problems*

GENITOURINARY
- ☐ Burning/Urgency/Frequency
- ☐ Blood in urine
- ☐ Recurrent UTI
- ☐ Kidney failure/Dialysis
- ☐ Kidney stones
- ☐ Prostate problems
- ☐ Incontinence
- ☐ Ostomy _____
- ☐ Other _____
- ☐ *No identified problems*

PSYCHOSOCIAL
- ☐ Alcohol use
  - Last alcohol use _____
  - Type/Amount _____
- ☐ Tobacco use
  - Last used _____
  - Type/Amount _____
- ☐ Drug use
  - Type/Amount _____
- ☐ Depression
- ☐ Panic/Anxiety attacks
- ☐ Bereavement
- ☐ Claustrophobia
- ☐ Physical/Psychological abuse
- ☐ Attention deficit disorder
- ☐ Other_____
- ☐ *No identified problems*

INTEGUMENTARY
- ☐ Pressure ulcers
  - location _____
  - stage _____
  - 2nd location _____
  - stage _____
- ☐ Multiple pressure ulcers
- ☐ Specialty bed
- ☐ Lower leg/foot wounds
  - ☐ Right ☐ Left ☐ Both
- ☐ Skin problems _____
- ☐ Dry skin
- ☐ Rash
- ☐ Old scars
- ☐ Tattoos/Body piercings
- ☐ Petechia/Bruising
- ☐ Other _____
- ☐ *No identified problems*

METABOLIC
- ☐ Diabetes type: _____
- ☐ Hypoglycemia
- ☐ Hypo/hyperthyroid
- ☐ Anemia
- ☐ Obesity
- ☐ Other_____
- ☐ *No identified problems*

GYN
- ☐ LMP _____
- ☐ Possibility of pregnancy
- ☐ Pregnant
- ☐ Breast feeding
- ☐ Breast Mass/Tenderness/Discharge
- ☐ Vaginal Discharge
- ☐ Pre/post menopausal
- ☐ Other_____
- ☐ *No identified problems*

CANCER/HEMATOLOGIC
Type of cancer _____

Prior Chemo/XRT _____
_____
PICC/PORTS
Location _____
- ☐ Blood/Bleeding Disorders
_____
- ☐ Immunosuppression
- ☐ Other _____
- ☐ Clinical Trial Experience
- ☐ *No identified problems*

SENSORY DEFICITS
- ☐ Vision Changes
- ☐ Glaucoma/Cataracts
  - ☐ Had surgery
- ☐ Hearing Deficit
- ☐ Other _____
- ☐ *No identified problems*

- ☐ Infectious Disease/STD
  - Type _____
- ☐ Sexually Transmitted Disease
  - Type _____

SLEEP HABITS
Usual bed time _____
Usual wake time _____
Sleepy during day   ☐ Yes   ☐ No
Trouble falling asleep ☐ Yes   ☐ No
Trouble staying asleep ☐ Yes   ☐ No
- ☐ Other _____
- ☐ *No identified problems*

COMMENTS
_____
_____
_____

ASSISTIVE DEVICES/PERSONAL ITEMS: *Check appropriate boxes*

☐ See personal belongings list, if applicable	PAT/POA	Brought to hospital	Left at home	NA
Glasses/Contacts				
Dentures ☐ Upper ☐ Lower ☐ Both ☐ Partial				
Jewelry: Type				
Crutches/Prosthesis/Cane/Walker				
Breathing devices: Type				
Wigs/Hairpieces				
Religious items				
Hearing Aid ☐ Right ☐ Left ☐ Both				

COMPLETE THIS SECTION FOR ALL PATIENTS

Patient I.D.

CULTURAL/RELIGIOUS/SPIRITUAL	ACTION TAKEN
Religious Preference: _____ □ NA Would like to see: □ Hospital Chaplain / Representative 　　　　　　　□ Personal Religious Leader 　　　　　　　(Name) _____ (Phone #) _____ 　　　　　　　□ No visits Any cultural, spiritual or religious requests while in the hospital? 　　□ No　□ Yes Specify: _____	□ Refer to Chaplain **Enter consult and place on pathway**

SOCIAL/DISCHARGE PLANNING	ACTION TAKEN
□ Lives Alone　□Lives with spouse/significant other/family/caretaker □ Stairs _____　　□ Bathroom on same level as living quarters □ Lives in nursing home/assisted living ❶ □ Unable to return to previous living arrangement ❷ □ Compromised in ADLs and /or lack of support network ❶ □ Insurance concerns ❶　□ Financial concerns ❷ □ Received services prior to admission: □unknown □home care □med equip ❶ □ Evidence of physical/emotional abuse or neglect or domestic violence ❷ □ Current substance abuse ❷ □ Special discharge needs _____ □ Patient plans to be discharged to: _____ □ Discharge Transportation 　　(Name) _____ (Phone #) _____ □ *No discharge planning needs identified*	□Assist With ADLs □Patient Education ❶ □ Refer to Case 　　Manager/Home Care ❷ □ Refer to Social Work **Enter consult and place on pathway**

NUTRITIONAL STATUS　□ No Identified Problems	ACTION TAKEN
Diet prior to admission _____ If any of the following are present, send computer order to Nutrition Services □ Unintentional weight loss/gain ≥10 lbs in the last 6 months ❶ □ Vomiting/diarrhea for the last 3 days or longer ❶ □ Poor appetite for the last 5 days or longer ❶ □ Reliance on Nutrition support/tube, feeding/TPN ❶ □ Newly diagnosed pt. with diabetes need for education ❶,❷ □ Pressure ulcer stage II or greater ❶ □ Pregnant or breastfeeding	❶ □ Nutrition Referral ❷ □ Community Educator/ 　　Diabetes Referral

SMOKING STATUS　　　□ No Identified Problems	
□ Smoking cessation information given □ Smoking cessation information declined □ Community Educator/Smoking Cessation Referral	**Enter consult and place on pathway**

EDUCATION NEEDS ASSESSMENT	ACTION TAKEN
Learning Readiness:　□ Willing to Learn　□ Unable to Learn　□ Resists/refuses at this time **Barriers to Learning:**　□ No Barriers　□ Cognitive　□ Cultural 　　　　　　　　　　□ Educational　□ Emotional　□ Language 　　　　　　　　　　□ Motivational　□ Financial　□ Physical　□ Religious 　　□ Comments/Other_____ **Plans to Overcome Barriers to Education:**□ Family involvement　□ Reinforcement 　　　　　　　　　　　　　　□ Written Materials　□ Audiovisual Aids 　　　　　　　　　　　　　　□ Interpreter 　　□ Other_____ **Specific Educational Needs:**　□ Disease Process　□ Activity Level　□ Diet 　　　　　　　　　　□ Procedures　□ Hygiene 　　　　　　　　　　□ Medications (including Drug and Food Interactions) 　　　　　　　　　　□ Medical Equipment/Assistive Devices 　　　　　　　　　　□ Skin/Ostomy　□ Pain Management 　　　　　　　　　　□ Other _____ **Teaching to be directed primarily to:**　□ Patient　□ Family 　　□ Other_____	□ Education Initiated □ Unable to initiate education

Information obtained from/completed by: _____ Date/Time:_____

Completed by: _____ Date/Time:_____

Reviewed by RN:_____ Date/Time:_____

**COMPLETE THIS SECTION FOR
INPATIENTS ONLY**

Patient I.D.

Patient Folder Given?   □ Yes   □ No

□ Patient Handbook/Patient's Rights and Responsibilities reviewed.
□ Patient/family oriented to room

**Patient Information May be Given
To/Emergency Contact:**
Name:_____
Phone Number:_____

RESPIRATORY STATUS □ No Identified Problems	ACTION TAKEN
□ Patient is pre-op for upper abdominal or thoracic surgery <u>and</u> has a history of Emphysema, Bronchitis, Asthma, or Pulmonary Fibrosis	**Requires Physician Order** □ Respiratory Care Referred **Enter consult and place on pathway**

PHYSICAL THERAPY/OCCUPATIONAL THERAPY/SPEECH THERAPY □ No Identified Problems	ACTION TAKEN
□ Recent loss of function affecting Activities of Daily Living (ADL) □ Decreased strength and/or range of motion that could be resolved with therapy □ Difficulty swallowing and/or signs of choking while drinking/eating	**Requires Physician Order** **Enter consult and place on pathway**

REMINDERS:

COMPLETE MEDICATION RECONCILIATION FORM FOR ALL MEDICATIONS

COMPLETE VACCINE SCREENING/STANDING ORDER FORM

<u>COMMENTS</u>

_____
_____
_____
_____
_____
_____
_____
_____
_____
_____
_____
_____
_____
_____
_____
_____
_____

Completed by RN _____ Date/Time _____

Appendix F
NCLEX® Practice Questions*

Note: Correct answers and rationales can be found on pages 294 to 297.

1. Which of the following play activities would be appropriate for a toddler?
   1. Musical mobile above bed
   2. Rattle
   3. Jigsaw puzzle
   4. Wagon

2. The nurse is assessing a client who is recovering from surgery that was performed under a local anesthetic. The client's speech has become very slurred. What would be the nurse's priority action?
   1. Check intravenous (IV) placement, blood pressure, pulse, and respiratory status.
   2. Recognize this as a symptom of anxiety, and encourage the client to sleep off the effect.
   3. Determine whether the client consumed a large quantity of alcohol before surgery.
   4. Do nothing because this frequently occurs in clients who receive large doses of local anesthetics.

3. Which of the following tasks should the charge nurse delegate to an experienced LPN working on the adult medical unit?
   1. Teaching a client about the preprocedure preparation for a gastric endoscopy
   2. Inserting a nasogastric (NG) tube for gastric acid analysis
   3. Administering IV midazolam hydrochloride (Versed) during endoscopy
   4. Developing a nursing care plan for a client having a cystoscopy

4. Which of the following clients is likely to be predisposed to an adverse reaction to a medication?
   1. A 5-year-old with an eye infection
   2. A 20-year-old with a fracture
   3. A 4-year-old with an upper respiratory tract infection
   4. A 70-year-old woman with liver disease

*Practice questions from the companion CD for Zerwekh, J., and Claborn, J. (2010). *Illustrated study guide for the NCLEX-RN Exam.* St Louis: Mosby. To order this book with companion CD, go to www.elsevierhealth.com or call (800) 545-2522.

5. A client is experiencing respiratory alkalosis as a result of hyperventilation. The nurse would expect the blood gas values to reflect what changes?
   1. Decreased pH, decreased Pco_2
   2. Decreased pH, increased Pco_2
   3. Increased pH, decreased Pco_2
   4. Increased pH, increased Pco_2

6. A client who is positive for the human immunodeficiency virus (HIV) has been receiving antiviral medication for the past 3 months. He calls the clinic complaining of polydipsia, polyuria, and polyphagia. The nurse understands that which of the following is most likely the reason for the symptoms?
   1. Pancreatic infiltration by HIV virus, which has led to diabetic-like symptoms
   2. Allergic reaction to the nonnucleoside reverse-transcriptase inhibitor medications
   3. Nonadherence with the antiviral medication regimen
   4. Hyperglycemia caused by the protease inhibitor

7. When assessing a client for possible side effects of vincristine, the nurse should observe for which toxic side effect?
   1. Diarrhea
   2. Alopecia
   3. Hemorrhagic cystitis
   4. Peripheral neuropathy

8. A 9-year-old client with leukemia asks, "Will I die?" What is an initial therapeutic response based on the needs of the dying child?
   1. "Think about getting well instead of dying."
   2. "Tell me what you are thinking about dying."
   3. "You need to ask your doctor."
   4. "I really don't know."

9. The nurse is assessing a client who may be experiencing auditory hallucinations. Which client activity would assist the nurse to confirm that a hallucination is occurring?
   1. Client mumbling to self, head is tilted, and eyes are darting back and forth.
   2. Client performing obsessive-compulsive rituals such as turning a radio off and on, and talking to self.
   3. Client is hyperactive, very easily distracted, and avoids contact with other clients.
   4. Client is cool, aloof, and unapproachable and avoids enclosed areas.

10. A client has extensive burns with eschar on the anterior trunk. What is the nurse's primary concern regarding eschar formation?
    1. It prevents fluid remobilization in the first 48 hours after burn trauma.
    2. Infection is difficult to assess before the eschar sloughs.
    3. It restricts the ability of the client to move about.
    4. Circulation to the extremities is diminished because of edema formation.

11.   The nurse is assessing the hearing of a client with Bell's palsy. What would be the best way to determine the hearing of the client?
    1.   Stand out of the client's sight and ask him to do something specific.
    2.   Use a tuning fork to test for lateralization of sound.
    3.   Stand in front of the client and whisper, "Raise your hand."
    4.   Snap your fingers next to the client's ear, and ask whether the sound was heard.

12.   The nurse is caring for a client postoperative thyroidectomy. What would be an important nursing intervention?
    1.   Have the client speak every 5 to 10 minutes if hoarseness is present.
    2.   Provide a low-calcium diet to prevent hypercalcemia.
    3.   Check the dressing at the back of the neck for bleeding.
    4.   Apply a soft cervical collar to restrict neck movement.

13.   A client in sickle cell crisis is admitted to the ED. What are the priorities of care in order of importance?
    1.   Nutrition, hydration, electrolyte balance
    2.   Hydration, pain management, electrolyte balance
    3.   Hydration, oxygenation, pain management
    4.   Hydration, oxygenation, electrolyte balance

14.   A client with chronic asthma develops Cushing's syndrome. Development of the complication can most likely be attributed to long-term use of:
    1.   Prednisone
    2.   Theophylline
    3.   Metaproterenol (Alupent)
    4.   Cromolyn (Intal)

15.   While discussing her diagnosis of hypertension, a client asks the nurse how long she will need to take all of the medications that have been prescribed. On what principle is the nurse's response based?
    1.   The client will be scheduled for an appointment in 2 months; the doctor will decrease her medications at that time.
    2.   As soon as her blood pressure (BP) returns to normal levels, the client will be able to stop taking her medications.
    3.   To maintain stable control of her BP, the client will have to take the medications indefinitely.
    4.   The nurse cannot discuss the medications with the client; the client will need to talk with the doctor.

16.   An older client is admitted for congestive heart failure. What observation by the nurse indicates that the client's condition is getting worse?
    1.   Arterial blood gases show a significant decrease in pH and Pco_2.
    2.   Blood pressure is 160/98 mm Hg; pulse is 110 beats/min.
    3.   Urinary output is 60 mL/hr; crackles are heard at the base bilaterally.
    4.   Irritability and confusion are increasing.

17.   A client returns to the unit after surgical creation of a continent (Kock's) ileostomy. What will care of the ileostomy include?

    1. Draining the reservoir or pouch with a soft catheter

    2. Irrigating it with normal saline solution after 24 hours

    3. Attaching an ostomy bag with careful checking for a watertight seal

    4. Assessing for skin excoriation and increased drainage caused by location of the stoma

18. A client is scheduled for paracentesis for ascites. Which statement by the client would indicate to the nurse that the preprocedure teaching has been successful?

    1. "I will need to lie flat in bed during the procedure."

    2. "The doctor will instill about 200 mL or normal saline into my abdomen and then drain it out."

    3. "I need to drink two glasses of water right before the procedure to maintain a full bladder."

    4. "The doctor will slowly remove fluid from my abdomen to relieve the pressure."

19. The nurse is administering mannitol (Osmitrol) to a client who had a craniotomy for a pituitary tumor the previous day. What nursing observation would indicate that the medication is having the desired effect?

    1. The serum blood glucose level is within normal range.

    2. A significant increase in urinary output has occurred.

    3. There has been a weight loss of 3 lb since the previous day.

    4. The neurologic signs indicate no evidence of intracranial pressure.

20. The nurse is preparing health teaching for adult women regarding the prevention of osteoporosis. What would be important to include in the teaching plan? **Select all that apply.**

    1. Walking for 15 to 30 minutes each day

    2. Supplemental calcium intake

    3. Reduced intake of caffeine

    4. Increased intake of water

    5. Avoiding sunlight because of photosensitivity

    6. Increased intake of fresh fruit and vegetables

21. After a transurethral resection of the prostate (TURP), a client has a three-way urinary catheter with continuous bladder irrigation. The nurse is preparing to hang a new container of the bladder irrigation solution. What type of solution will the nurse hang?

    1. Isotonic sterile irrigating solution

    2. Distilled sterile water

    3. Normal saline solution with 2000 units of heparin

    4. Nonsterile saline irrigating fluid

22. What specific directions are given to the client who is taking phenazopyridine (Pyridium)?

    1. The medication may discolor contact lenses; if the sclera begin to turn yellow, return to the clinic.

    2. Always take the medication on an empty stomach to increase absorption.

    3. Do not take any medication containing aspirin or salicylates while taking phenazopyridine.

    4. The medication may interfere with the effectiveness of birth control pills.

23. The nurse understands that combination oral contraceptive pills prevent pregnancy primarily by:
    1. Decreasing fallopian tube motility
    2. Thinning of cervical mucus
    3. Suppressing ovulation
    4. Causing inflammation of the endometrium

24. The nurse admits a client in active labor. Her assessment reveals 9 cm dilation with complete effacement, +2 station. The woman asks the nurse to give her something for pain. The best nursing action would be to:
    1. Administer a placebo and tell her it's for pain control.
    2. Tell the woman to wait just a little bit longer.
    3. Call the anesthesiologist to insert an epidural.
    4. Stay with the woman and assist her to breathe with the contractions.

ANSWERS TO NCLEX® PRACTICE QUESTIONS

1. **Correct answer:** 4
   Rationale: Toddlers enjoy motion toys, such as pull toys, riding toys, and wagons. Play activities such as finger paints, interlocking blocks, and puzzles with large pieces would help with refining fine motor movement. Musical mobiles and rattles are better suited as toys for infants.

2. **Correct answer:** 1
   Rationale: It is important for the nurse to recognize that this is an abnormal symptom. The nurse should check the IV for patency in case rapid treatment is needed and should obtain a complete set of vital signs to assess for cardiovascular effects. The nurse should complete the appropriate assessments, given the change in the client's condition. Client alcohol consumption should be determined before the procedure. The client's change in condition should be assessed appropriately, and the nurse should contact the health care provider and provide a condition report after the assessment.

3. **Correct answer:** 2
   Rationale: NG tube insertion is included in LPN education and is an appropriate task for an experienced LPN. Client teaching, administration of IV conscious sedation medications, and developing the plan of care are all parts of the (RN) scope of practice.

4. **Correct answer:** 4
   Rationale: The 70-year-old woman has multiple factors that can predispose her to an adverse reaction, including age and liver disease. The kidneys are the primary organ for medication excretion, but liver malfunction and disease will affect how rapidly the medications are metabolized for renal excretion. The 20-year-old and 40-year-old have no identified predisposing risk factors, such as genetics, pathophysiologic dysfunction, or drug allergies. A 5-year-old may have an adverse reaction

to topical eye medication but is not as likely as an older adult to have such a reaction.

5. **Correct answer: 3**
   Rationale: The blood gas indications for respiratory alkalosis are increased pH and decreased Pco_2. With excessive hyperventilation, there is excessive loss of Pco_2. The loss of Co_2 with hyperventilation causes a decrease in the pH, resulting in respiratory alkalosis. (Hint: Use this mnemonic to remember the direction of pH and Pco_2: "respiratory opposite, metabolic equal.")

6. **Correct answer: 4**
   Rationale: Protease inhibitors have been associated with hyperglycemia, new-onset diabetes, abrupt exacerbation of existing diabetes, and diabetic ketoacidosis. This usually occurs after 2 months of use. Polydipsia, polyuria, and polyphagia are symptoms attributed to diabetes, rather than to an allergic reaction. These symptoms are not an indication of nonadherence to the antiviral regimen, although nonadherence can be attributed to many factors, including the complexity of the treatment regimen.

7. **Correct answer: 4**
   Rationale: Peripheral neuropathy is toxic, has long-term consequences, and is specific to vincristine. This is a good example of how a test question asks for a distinction between a toxic effect and a side effect. The other options all occur, but they are adverse side effects with the majority of chemotherapy drugs.

8. **Correct answer: 2**
   Rationale: The child usually has a fairly accurate evaluation of a situation. The nurse needs to respond to his questions about dying in a way that allows him a chance to express his concerns, which would be by making an open-ended statement. The other options do not answer the child's question or encourage him to express his feelings.

9. **Correct answer: 1**
   Rationale: The client experiencing the auditory hallucination will often look out into space and act as if he is listening to someone talking. This is associated with behaviors such as tilting the head, mumbling, and eye movement. There may be times the client actually responds verbally to the auditory hallucination.

10. **Correct answer: 2**
    Rationale: The burns are on the anterior trunk and do not involve extremities; hence the problem would be in watching for infection, because the eschar makes it difficult to visually examine the healing skin. Removal of the eschar enhances healing and prevents infection, which occurs because of the moist, enclosed area under the eschar.

11. **Correct answer: 1**
    Rationale: Bell's palsy involves sensorineural hearing loss. For an accurate assessment, the client must be able to hear the direction of sound without any visual prompting. The tuning fork assists in differentiating between air and bone conduction of sound. Standing in front of the client would allow him to

read lips, and snapping fingers beside the ear is not a valid assessment tool for hearing.

12. **Correct answer: 3**

Rationale: If bleeding occurs, the blood will drain posteriorly, or behind the client's neck. Serum levels of calcium are important to monitor because of possible damage to the parathyroids during surgery. Oral intake of calcium is not immediately significant. The client is often hoarse; it is important to monitor for increasing hoarseness that would be indicative of edema. A cervical collar is not indicated.

13. **Correct answer: 3**

Rationale: The priorities for care of a client in sickle cell crises are providing fluid, administering oxygen, and controlling pain (in that order) during the crisis. Electrolyte management is not a priority, nor is nutrition.

14. **Correct answer: 1**

Rationale: Cushing's syndrome results from excessive use of glucocorticoids. This can occur from frequent or long-term use of corticosteroids such as prednisone. Theophylline, metaproterenol, and cromolyn do not cause Cushing's syndrome.

15. **Correct answer: 3**

Rationale: Noncompliance with blood pressure medications is a common problem in the treatment of hypertension. The client must understand that the only way to keep her blood pressure under control is to continue to take her medications. She will not be able to discontinue the medications unless there is a significant change in her condition as a result of weight loss, an exercise program, and/or decreased stress.

16. **Correct answer: 4**

Rationale: Increasing irritation and confusion are early indications of hypoxia. The Pco_2 usually goes up, and the blood pressure and pulse are within expected levels. Crackles at the base of the lungs are a common finding in this client.

17. **Correct answer: 1**

Rationale: The reservoir will initially need to be drained by insertion of a soft catheter or by a continuous drainage system. As the pouch increases in size, the client is taught how to catheterize his stoma whenever he feels any dilatation. The potential for fluid and electrolyte imbalance is decreased, the stoma is not pouched on a continuous basis, and the stoma should not leak.

18. **Correct answer: 4**

Rationale: After signing an informed consent form for the procedure, the client will need to sit upright at the side of the bed, with feet propped on a stool, while fluid is removed to relieve acute symptoms of ascites. The fluid is drawn out slowly and checked for amount, color, and characteristics of drainage. Rapid removal can lead to decreased abdominal pressure, which can contribute to shock and vasodilation. The puncture site will need a compression bandage, and the site must be monitored. Fluid instilled into the abdomen is a diagnostic peritoneal lavage to determine internal injuries.

19. **Correct answer:** 4

    Rationale: Mannitol is an osmotic diuretic and is given to clients who have undergone a craniotomy to decrease or to prevent an increase in cerebral pressure. Normal neurologic signs would indicate that the medication is achieving the desired effects. An increase in urine output and the weight loss may occur, but these findings have no specific neurologic implications.

20. **Correct answers:** 1, 2, and 3

    Rationale: These are the most common preventative measures in women at increased risk for osteoporosis. Some sunlight is encouraged to facilitate utilization of vitamin D and absorption of calcium intake. Drinking more water and eating more fresh fruits and vegetables are health measures, but they are not specific to the prevention of osteoporosis.

21. **Correct answer:** 1

    Rationale: The isotonic sterile irrigating solution is critical to prevent absorption of the irrigation fluid, which could result in fluid overload. Distilled water should never be used for irrigations, and the solution for a continuous bladder irrigation should always be sterile. Heparin would not be used.

22. **Correct answer:** 1

    Rationale: The nurse should advise the client that if she notices yellow discoloration of the sclera while taking phenazopyridine (Pyridium), she should return to the office immediately. This may indicate poor renal excretion and requires follow-up with the physician. The medication should be administered with food, and there is no drug interaction with aspirin or birth control pills.

23. **Correct answer:** 3

    Rationale: The primary mechanism of action of oral contraceptives is suppression of ovulation. Ovulation is suppressed in 95% to 98% of clients taking the pill. Should ovulation occur, the combination pills may also prevent pregnancy by thickening the cervical mucus, causing the endometrium to become atrophic, and making the uterine environment unfavorable for implantation.

24. **Correct answer:** 4

    Rationale: The woman is too far along in the labor process to be given any pain medication; it would significantly depress the neonate. The best approach is to stay with her and coach her through breathing and relaxation techniques during the contractions. The delivery of this infant will most likely occur within the next hour.

Glossary

accountability The state of being responsible or answerable for something. Nurses, as members of a knowledge-based health profession and as licensed health care professionals, must answer to patients, nursing employers, the board of nursing, and the civil and criminal court systems when the quality of patient care provided is compromised or when allegations of unprofessional, unethical, illegal, unacceptable, or inappropriate nursing conduct, actions, or responses arise.

assignment The distribution of work that each staff member is responsible for during a given work period.

advanced practice nurse A nurse who, by virtue of credentials (usually completion of a master's program and certification), has a wide scope of authority to act (may include treating medical problems and prescribing medications).

air embolism An air bubble that gets into the bloodstream. Can be fatal.

analysis A mental process in which one seeks to get a better understanding of the nature of something by carefully separating the whole into smaller parts. For example, if you want to know more about someone's physical health, each organ and system separately is examined separately.

anaphylactic shock Extreme hypotension caused by an allergic reaction; requires immediate treatment or can be fatal.

assessment tool A printed or electronic form used to ensure that key information is gathered and recorded during assessment.

assumption Something that is taken for granted without proof. (*Compare with* Hypothesis and Inference.)

attitude A way of acting, feeling, or thinking that shows one's disposition, opinion, and so forth (e.g., a threatening attitude).

baseline data Information that describes the status of a problem before treatment begins.

benchmark A standard or point in measuring quality. In health care, benchmarks are determined by analyzing the data collected over a period of time.

best practices A term referring to ways certain problems are best prevented and managed from an outcome and cost perspective.

care variance When a patient has not achieved activities or outcomes by the time frame noted on a critical path.

caring behavior Actions that show understanding and respect for another's perceptions, feelings, needs, and desires.

circumstances The conditions or facts attending an event or having some bearing on it.

classify To arrange or group together data according to categories, thereby increasing understanding because relationships become more obvious.

competence The quality of having the necessary knowledge, skill, and attitude to perform an action under various circumstances.

critical Characterized by careful and exact evaluation; crucial.

cues *See* Data.

data Pieces of information about health status (e.g., vital signs).

data base form *See* Assessment tool.

database assessment Comprehensive data collected when a client first enters the health care facility in order to gain information about all aspects of the health status.

deductive reasoning Drawing specific conclusions from general principles and rules; for example, "Because it is true that bacteria are killed by antibiotics, bacterial infection requires treatment with antibiotics." (*Compare with* Inductive reasoning.)

defining characteristics Signs and symptoms usually associated with a specific nursing diagnosis.

definitive diagnosis The most specific, most correct diagnosis.

definitive interventions The most specific actions required to prevent, resolve, or control a health problem.

diagnose To identify and name health problems after careful analysis of evidence from an assessment.

diagnostic error When a health problem has been overlooked or incorrectly identified.

diagnostic reasoning A method of thinking that involves specific, deliberate use of phases of the nursing process to reach conclusions about a patient's health status, risk factors, and current health problems.

diaphoretic The condition of being sweaty, usually suspected to be a sign of a health problem (e.g., shock, disease).

disposition One's attitude, customary frame of mind, or manner of response.

diuretic A drug given to enhance kidney function, thereby increasing fluid elimination from the body.

efficiency The quality of being able to produce a desired effect safely, with minimal risks, expense, and unnecessary effort.

emboli More than one embolus. (*See* Embolus.)

embolus A clot that has moved through one vessel and lodged in another, reducing or totally blocking blood supply to tissues usually nourished by the vessels involved. (*Compare with* Thrombus.)

empathy Understanding another's feelings or perceptions but not sharing the same feelings or point of view. (*Compare with* Sympathy.)

empiric Relying solely on practical experience and ignoring science.

epidemiology The body of knowledge reflecting what is known about a specific health state.

esthetics A sense of what is pleasing to the eye.

ethics The study of the general nature of morals and of the specific moral choices to be made by individuals in relationships with others.

etiology The cause or contributing factors of a health problem.

expedite To make something happen in a quick fashion.

explicit Clearly and specifically expressed or described.

focus assessment Data collection that aims to gain specific information about a certain aspect of health status.

guidelines Documents that delineate how care is to be provided in specific situations.

habits of inquiry Habits that enhance the ability to search for the truth (e.g., verifying that data is correct and following rules of logic).

hospitalist A medical doctor trained to manage hospital care. Hospitalists take over care management of hospitalized patients.

humanistic A way of thought or action concerned with the interests or ideals of people.

hypothesis (1) A hunch. (2) An assertion subject to verification or proof. (*Compare with* Assumption and Inference.)

imply To suggest by logical necessity.

inductive reasoning Drawing general conclusions by observing a few specific members of a class; for example, "Since everyone I ever knew with a bacterial infection required an antibiotic, and Jane has a bacterial infection, Jane requires an antibiotic." (*Compare with* Deductive reasoning.)

infer To suspect something or to attach meaning to information; for example, if someone is frowning, one may infer that he or she is worried.

inference Something suspected to be true, based on a logical conclusion after examination of the evidence. (*Compare with* Assumption and Hypothesis.)

intervention Something done to prevent, cure, or manage a health problem (e.g., turning someone every 2 hours to prevent skin breakdown).

informatics The use of computers and other health information technology (HIT) to facilitate the acquisition, storage, retrieval, and use of information by all healthcare professionals.

intubation The process of inserting a tube into an individual's bronchus to facilitate breathing.

intuition Knowing something without evidence.

irrigate To flush a tube (with normal saline solution or water) to keep it patent (open and flowing).

life processes Events or changes that occur during one's lifetime (e.g., growing up, getting married, losing someone).

malpractice The negligent conduct of a person acting within his or her professional capacity.

measurable Capable of being clearly observed so that the quality and quantity of something can be determined.

medical domain Actions a physician is legally qualified to perform.

mentor A knowledgeable, insightful, and trusted person who helps someone else clarify his or her thinking.

moral Concerned with the judgment of whether a human action or character is right or wrong.

myocardial infarction Partial or complete occlusion of one or more of the coronary arteries, causing the death of coronary tissue.

nasogastric tube A tube inserted through the nose, down the esophagus, and into the stomach.

negligence Failure to provide the degree of care that someone of ordinary prudence would provide under the same circumstances. To claim negligence, it is necessary that there be a duty owed by one person to another, that the duty be breached, and that the breach cause harm.

nursing actions Something done by a nurse to achieve an outcome.

nursing assistive personnel (NAP) Individuals who are trained to assist licensed registered nurse in providing patient care, as delegated by the registered nurse. The term includes, but is not limited to, nurses' aides, medication aides, and other licensed or certified workers.

nursing intervention An action taken by a nurse to produce a nursing outcome.

nursing domain Actions a nurse is legally qualified to perform.

objective data Information that one can clearly observe or measure (e.g., a pulse of 140 beats per minute).

outcome The result of interventions.

paradigm A model or way of doing things.

patent Open, so as to allow the flow of fluid or air.

phenomena Observable occurences that are concerns of nursing; often considered "human experiences" (e.g., pain, anxiety).

policies *See* Guidelines.

preceptor An experienced, more qualified nurse assigned by a facility to facilitate learning for a less experienced nurse.

proactive A way of thinking and behaving that accepts responsibility for one's actions and takes initiative to plan ahead to anticipate and prevent problems before they happen.

procedures *See* Guidelines.

protocols *See* Guidelines.

pulmonary embolus A clot that has blocked off circulation and oxygenation to lung tissue; considered to be life-threatening.

QA *See* Quality assessment.

QI *See* Quality improvement.

qualified Having the competence and authority to perform an action.

quality assessment (QA) Ongoing studies designed to evaluate the quality of patient care and services. Just as assessment is the first step of the nursing process, QA is the first step of QI (quality improvement).

quality care Health care services that increase the probability of achieving desired results with decreased probability of undesired results.

quality improvement (QI) Ongoing studies designed to identify ways to promote achievement of desired outcomes in a timely, cost-effective manner while decreasing the risks for undesired outcomes.

rales Abnormal breath sounds (crackles) caused by the passage of air through bronchi containing fluid. This sign is frequently associated with congestive heart failure.

related factor *See* Risk factor.

response A reaction of an organism or person to a specific mechanism.

risk factor Something known to contribute to (or be associated with) a specific problem. (*See also* Etiology.)

signs Objective data that cause one to suspect a health problem. (*Compare with* Symptoms.)

somnolent Overly sleepy; difficult to arouse.

stakeholders The people who will be most affected by care (e.g., patients, families) or from whom requirements will be drawn (e.g., caregivers, third-party payers, healthcare organizations).

standard of nursing care The degree of skill, care, and diligence exercised by the members of the nursing profession practicing in the same or a similar locality. Many states refer to standards in their nurse practice acts.

standards Authoritative statements that describe the responsibilities for which its practitioners are accountable.

subjective data Information the patient states or communicates; the patient's perceptions (e.g., "My heart feels like it's racing").

surveillance The close observation of patients and their surroundings for the purpose of preventing complications or injury.

sympathy Sharing the same feelings as another. (*Compare with* Empathy.)

symptoms Subjective data that cause one to suspect a health problem. (*Compare with* Signs.)

synthesis The process of putting pieces of information together to make a whole; for example, nurses put individual signs and symptoms together to make a diagnosis.

thrombi More than one thrombus (clot). (*See* Thrombus.)

thrombus A clot that threatens blood supply to tissues. If the clot moves, it becomes an embolus. (*Compare with* Embolus.)

tubal ligation Surgery performed to sterilize a woman by cutting and suturing her fallopian tubes.

unlicensed assistive personnel (UAP) Workers who are not licensed by the state but are trained to help with care of patients.

validity The extent to which something can be believed to be factual and true.

variance in care *See* Care variance.

Index

Page numbers followed by *b*, *t*, and *f*
indicate boxes, tables and figures,
respectively.

ABOUT THE AUTHOR

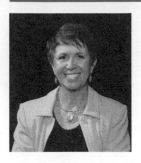 Known for making difficult content easy to understand, **Rosalinda Alfaro-Lefevre, RN, MSN, ANEF**, is a National League for Nursing Academy of Nursing Education Fellow. She is an energetic presenter and an *AJN Book of the Year* and *Sigma Theta Tau Best Pick* award recipient, and her work is used throughout the world. Rosalinda has over 20 years of clinical experience—mostly in ICU, CCU, and ED—and has taught in associate degree and baccalaureate nursing programs. She is the president of Teaching Smart/Learning Easy in Stuart, Florida, a company dedicated to helping people to acquire the intellectual and interpersonal skills needed to deal with today's personal and workplace challenges. Born in Buenos Aires, Argentina, to a British mother and an Argentine father, Rosalinda immigrated to the United States from Argentina via Canada as a child. Although Rosalinda says she's an American at heart, she points out that she is blessed with multicultural experiences, presenting nationally and internationally and enjoying close relationships with her family in Spain, Argentina, and the United Kingdom. You can learn more about Rosalinda at www.AlfaroTeachSmart.com.